Oxytocin: The Biological Guide To Motherhood

By Kerstin Uvnäs-Moberg, M.D., Ph.D.

Oxytocin: The Biological Guide to Motherhood

Kerstin Uvnäs-Moberg, M.D., Ph.D.

Praeclarus Press, LLC

2504 Sweetgum Lane

Amarillo, Texas 79124 USA

806-367-9950

www.PraeclarusPress.com

DISCLAIMER

The information contained in this publication is advisory only and is not intended to replace sound clinical judgment or individualized patient care. The author disclaims all warranties, whether expressed or implied, including any warranty as the quality, accuracy, safety, or suitability of this information for any particular purpose.

ISBN: 978-1-939807-80-9

Acknowledgements

I have been very fortunate to have many fantastic collaborators over the years, some of them Ph.D. students or Post Docs, and some of them simply wonderful and skilled collaborators. I am very grateful to all of them, because without their help, it would not have been possible to perform this work. I still have a fruitful and stimulating collaboration with some of them.

In this context I would, in particular, like to mention the late professor in pediatrics at the Karolinska Hospital, professor Jan Winberg. Without his willingness to accept the concept of biology in the context of motherhood and interaction between mothers and their infants and without his generous support of my research in its early stages at a time when these ideas were not considered to be politically correct, I would not have dared to go on pursuing research along these lines.

I would also like to extend my thanks to the late professor James P. Henry for so many fruitful scientific discussions and, of course, to my dear friends Professor Marshal Klaus and his wife Phyllis for sharing their enormous and broad knowledge about the clinical aspects of interaction between mothers and infants and for their supportive friendship over the years.

Dedication

I dedicate this book to my family:

My children — Jenny & Dimitiri, Anders & Johanna, Wilhelm, and Axel

My grandchildren — Maja, Theodora, Alexandra, Theodor, Hjalmar, and Hector

My parents — Brita and Börje

My grandparents — Jenny & Oscar and Deborah & Lorenz

My sister — Anna

My brother — Magnus

Preface

Why I Wrote This Book

In Search of the Inner Roots of Motherhood

There are always personal reasons behind the decision to write a book. You may have experienced something that you want to tell others about or you may simply have a deep knowledge about something that you want to share. In my case, it is a little of both.

When I had my first child, I knew nothing about babies. Still, I managed and found the experience of giving birth and caring for children absolutely wonderful. Much to my own surprise, I found that without previous experience I often knew how to hold and what to do with the baby. Later on, after having three more children, I also noted that something happened to me during pregnancy. I never had any problems with being sick, but I became extremely tired during the first months of pregnancy, and I had to rest after eating because I felt so sleepy. My mood also changed; I became more emotional, in fact, I felt both happier and unhappier. In spite of not eating more than usual, kilos started to appear all over my body. Thinking of and planning for the unborn child took more and more time, in spite of my initial plans of really using my time in an optimal and maximal way for my work.

But the changes that occurred during pregnancy were nothing compared to those appearing during breastfeeding. In the midst of happiness, joy, pride, and contentment, an even greater sensitivity appeared and tears were close the days after birth. Also, a new anxiety occurred. I did not like to be alone, the darkness was darker and unknown places and people became even more unknown and strange. I withdrew to my home and family, where I felt calmer and safer than at any time before. If I had to leave home without the baby, I felt not only unhappy, but also anxious and incomplete, as if I had lost a leg or my handbag.

At the same time, I felt I desperately needed time for myself and tried to do some writing for work. To my despair I found this was very difficult, particularly writing texts based on logic and order, such as abstracts for scientific papers. The different threads of scientific material that I had been able to organize so well started to float and mingle, and I could not get anything out of it. I had to ask for help. I was terrified, would I ever be capable of being able to think and write clearly again? In time the scientific work, the teaching and writing that previously had occupied 200% of my time, gradually became distant and even uninteresting.

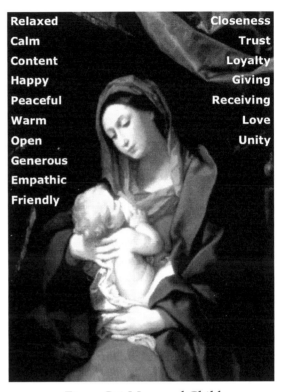

Figure P. 1 Mary and Child

In contrast, I noted that I got better at other things, such as writing up new ideas and applications. I started to dream in an entirely different way and often remembered the "images" in the morning and tried to understand what meaning they conveyed. "Real" pictures and paintings started to attract my attention—it was almost as if they looked at me and talked to me. Three classical religious motives, i.e., Mary and Child, Mary, the Child, and Mary's mother Anna, and Mary and her relative Elizabeth telling each other that they were pregnant, suddenly had a new meaning, not in the sense of being religious motives, but as timeless symbols and representations of motherhood and the increased need of support and social communication women experience during these periods. The more I looked at them, the more knowledge and messages I got from them. The picture of Mary and Child became a timeless representation of breastfeeding women, depicting not only transfer of milk, but also increased social skills, happiness, joy, and contentment, as well as calm and relaxation. The picture of Anna, Mary's mother, standing behind her daughter, symbolized the presence of a supportive woman during birth, a midwife or a doula, or even an internalized picture of Mary's own loving mother. I could "see" how Anna's hands touching Mary not only calmed her, thereby promoting labor, but also reduced her pain. Pictures of the pregnant Mary touching and holding

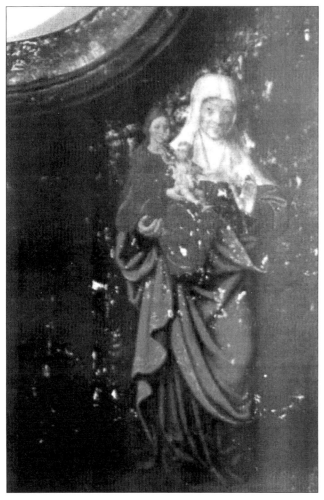

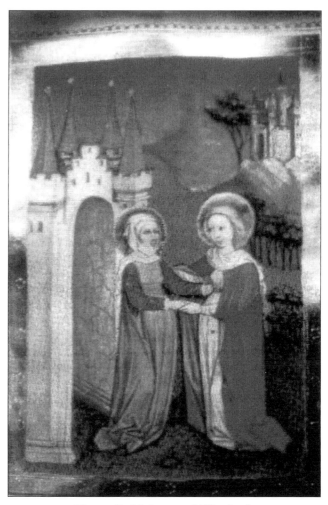

Figure P. 2 Mary, Child, and Anna

Figure P. 3 Mary and Elizabeth

hands with her pregnant cousin Elizabeth represented the need for communication between women and transfer of information about female competence from one woman to another (Figures P.1, P.2, and P.3; Uvnäs-Moberg, 1985).

From Intuition to Evidence-Based Research

At that time I was a physician (MD) with a Ph.D. in pharmacology, and I had performed research within the field of gastrointestinal physiology for ten years. Using my medical training and my competence as a researcher, I started to translate the nonverbal message of these archetypal images into the language of medical sciences. I soon realized that the hormone oxytocin, long known to promote labor and breastfeeding, might play a much more important role than previously thought during motherhood. By exerting effects in the brain, oxytocin might induce the vast spectrum of physiological and psychological adaptations and effects depicted in the archetypal images. I initiated animal experiments and clinical studies based on these ideas.

Piece by piece, the contours of the Growth and Relaxation

System (Uvnäs-Moberg, 1997, 1998b) or the Calm and Connection System started to materialize, which I described in my book *Lugn och Beröring* (Uvnäs Moberg, 2000) or in English, *The Oxytocin Factor* (Uvnäs-Moberg, 2003). After 30 years, I'm still performing research along these lines, but the studies now include more generalized aspects of the oxytocin system. It soon became apparent that oxytocin release is stimulated and exerts effects not only in mothers, but also in females and males of all ages in response to various types of positive interaction. The oxytocin system is even activated during loving interaction between humans and animals. This extended view on the oxytocin system and its effects has been described in a second book, *Närhetens hormon* (Uvnäs Moberg, 2009) or in English, *The Hormone of Closeness* (Uvnäs-Moberg, 2012). Altogether I have published around 450 original scientific papers and supervised 30 PhD students.

By writing this book, I wish to help mothers become aware of their inborn oxytocin-linked maternal competencies. By "listening" to and allowing their inner guide to come into play, they can access an inborn female competence aimed at helping them during the transition to motherhood. In this way, women may not only give birth more easily, they may also feel better after birth, find it easier to breastfeed and to establish a good connection with their children, and become more secure and confident in their role as a mother. In the long run, their children may develop a better relationship, not only with their own mothers, but also with other people, including their own children. The children may become better at handling stressful situations and enjoy better health in the future. Possibly, their children will, in turn, enjoy the same advantages. I would definitely have profited if I had known this information before I had my own children!

The Aim and Contents of This Book

The aim of this book is to provide scientific data to demonstrate that oxytocin plays an important role far beyond stimulation of uterine contractions during birth and milk ejection during breastfeeding.

Oxytocin is not only a hormone, but also a signaling substance in the brain that when released during birth, skin-to-skin contact, and breastfeeding induces important physiological and psychological adaptations in the mother and infant. Basically, oxytocin stimulates the mother's and baby's ability for social interaction, decreases the levels of anxiety and stress, and stimulates functions related to growth, restoration and health.

The way we give birth, handle, feed, and interact with our infants may influence the release of oxytocin and the development of the oxytocin-linked effects not only in the shorst-term, but possibly also in a long-term perspective in both mothers and infants.

Medical interventions in connection with vaginal birth may influence the release of oxytocin and the development of the oxytocin-linked effects.

The book is written out of the perspective of oxytocin as an important integrative principle in both physiological and psychological functions and effects taking place during birth, in the period, and during breastfeeding. This does not by any means exclude an important role for many other hormones and transmitters. I have tried to include as much information as possible, but there is a limit to what you can achieve in a book like this.

Contents of the Individual Chapters

Chapter 1 introduces oxytocin. To facilitate an understanding of how oxytocin works, a mini review of the nervous and hormonal mechanisms by which the brain influences the body, and the body and environment influence the brain will be presented. The role of the nervous system and the neuroendocrine system are described in chapters 2 and 3, respectively.

Chapter 4 is devoted to basic aspects of oxytocin. In chapter 5, the effects following administration of oxytocin are described. Chapter 6 describes the mechanisms by which oxytocin is released.

Chapters 7 - 10 are devoted to the processes of milk production and milk ejection as they occur in animals and women. In chapters 11 - 16, the different components of maternal behavior as they are displayed in animals and humans will be described. Also, the mechanisms involved in activation of maternal behavior will be covered.

Anti-stress and growth-promoting effects during breastfeeding in mothers and infants are described in chapters 17 - 21. In chapters 22 - 24, different factors that promote and facilitate breastfeeding and bonding between mother and infant will be discussed.

Chapters 25 - 27 describe the effects caused by medical interventions during birth on oxytocin release and oxytocin effects. In the final chapter, chapter 28, called Closeness and Support: The Gateway to Oxytocin, the consequences of exposure to too little or too much oxytocin after birth in a long-term perspective are discussed, as well as different ways to optimize oxytocin production in a more long-term perspective.

Table of Contents

Chapter 1

Oxytocin: The Biological Guide to Motherhood

The Inner Guide to Motherhood

We are well aware that other mammalian mothers instinctively know how to care for their newborns. They may build nests for their offspring before they give birth, and after birth, they provide them with milk, warm them, and care for them in every way. They also protect them from strangers and other potentially dangerous situations.

What is less well known is that human mothers also have an inborn competence as to how to give birth, breastfeed, and care for their children. It is not as strong and imperative as in other mammals. Humans have developed outstanding social, communicative, and cognitive skills, which normally override the more ancient and unconscious knowledge based on our instinctual mammalian heritage. The intuitive capacities are still there and may operate behind the scenes to help mothers become mothers. However, the inborn knowledge or competence needs to be stimulated in the right way in order to be fully expressed.

Integrative Role of Oxytocin

Oxytocin plays a major integrative role in the expression of innate maternal competencies. It is a small substance produced in the hypothalamus, an old part of the brain. The ability of oxytocin to stimulate uterine contractions and milk ejection were discovered in the beginning of the 20th century. Oxytocin was introduced as a clinical treatment for stimulation of contractions during labor and for facilitation of milk ejection during breastfeeding in the 1950s. These effects of oxytocin are exerted via hormonal or blood-borne effects.

More recently, it has been discovered that oxytocin plays a major organizing and integrating role in the brain during labor and breastfeeding, a role far beyond stimulation of uterine contractions and milk ejection, to adapt the mother for motherhood. In these cases, oxytocin is released from oxytocin-containing nerves in the brain and acts as a signaling substance. For example, oxytocin increases the mother's "social intelligence" and facilitates her contact with and bonding to her newborn. It makes her feel well and calm. It may help to reduce pain during labor and stress levels during breastfeeding. It even increases the mother's capacity for digestion and handling of ingested nutrients in a more efficient way.

Oxytocin released in the newborn's brain during skin-to-skin contact with the mother and in response to suckling influences the infant in a corresponding way. The newborn approaches and seeks contact with the mother, and attachment to the mother is facilitated. The baby becomes calmer, has less pain, and handles stress more easily. The baby even increases in weight and grows more quickly.

The release of oxytocin is increased in women during pregnancy due to the high levels of the sex hormone estrogen. During labor and breastfeeding, maternal oxytocin is released in response to activation of sensory nerves induced by the baby's head pushing against the cervix of the uterus (the Ferguson reflex) or by sucking of the nipple of the breast (the milk ejection reflex). In addition, oxytocin is released into the brain by close contact, e.g., skin-to-skin contact, in both the mother and infant, and later on in response to the sight, sound, and even thoughts of the mother and infant, respectively. Maternal oxytocin release within the brain may also be induced by the touch or mere presence of warm and supportive persons during labor.

The period during and just after birth (the early sensitive period) is extremely important for the development of oxytocin-related effects on social interaction and ability to handle stress, as the oxytocin-mediated effects induced at this time tend to be extremely long lasting. In this way, early closeness has a positive impact on future physical and mental health.

Since closeness and positive, supportive social interaction influences oxytocin release in connection with birth and breastfeeding, thereby inducing long-lasting oxytocin-related effects, the future wellbeing and health of both mothers and children, and their ability to interact socially, are influenced by the amount of closeness and support they receive in connection with birth. These long-lasting effects depend on how the mothers give birth, whether mother and baby are close to each other or separated after birth, and whether the mother breastfeeds. The care, understanding, and support the mother receives from her family and healthcare providers may also play an important role in the development of oxytocin-related functions.

Changes in Society That May Disturb the Expression of Oxytocin-Mediated Effects

Our Western society has been and is still undergoing dramatic social changes. The extended family is gradually disappearing and has been substituted with the smaller nuclear family. Grandparents, parents, and children do not live together any longer and the "village community" is often lost. In some western countries, the classical nuclear family is also on its way out. Men and women often have several relationships during their life and may actually live in "mixed" families of various types. Others prefer to live as singles.

Loss of Information

The transfer of experiences and knowledge from one generation of women to the next, which occurred naturally when all generations lived together or at least lived close by, has to a great extent disappeared as a consequence of the disruption of family structures. It was by listening to the older female relatives that young women were taught everything about motherhood. They learned about pregnancy and morning sickness, about the pain and joy of labor, and about the pleasure and anxiety of breastfeeding. They always had somebody to talk to and ask the questions that inevitably come into a woman's mind during the fantastic, but also upsetting experience of expecting, having, and nurturing a child. Today, women often get information on these issues from books, brochures, the staff at the maternity clinics, or even from the Internet. It is, however, much easier and quicker to learn and "take in and digest information in a positive way," if it is given by someone you like and trust.

No wonder women of today, having lost the natural ties to the female tradition of knowledge and support, are afraid of giving birth and become easy prey of the recommendations and interventions formulated and created by the medical establishment and other forces in modern society.

Changes Around Childbirth That May Disturb the Expression of Oxytocin-Mediated Effects

Routines around birth and breastfeeding have differed greatly over time. They are still changing and will probably always change. We easily forget that the era during which birth has taken place in hospitals is short. Until the beginning of the twentieth century babies were born at home, with the assistance of midwives and/or other competent women.

Loss of Support

When birth took place in homes, female relatives and other wise women were often present to help and support the woman giving birth. After birth, they helped the new mother in every way and showed her how to breastfeed. When birth was moved from homes to hospitals, the support given by female relatives or other supportive women to the women giving birth was lost. Instead, staff from the hospitals, most often unknown to the birthing mother, took over. To have access to more experienced relatives or close friends is not only a way of receiving information, it is also about receiving both physical and mental support. As will be described later on in this book, the mere presence of supportive women makes labor quicker and less painful, and makes breastfeeding easier and more successful. When mothers feel better and more confident, they interact in a more positive and secure way with their newborn child.

Vaginal Birth No Longer a Necessity

Cesarean Section

Today, at least in the Western civilization, an increasing number of women give birth by Cesarean section. In Sweden, around 20% of all primiparas (first-time mothers) give birth by Cesarean section, whereas in some Western countries the figures are even higher.

There are many and complex reasons behind the increased use of Cesarean sections. The surgical techniques have been substantially improved, reducing possible risks associated with the surgical intervention. The need for quick deliveries and cost-effective care in the labor and maternity wards, the lost competence of midwives and physicians to deliver babies in breech position, and the increased tendency to blame the hospital/staff if something goes wrong with mother or baby during birth are some of the reasons why the incidence of Cesarean section is on the increase. But mothers also contribute to the increased use of Cesarean section by demanding it. They are afraid of giving birth in a natural way because of the pain and the loss of control associated with vaginal birth. They may also be afraid of physical damage to their body as a consequence of vaginal birth.

A consequence of Cesarean section is that less oxytocin is released than in mothers giving birth vaginally. In the case of elective Cesarean section, no oxytocin at all is released during labor since there are no contractions. In the case of emergency Cesarean sections, the amount of oxytocin released depends on the duration of contractions preceding the intervention.

Pain Relief

If mothers give birth vaginally, they may receive different kinds of medical pain relief, such as injection of opioids, a pudendal block, or an epidural analgesia. The use of epidural analgesia is becoming increasingly common. Fifty percent of the primiparas giving birth in Sweden today receive epidural analgesia during labor. In fact, there is a Swedish law that gives women the right to receive pain relief during labor, if they so wish.

Administration of Oxytocin

Synthetic oxytocin is often given as an intravenous infusion to initiate or to augment labor. Fifty percent of the women giving birth in Sweden receive infusions of oxytocin during labor, and the use of oxytocin is increasing. Almost all women receive an injection of oxytocin after birth to help contract the uterus and prevent unnecessary bleeding.

Administration of synthetic oxytocin is often associated with very painful contractions, which increases the need of pain relief, such as epidural analgesia, during labor. Administration of epidural analgesia often results in less efficient contractions, which increases the need for infusion of synthetic oxytocin to augment labor. In this way, a vicious circle is created, leading to more and more medical interventions.

Loss of Closeness

When babies were born at home, the newborn babies were immediately put to the mother's breast after birth. Afterwards, mother and baby spent most of their time close together, both day and night, for a long time.

When birth was moved to hospitals, mothers and babies were separated from each other. Babies were taken from their mothers when they were born and placed in a cot in a nursery, while the mothers stayed in the maternity ward. Staff brought the babies to their mothers every four hours, when the mothers were supposed to breastfeed their babies. As early closeness is important for the release of oxytocin and bonding between mothers and infants, as well as for the infant's ability to handle stress in the future, separation of mothers and infants after birth may have a negative impact on the development of these variables.

Today, most mothers in Sweden are allowed to have their babies in skin-to-skin contact immediately after birth and to be with them in the maternity ward (rooming in). In many other countries, mothers and infants are still often separated from each other in the labor and maternity wards.

Breastfeeding No Longer a Necessity

Today, breastfeeding is often replaced by bottle feeding in large parts of the world, as artificial milk or formula is widely available. Formula is based on cows' milk. Although it has been much refined over the years, it is still far from identical to mothers' milk. An additional difference between breastfeeding and bottle-feeding is that oxytocin is released in breastfeeding mothers when the infants are suckling, whereas this is not the case during bottle-feeding.

Unfortunately, the use of formula has spread to countries where breastfeeding is both healthier and a more economical alternative for mothers to feed their infants. It has been proposed that unethical advertising and economic interests may lie behind this misconception.

In Sweden, the rate of breastfeeding is high. Ninety percent of the newly delivered mothers are breastfeeding when they leave the maternity ward, and about 60% breastfeed exclusively for six months. In many other Western countries, the breastfeeding frequency is much lower.

Much energy is spent informing mothers of the physiological and psychological advantages of breastfeeding. Still, it is often difficult to convince mothers to breastfeed because they find bottle-feeding easier and more practical. It gives them more freedom and may be the only solution if they have to work.

Some women choose to express their milk using a breast pump. In this way, they can give their own milk to their infant. This is a solution for many mothers with premature infants in the hospital and mothers who want to go back to work, but can't go home to breastfeed during the day or bring their babies to the work place.

Impact on Release of Oxytocin Following Interventions During Birth

Since oxytocin exerts such vital effects in both mother and infant, it is important they are exposed to routines in the labor and maternity wards that are consistent with maximal stimulation of oxytocin release. As mentioned above, oxytocin is released during vaginal birth, skin-to-skin contact between mother and infant, and breastfeeding to help the mother adapt to motherhood. Less oxytocin is released in mothers who have a Cesarean section, are separated from their infants after birth, or bottle-feed their infants than in those giving birth vaginally, have skin-to-skin contact with their babies after birth, and breastfeed.

An important question is whether the maternal adaptations are less well developed in mothers who have a Cesarean section instead of a vaginal birth, are separated from their infants immediately after birth instead of having skin-to-skin contact, and who are bottle-feeding instead of breastfeeding. What happens in mothers who have given birth vaginally, but have an epidural analgesia or received exogenous (synthetic) oxytocin during labor?

All these interventions can be expected to influence the release of endogenous (natural) oxytocin normally occurring in labor. Recent scientific data suggests that the release of endogenous oxytocin and the effects mediated by oxytocin are influenced under these circumstances.

If so, what are the consequences for mothers and children on their ability to interact socially, handle stress, and their future health in a short and long-term perspective? What are the consequences for the next generation?

Need of Information to Make Decisions

There are many obvious advantages of Cesarean sections, pain relief during birth, and bottle-feeding, which may be the reason why so many mothers choose or accept these solutions. But would all these women have done so if they had known about oxytocin, its positive effects for both mother and child, and the link between oxytocin release in natural birth, skin-to-skin contact, and breastfeeding? Would they have made the same choices or accepted the recommendations if they had known that Cesarean section, epidural analgesia, separation of mother and infant after birth, and bottle-feeding reduce oxytocin release in themselves and sometimes in the infant, and thereby the future expression of the oxytocin-related effects?

In the future women should be informed during pregnancy about oxytocin and its positive effects, since this knowledge may be important in their decisions as to what kind of birth they want and whether they want to breastfeed their baby. The choices they make may not only be important for them, but also for their children.

Chapter 2

Brain-Body and Body-Brain Connections: The Nervous System

In order to make it easier for readers to understand the parts in the book in which the many and diverse functions of oxytocin will be described, a short and simplified summary of the structure and function of the brain, the peripheral nervous system, and the neuro-endocrine system will be given. The basic information on the nervous and endocrine systems in this chapter and in the following chapter can be obtained from any textbook on medical physiology or endocrinology unless specific references are given (Guyton, 2002; Hadley, 2000). Figure 2.1 identifies the different parts of the brain.

The Nervous System

We normally consider the brain as the site where all our functions are controlled. It should be remembered that our inner organs and the outside world provide the brain with an enormous amount of information via our sensory organs and nerves. This information is then integrated in the central nervous system to exert important regulatory effects on the function of the brain.

The nervous system can be divided into two main parts: *the central nervous system*, which consists of the brain and the spinal cord, and *the peripheral nervous system*, which consists of nerves that connect the brain with different parts of the body.

The Nerve Cells

The nervous system, the brain, and the peripheral nervous system are mainly made up of nerve cells (neurons) and cells that support the nerve cells—the glia cells. Nerve cells differ in shape and size, but are often elongated. In principle, each nerve cell consists of a cell body, with thin extensions running in opposite directions. The shorter ones are called dendrites and receive information from other nerve cells, whereas the longer extensions, called axons, transfer information to other nerve (or endocrine) cells.

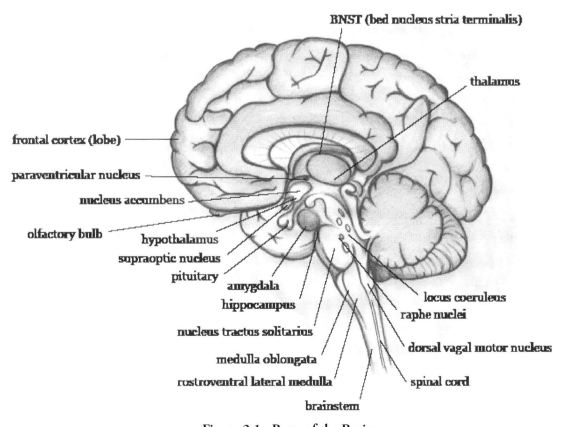

Figure 2.1. Parts of the Brain

Nerve cells transmit information to other cells via chemical messengers (neurotransmitters or signaling substances), which are released into a small space between cells called the synaptic cleft. The chemical messengers then bind to receptors on the receiving cells to induce a new cascade of events.

The chemical messengers can be very different from a chemical point of view. They are often amino acids or slightly modified amino acids. Small peptides (substances consisting of several linked amino acids), gases, such as nitric oxide, and certain fat molecules may also serve as signaling substances.

The Central Nervous System

The central nervous system consists of the brain and the spinal cord. The brain consists of several layers, which from an evolutionary perspective are of different ages. The modern brain or the neocortex lies on top of older parts of the brain, such as the limbic system, the brainstem, and the spinal cord. Our conscious intellectual functions are located in the part of the modern brain called the frontal cortex. This is where evaluation and interpretation of information and conscious strategic thinking take place. This part of the brain is much more developed in humans than in other mammals.

The limbic system, located underneath the cortex, is an important center for emotions and emotional reactions, memory, and learning. In the hypothalamus—an important part of the limbic system—basal functions, such as reproduction, food and water intake, aggression, and sexuality, are controlled.

Centers for control of basic functions, such as breathing, blood pressure, pulse rate, and digestion, are located in the brainstem, an even older part of the brain from an evolutionary viewpoint. Finally, even more primitive reflexive functions take place in the spinal cord.

Both the modern and the older parts of the brain contain areas that may relate to specific brain functions. Knowledge about the activity in such areas has increased dramatically during the last decades because the development of new brain imaging techniques now allow studies of the activity in specific areas in the brain in specific situations.

The Peripheral Nervous System

The peripheral nervous system can be divided into two major parts—the *somatic* and the *autonomic nervous system.*

The Somatic Nervous System

The function of the somatic nervous system can be controlled by our will.

The Autonomic Nervous System

Normally, we cannot consciously control the function in the autonomic nervous system, since it is regulated from areas located in older parts of the brain.

The Sympathetic and the Parasympathetic Nervous System

The autonomic nervous system is normally divided into the *sympathetic* and the *parasympathetic nervous system.* A subpopulation of the sympathetic nerves innervates the adrenal medulla, the *sympatho-medullary axis.* The remaining part of the sympathetic nervous system is sometimes referred to as *the sympatho-neural system.* The sympathetic nerves originate in the thoracic and lumbar regions of the spinal cord. The big vagal nerve that links the gastrointestinal tract, the heart, and the lungs with the brain is a part of the parasympathetic nervous system that leaves the brain at the level of the medulla oblongata (the lowest part of the brain stem). A second part of the parasympathetic nervous system emanates from the sacral region of the spinal cord.

Greatly simplified, the sympathetic and the parasympathetic parts of the autonomic nervous system act in opposite directions. The sympathetic nervous system is activated during physical activity, in situations of defense, and during stress. Activation of the sympathetic nervous system leads to arousal, increased blood pressure and heart rate, and mobilization of energy, which, e.g., gives rise to elevated glucose levels.

The parasympathetic nervous system is activated during feeding, breastfeeding, close contact, and situations of relaxation. It stimulates digestion, storage of nutrients, healing, and growth.

Both the sympathetic and parasympathetic nervous systems innervate the uterus, and both are involved in the birth process. The mammary glands lack parasympathetic innervation and, therefore, only the sympathetic nervous system influences milk production and milk ejection.

Motor Nerves or Efferent Nerves

The outgoing nerves (the nerves that leave the brainstem or spinal cord to reach different organs in the body) are called motor or efferent nerves. The motor nerves that belong to the somatic nervous system control the movement of our muscles. The motor nerves that belong to the autonomic nervous system control the activity of our inner organs, such as the cardiovascular system, the lungs, and the gastrointestinal tract.

Signaling Substances

Acetylcholine is the main neurotransmitter or signaling substance of the somatic motor fibers innervating the muscles. The motor fibers of the parasympathetic nervous system use acetylcholine as a neurotransmitter, whereas noradrenaline is the main neurotransmitter in the sympathetic branches of the autonomic nervous system.

Adrenaline is released into the circulation in response to activation of the sympathetic fibers that innervate the adrenal medulla.

Sensory Nerves or Afferent Nerves

The brain is continuously being provided with information via our senses, which relay information from the surrounding environment and our inner organs to the brain. The peripheral sensory nerves emanate from the skin, muscles, joints, and sinews, and inform our brains about what is going on at the level of the skin and also about our movements and position (proprioception). The sensory nerves are organized in a more or less segmental way.

The sympathetic and parasympathetic nervous systems also have a sensory component. These fibers convey information to the brain about the function of our inner organs—the cardiovascular system, lungs, gastrointestinal tract, and reproductive organs. A subpopulation of sensory fibers from the vagina, uterus, and mammary glands bypass the spinal cord and travel with the vagal nerves via the nodose ganglion and the nucleus tractus solitarius (NTS) in the medulla oblongata (Adams, Grummer-Strawn, & Chavez, 2003; Eriksson, Lindh, Uvnäs-Moberg, & Hokfelt, 1996; Komisaruk & Sansone, 2003).

The Skin as a Sensory Organ

The importance of the skin as a sensory organ is often forgotten, but it is the largest sensory organ in the body. It occupies an area of about two square meters in adult humans. It is the first of our senses to develop. The fetus may respond to touch at the age of two months.

Sensory Innervation of the Skin

The skin is richly provided with receptors, which are linked to cutaneous sensory nerves. These nerve fibers convey information to the spinal cord where a second neuron is activated, which then transfers the information to the thalamus in the brain. Activation of skin receptors may be induced by physical or chemical damage to the skin. They may also be induced by light and deep pressure, touch, stroking, and cold and warm temperatures.

Sensory fibers from the skin are divided into different subtypes—A, B, and C-fibers, depending on whether they are covered by myelin and how thick they are. The thinner, unmyelinated C-fibers are older from an evolutionary point of view. They transmit nerve impulses at a slower pace than the thicker, myelinated sensory fibers in the A or B subgroups.

Touch and acute pain are mediated via the myelinated fibers belonging to the A and B fiber subgroups, whereas activation of C-fibers gives rise to pain, which is often chronic and diffuse as to its localization. Recently, a special type of C-fibers, the C-Tactile (CT) fibers, activated by stroking the skin in humans, has been demonstrated (Olausson, Wessberg, Morrison, McGlone, & Vallbo, 2010; Vallbo, Olausson, Wessberg, & Norrsell, 1993).

When the CT fibers are stimulated, areas in the insular cortex related to the sensation of wellbeing are activated (Craig, 2003; Olausson et al., 2002; Vallbo, Olausson, & Wessberg, 1999).

Noxious and Non-Noxious Stimulation

Sensory stimulation from the skin by painful (noxious) stimuli or by touch or other types of pleasant (non-noxious) stimuli, not only reaches the thalamus and sensory cortex in the brain to give rise to a localized perception of pain or touch, but also gives rise to emotional, behavioral, and physiological effects. Noxious stimulation may be associated with pain, anxiety, activation of the sympathetic nervous system, and increased cortisol levels. Non-noxious stimulation may be associated with wellbeing, reduced stress levels, and increased activity in the parasympathetic nervous system (Uvnäs-Moberg, 1998a; Uvnäs-Moberg & Petersson, 2011).

Reflexes

On their way to the thalamus and sensory cortex, the sensory nerves may influence functions at many levels—the hypothalamic level, the brainstem level, and also at the level of the spinal cord. Normally, the effect exerted at the "highest" levels override the effects exerted at the "lower" levels, which they may antagonize or reinforce.

Sensory nerves emanating in the skin may also exert local effects via axon reflexes at the site of origin of the nerve, in addition to transferring information from the skin to the spinal cord. The axon reflexes are mediated via extensions of the nerve fibers, which run backwards or in an opposite direction to the main nerves.

Coexistence of Neurotransmitters

Many nerve fibers, both motor and sensory, contain several other transmitter substances that modulate the effects of the main signaling substance (Björklund, Hökfelt, & Owman, 1988; Salt & Hill, 1983). There are numerous examples of coexistence between neurotransmitters, but only a few relevant to the content in this book will be mentioned here.

For example, the peptide Neuropeptide Y (NPY) is present and coexists with noradrenaline in the motor neurons of the sympathetic nervous system (Lundberg, Terenius, Hokfelt, & Goldstein, 1983). Axon reflexes may be induced in response to activation of sensory nerves. The effects induced by axon reflexes are often induced by peptides that are co-localized with the main neurotransmitter of the sensory neurons, which is often glutamate. Calcitonin gene-related peptide (CGRP), substance P (SP), and vasoactive polypeptide (VIP) are examples of peptides which can be released locally via axon reflexes in the skin (Gibson et al., 1984; Hokfelt, Kellerth, Nilsson, & Pernow, 1975; Shehab & Atkinson, 1986).

<h1 style="text-align:center">Chapter 3</h1>

Brain-Body and Body-Brain Connections: The Neuroendocrine System

The brain can control the function of the body and its organs via the autonomic nervous system as described in the previous chapter and via hormones, which will be described in this chapter. The function of the autonomic nervous system and the neuroendocrine system are, in part, coordinated by the regulatory systems in the hypothalamus.

Hormones

Hormones or endocrine substances are produced in special endocrine glands in the body. They are released into the circulation to reach their target organs. In the target organ, they bind to specific receptors to induce their effects.

There are different types of hormones. Some are derivatives of the cholesterol molecule—the steroid hormones. Others consist of chains of amino acids—the peptide hormones.

Steroid Hormones

The stress hormone cortisol, produced in the adrenal cortex, the female sex hormones estrogen and progesterone, produced in the ovaries, and the male sex hormone testosterone, produced in the testes, are all steroid hormones. The steroid hormones are fat molecules. They easily penetrate biological membranes, such as the blood-brain barrier or gastrointestinal mucosa. These hormones can be given orally, they are secreted into saliva and urine, and they may exert functions within the brain. The onset of action is relatively slow since they exert their effects on specific receptors located in the nucleus of the cells.

Peptide Hormones

Most of the hormones produced in the pituitary (e.g., growth hormone, adrenocorticotrophic hormone [ACTH], oxytocin, and prolactin) and most of the gastrointestinal and pancreatic hormones (e.g., gastrin, cholecystokinin, and insulin) are often peptide hormones. These hormones do not easily pass biological membranes because they are often quite big and electrically charged. Peptide hormones can't be administered orally because they will not be absorbed from the gastrointestinal mucosa. They do not normally pass from the circulation into urine or saliva, making them difficult to measure in urine or saliva. Finally, they do not pass from the circulation into the brain unless administered in extremely high doses or if special transport systems exist. The onset of action of peptides is most often immediate, since the peptide hormones usually activate receptors located in the membranes of the cells.

The Pituitary

The pituitary is the most important endocrine gland in the body. It controls the function of most other endocrine glands.

The Anterior Pituitary

The hormones produced and released from the anterior pituitary control the activity in most of the peripheral hormone-producing glands. Follicle stimulating hormone (FSH) and luteinizing hormone (LH) control the secretion of the sex hormones, estrogen, progesterone, and testosterone, from the ovaries and testes, respectively. Thyroid stimulating hormone (TSH) regulates the production of thyroid hormones in the thyroid gland.

Two other important, and from a chemical point of view related, hormones are produced in the anterior pituitary—growth hormone and prolactin. Growth hormone stimulates growth in most tissues, either directly or via release of insulin-like growth factor. Prolactin, produced in special cells called lactotrophs, stimulates milk production from the milk-producing cells (the lactotrophs) in the mammary gland.

ACTH controls the secretion of cortisol from the outer layer of the adrenal gland—the adrenal cortex. Cortisol recruits energy from the stores in the body and reinforces the activity of the sympathetic nervous system. It is necessary for any energy-demanding activity and also during stress.

The Regulatory Role of the Hypothalamus

The secretion of the hormones in the anterior pituitary is controlled from the hypothalamus by specific regulatory substances, such as thyroid-releasing hormone (TRH), gonadotrophin-releasing hormone (GNRH), and corticotrophin-releasing hormone or factor (CRF). These hormones are secreted from neurons in the hypothalamus into the median eminence and reach the anterior pituitary via a small network of blood vessels.

Feed Back Inhibition

The levels of peripheral hormones are kept under control by a feed back inhibitory system. The circulating cortisol, estrogen, testosterone, and thyroid hormones inhibit the secretion of the hormones from the pituitary that stimulate their release and inhibit the secretion of their respective hypothalamic regulatory factors when the levels of the respective circulating hormones get too high.

The Posterior Pituitary

The hormones vasopressin and oxytocin are released into the circulation from the posterior pituitary or neurohypophysis. In contrast to the hormones released from the anterior pituitary, these hormones are produced in neurons, which have their cell bodies in the supraoptic and the paraventricular nuclei (SON and PVN) of the hypothalamus. The hormones are then transported to the posterior pituitary via long axons to be secreted into the circulation. The neurons that secrete oxytocin and vasopressin into the blood stream are labeled magnocellular neurons, as they are larger than the parvocellular neurons, which project to other areas in the brain. More information about oxytocin will be given in the next three chapters.

Circulating vasopressin exerts anti-diuretic effects in the kidney. It also increases blood pressure. Vasopressin stimulates the activity of the HPA axis as vasopressin released into the median eminence from the PVN reaches the anterior pituitary. In the anterior pituitary, it stimulates ACTH release and activity in the HPA axis, particularly during chronic stress.

The Endocrine System of the Gastrointestinal Tract

Another important site of production for hormones is the gastrointestinal tract. The endocrine system of the gastrointestinal tract is the largest endocrine gland in the body (Uvnäs-Moberg, 1989). More than a hundred peptides have been shown to be produced in a special type of endocrine cells located in the mucosa of the gastrointestinal tract, but only of few of them relevant for the content in this book will be mentioned here.

The endocrine cells where the hormones are produced are in open contact with the gastrointestinal lumen. The hormone-producing cells sense or "taste" the contents of the gastrointestinal tract via receptors located on microvilli that project into the lumen. In this way, the cells can release hormones into the circulation depending on the amount of food that is present in the stomach and the intestine, the pH of the contents, and the type of nutrition present—fat, protein, or carbohydrates.

The release of gastrointestinal hormones is not only controlled by the contents in the gastrointestinal tract, but also by the autonomic nervous system. The vagal nerves (part of the parasympathetic nervous system) have an important stimulatory effect on the release of these hormones and on the pancreatic hormones (insulin and glucagon) involved in the control of blood sugar levels. Inhibitory effects on the release of these hormones may be exerted by the sympathetic nervous system, as well as by specific inhibitory vagal mechanisms (Uvnäs-Moberg, 1994).

Gastrointestinal and Pancreatic Hormones

The hormones produced in the gastrointestinal mucosa influence the digestive function of the gastrointestinal tract. The hormone gastrin stimulates the secretion of gastric acid, cholecystokinin (CCK), and secretin, stimulating the secretion of pancreatic juices. CCK empties the gall bladder and closes the duodenal sphincter—the ring-shaped muscles separating the stomach and the duodenal part of the small intestine.

Insulin is produced in the pancreas and stimulates the uptake of nutrients, particularly glucose, into the cells. Insulin is the only hormone that lowers blood glucose levels and is very important for the regulation of blood sugar. Another pancreatic hormone, glucagon, has the opposite effect. It recruits glucose from its stores in the liver and elevates blood glucose levels.

Somatostatin is a hormone that was originally described as the substance in the hypothalamus that inhibits the secretion of growth hormone from the anterior pituitary. However, this substance is also produced in the stomach, intestine, and pancreas, where it inhibits both the function of the gastrointestinal tract and the release of gastrointestinal and pancreatic hormones. By these inhibitory actions, somatostatin counteracts growth in a broad sense, since the availability of nutrients needed for growth is diminished. The vagal nerve inhibits the release of somatostatin, whereas sympathetic nerve activity increases the levels of this hormone (Uvnäs-Moberg, 1989).

The Incretin Effect

The gastrointestinal hormones also have a broader effect pattern, since they influence metabolism and stimulate anabolic metabolism and growth by promoting the release of insulin.

Indirect Effect on the Central Nervous System

Some gastrointestinal hormones influence brain function indirectly via activation of sensory fibers in the vagal nerves. CCK is released after ingestion of food, particularly if the food contains fat and proteins. It causes satiety, feelings of wellbeing, and sedation via activation of the vagal nerves. It also stimulates social interaction and bonding by releasing oxytocin (Uvnäs-Moberg, 1989, 1994).

Coordination of Stress Responses

The HPA Axis

The HPA axis consists of several neurogenic and hormonal mechanisms in the brain and in the body. Corticotrophin-releasing factor (CRF) is produced in the paraventricular nucleus of the hypothalamus (PVN). It is secreted into the median eminence and transported to the anterior pituitary via local blood vessels (the portal system). When CRF reaches the anterior pituitary, it stimulates the release of ACTH into the blood stream. ACTH, in turn, stimulates the release of cortisol from the adrenal cortex.

The function of the HPA axis is influenced from several areas in the brain, such as the prefrontal cortex, the hippocampus, the amygdala, the Locus Coeruleus (LC), and the Nucleus Tractus Solitarius (NTS; Herman, Ostrander, Mueller, & Figueiredo, 2005; Herman, Prewitt, & Cullinan, 1996). These pathways are important for the mechanisms in which oxytocin exerts anti-stress effects.

Both the release of CRF and ACTH is under "feed-back" inhibitory control by cortisol, which due to its chemical properties, easily penetrates into the brain. Cortisol also inhibits the activity of the HPA axis by activation of special corticoid (GR and MR) receptors in the hippocampus, which via a neurogenic mechanism inhibits the release of CRF in the PVN.

Fear and Activation of the Amygdala

The amygdala is activated in response to fearful situations via impulses from the different sensory systems (visual, auditory, olfactory, gustatory, and tactile), inducing adaptive reactions involving behavior and autonomic and endocrine functions (LeDoux, 2012). Activation of the amygdala results in activation of the sympathetic nervous system and the HPA axis, which are the main regulators of stress responses in the body. The sympathetic nervous system, which emanates from the ventral side of the spinal cord, reaches the cardiovascular system, the lungs, and the gastrointestinal and genitourinary organs via different nerve branches, and stress hormones, such as cortisol, reach their targets via the circulation. The neurogenic sympathetic nervous system can induce very quick responses, whereas the endocrine HPA axis reacts more slowly. Still, the two systems are not completely independent of each other, as they share some regulatory mechanisms.

Link Between the Amygdala and the Locus Coeruleus

When the amygdala is activated in response to different kinds of fear or stressors, CRF-containing nerve fibers, which project to the LC, are activated and the release of noradrenaline is triggered (Van Bockstaele, Colago, & Valentino, 1998).

Noradrenergic Fibers from the Locus Coeruleus Activate Both the Sympathetic Nervous System and the HPA Axis

Noradrenergic fibers from the LC and adjacent areas in the brainstem play an important regulatory role for the activity of the sympathetic nervous system and in centers in the forebrain causing wakefulness and aggression. Noradrenergic fibers from the LC control the function of the HPA axis by stimulating the release of CRF. The noradrenergic control of the function of the CRF neurons in the PVN is of great importance in the function of the HPA axis. The levels of noradrenaline in the PVN are strongly correlated to the levels of CRF in the PVN and

ACTH in the circulation (Liu, Caldji, Sharma, Plotsky, & Meaney, 2000).

Noradrenergic Fibers from the NTS Activate the Sympathetic Nervous System and the HPA Axis

Noradrenergic neurons projecting from the NTS to the PVN contribute to the control of the HPA axis. Noxious (painful, unpleasant) sensory stimulation from the skin or the viscera, which activate noradrenergic neurons in the NTS, contribute to the release of CRF from the PVN and, hence, the release of ACTH and cortisol into the circulation (Sato, 1987; Tsuchia, 1994).

CRF and Vasopressinergic Neurons from the PVN Influence the Activity of the LC and the NTS

CRF and vasopressin from the PVN are part of the HPA axis, and they both stimulate the release of ACTH from the anterior pituitary. CRF and vasopressin produced in the PVN contribute to adaptations to stress in yet another way. Neurons emanating from parvocellular (small) neurons in the PVN containing CRF and vasopressin (and also oxytocin) project to areas in the brainstem involved in the control of the autonomic nervous system, such as the Locus Coeruleus (LC), the vagal motor (DMX) and sensory nucleus (NTS), the rostroventral lateral medulla (RVLM), and sympathetic ganglia, where they induce stress-related effects (Buijs, 1983).

CRF and Vasopressinergic Neurons from the PVN and Noradrenergic Neurons from the LC and NTS Exert Reciprocal Effects

In this way, a reciprocal effect on stress reactions is exerted by hypothalamic and brainstem structures. The activity of the CRF and parvocellular neurons in the PVN is stimulated by noradrenergic neurons emanating in the LC and the NTS. At the same time, CRF and vasopressin neurons, originating from the parvocellular neurons of the PVN, stimulate noradrenergic centers in the brainstem involved in stress regulation, such as the LC, the RVLM, and the NTS.

CRF and Vasopressinergic Neurons from the PVN
Influence the Activity of the Gastrointestinal Tract

CRF and vasopressin released from parvocellular neurons emanating in the PVN decrease the activity in the gastrointestinal tract by actions in the DMX and NTS. CRF, for example, stimulates the release of somatostatin, which exerts an inhibitory effect on gastrointestinal and pancreatic function by activating sympathetic nerves or vagal inhibitory fibers. In this way, CRF inhibits digestive and metabolic function.

Chapter 4

Oxytocin: General Aspects

As early as the beginning of the 19th century, it was found that extracts from the posterior pituitary (neurohypophysis) of cats could induce uterine contractions (Dale, 1906, 1909). The substance was named oxytocin, which means quick birth. A few years later, it was found that these extracts also induced milk flow, and this effect was induced by contraction of the myoepithelial cells of the mammary gland (Gaines, 1915; Ott & Scott, 1910). Oxytocin was the very first hormone in which the chemical identity was established. It was synthesized in the 1950s, which made the clinical use of oxytocin during labor and breastfeeding possible (Du Vigneaud, Ressler, & Trippett, 1953).

The Chemical Structure of Oxytocin

Oxytocin is a polypeptide hormone, which consists of nine amino acids. It has a disulfide bridge between positions 1 and 6, giving rise to a six-amino-acid ring structure (Figure 4.1).

Vasopressin is related to oxytocin from a chemical point of view, but differs from oxytocin by an exchange of the amino acids in positions 3 and 8 (Burbach, Young, & Russell, 2006).

The oxytocin/vasopressin molecules are well conserved from an evolutionary perspective. The structure of oxytocin is the same in all mammals. Vasotocin, which is a hybrid between oxytocin and vasopressin and an evolutionary precursor of both these molecules, has been demonstrated in non-mammalian vertebrates and in mammalian fetuses. The related peptides isotocin and mesotocin are found in bony fish, reptiles, and birds, respectively (Acher, Chauvet, & Chauvet, 1995; Sawyer, 1977).

Production of Oxytocin Within the Hypothalamus

Magnocellular and Parvocellular Neurons

Oxytocin is produced in two large cell groups in the hypothalamus, the supraoptic nucleus (SON) and the paraventricular nucleus (PVN). Within these cell groups, oxytocin is produced in two different types of cells, the big cells or the magnocellular neurons, which send their nerve endings (axons) down into the posterior pituitary where oxytocin is released into the blood circulation, and the small or parvocellular neurons, which send oxytocin-containing nerves to several important regulatory areas within the brain. The SON contains magnocellular oxytocin neurons alone, whereas the PVN contains both magno- and parvocellular oxytocin-producing cells (Figure 4.2; Richard, Moos, & Freund-Mercier, 1991).

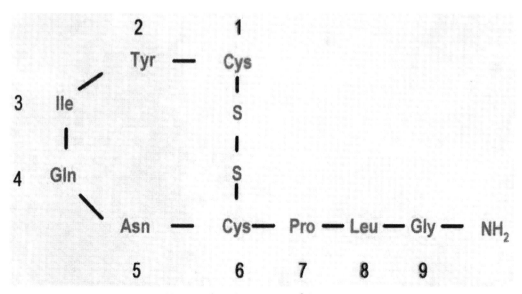

Figure 4.1. Structure of Oxytocin

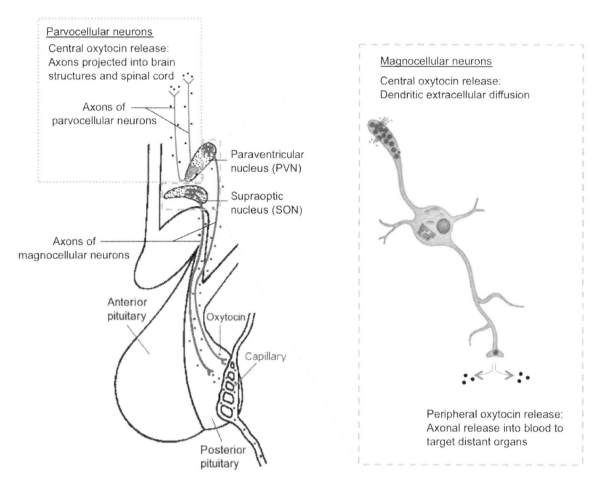

Figure 4.2. Magno- and Parvocelluar Oxytocin-Producing Cells

Source: Uvnäs-Moberg & Prime, 2013. Reprinted with permission.

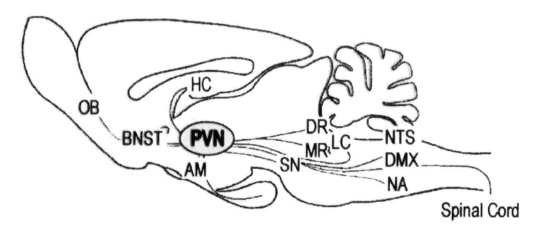

Figure 4.3. Projections of Oxytocinergic Nerves in the Brain

Projections of Oxytocinergic Nerves in the Brain

The parvocellular oxytocin neurons project to many different areas in the brain. Oxytocin-containing nerves reach the frontal cortex, the amygdala (important regulatory center for social interaction and fear), the olfactory bulb, the hippocampus (center for memory and learning), other areas within the hypothalamus (control of hypothalamo-pituitary-adrenal axis—HPA axis), anterior pituitary (control of pituitary hormone secretion), the Locus Coeruleus (LC, control of aggression and wakefulness, autonomic nervous tone, noradrenergic neurons), the raphe nuclei (RN, control of mood, serotonergic neurons), the striatum and the nucleus accumbens (NA, control of motor functions, wellbeing and reward, dopaminergic neurons), the periaqueductal grey (PAG, control of pain), and areas in which the activity of the autonomic nervous system is controlled, such as the vagal motor nucleus (DMX, cholinergic neurons) and the nucleus tractus solitarius, (NTS, noradrenergic neurons), the rostroventrolateral medulla (RVLM, important center for cardiovascular control), and the spinal cord (pain control, opioidergic neurons, sympathetic ganglia, and parasympathetic neurons) (Buijs, 1983; Buijs, De Vries, & Van Leeuwen, 1985; Sofroniew, 1983).

Not only the oxytocinergic nerves originating from parvocellular neurons of the PVN, but also a subpopulation of the magnocellular neurons originating in the PVN, which project to the posterior pituitary, may influence brain function. These magnocellular neurons are provided with axon-collaterals that reach several important regulatory areas within the brain, for example, the frontal cortex, the amygdala, and the anterior pituitary. In this way, these magnocellular neurons influence certain brain functions by acting as a neurotransmitter in the brain and, at the same time, exerting hormonal actions in the circulation, coordinating behavioral and physiological effects (Figure 4.3; Knobloch et al., 2012; Mason, Ho, & Hatton, 1984).

Morphological and Functional Changes of Oxytocin Neurons in Response to Strong Stimulation

When oxytocin release is intensely stimulated, for example, during labor and breastfeeding, morphological changes occur in the structure of the oxytocin-producing areas in the supraoptic and paraventricular nuclei of the hypothalamus. The oxytocin-producing cells actually come closer to each other because the surrounding supportive cells, the glia cells, withdraw. This change has functional consequences since the different oxytocin-producing cells start to act together, as if they were all one giant cell. As the electrical activity of the different oxytocin-producing cells becomes synchronized, big bursts of electrical activity are induced. Oxytocin is released in response to each "burst," which

will be reflected by a pulse or a peak of oxytocin into the circulation. The oxytocin pulses in the circulation may then cause contractions of the uterus during labor or contractions of the alveolar cells in the mammary gland and milk ejection during breastfeeding (Hatton & Tweedle, 1982; Poulain & Wakerley, 1982; Theodosis, 2002; Theodosis, Chapman, Montagnese, Poulain, & Morris, 1986; Wakerley, Poulain, & Brown, 1978).

Synthesis of Oxytocin

The Oxytocin Gene

The structure of the oxytocin gene has been elucidated in rats and humans. The gene contains three exons. The first exon includes the code for oxytocin, a spacer sequence, and part of the oxytocin-associated neurophysin. The second and third exons code for the rest of the neurophysin molecule (Burbach et al., 2006). The oxytocin gene contains response elements for estrogen, glucocorticoids, thyroid hormones, and retinoids (Burbach et al., 2006).

Larger Precursor Molecules

Like all peptide hormones, oxytocin is produced as a large precursor molecule, which includes a specific part called neurophysin. An important part of the synthesis of oxytocin takes place in the endoplasmic reticulum, where the disulphide bond of the six-amino-acid ring structure is formed. The prohormone is then packed into small vesicles or secretory granules within the Golgi apparatus. The neurophysin part of the prohormone is clipped off during the transport within the axons of the oxytocin-producing cells. The remaining extended oxytocin molecule is then gradually broken down to the final molecule, the nonapeptide, within the oxytocin-producing cells (Burbach et al., 2006). Sometimes the breakdown of oxytocin to the nonapeptide is not completed within the oxytocin-producing cells, and then elongated pre-oxytocin molecules are released into the circulation. The more intense and the more long lasting the stimulation of oxytocin release is, the more likely it is that elongated forms of oxytocin will be released into the circulation, giving rise to a mixed pattern of oxytocin molecules (Amico & Hempel, 1990; Green et al., 2001).

Hormone, Neurotransmitter, or Paracrine Substance

After being released from the oxytocinergic neurons, oxytocin may exert effects in different ways. When oxytocin is released from the posterior pituitary into the circulation and reaches its targets via the blood stream, it acts as a hormone or an endocrine substance. The effects of oxytocin on labor and milk letdown are examples of hormonal actions of oxytocin.

When oxytocin is released from parvocellular oxytocinergic nerves within the brain, which originate from the PVN, it acts as a signaling substance or a neurotransmitter. The effect of oxytocin on maternal behavior is induced by oxytocin acting as a neurotransmitter. Oxytocin may also be released from swellings on axons of magno- and parvocellular neurons into the median eminence, and further on transported to the anterior pituitary to influence the release of hormones in the anterior pituitary (Burbach et al., 2006).

When oxytocin secretion is intensely stimulated, as during labor and suckling, oxytocin may also act by local or paracrine effects, since oxytocin is then not only released from the axons of the oxytocin-producing neuron, but also from the dendrites and the cell body itself. Large amounts of oxytocin may be released directly into the areas surrounding the oxytocin-producing cells. In this way, oxytocin may, by diffusion, reach nearby and even distant areas in the brain, which lack oxytocin-containing nerves to exert effects via oxytocin receptors located in these areas (Ludwig & Leng, 2006).

Oxytocin of Non-Hypothalamic Origin

It is becoming increasingly clear that the hypothalamus is not the only site of production for oxytocin. Production of oxytocin has been demonstrated in the uterus, ovaries, amniotic fluid, and placenta. Recently, a substantial synthesis of oxytocin has been demonstrated to occur in the heart, blood vessels, and gastrointestinal tract (Gutkowska & Jankowski, 2008; Lefebvre, Giaid, Bennett, Lariviere, & Zingg, 1992; Lefebvre, Giaid, & Zingg, 1992; Lefebvre, Lariviere, & Zingg, 1993; Ohlsson, Truedsson, Djerf, & Sundler, 2006; Wathes & Swann, 1982).

Oxytocin produced in other organs in the body, such as the uterus, the cardiovascular system, or the gastrointestinal tract, may exert endocrine effects, but is most likely to exert paracrine (local) effects. It may also influence the activity within the oxytocin-producing cells themselves by autocrine effects.

Metabolism of Oxytocin

Circulating oxytocin is metabolized and degraded in the liver and kidney. It is also degraded by placental oxytocinases in the circulation and other tissues, in particular during pregnancy (Ito et al., 2003; Naruki et al., 1996). The half-life of oxytocin in the circulation is around 90 seconds in rats and has been claimed to be around three to four minutes in women (Richard et al., 1991; Ryden & Sjoholm, 1969). In the study by Rydén and Sjöholm, tritium-labeled oxytocin was used to determine the plasma half-life in women. In another study, in which 1 I.U. (1.71 micrograms) of oxytocin was injected intravenously in men and oxytocin levels were measured with radioimmunoassay, the half-life was found to be considerably longer. Oxytocin levels fell rapidly during the first minutes after administration

of oxytocin, reflecting distribution of the peptide within the organism. The initial fall was followed by a period of slower elimination, with a half-life of 20-30 minutes (De Groot et al., 1995). A similar half-life of oxytocin has been demonstrated in non-pregnant women (Uvnäs-Moberg, Nielsen, Ahmed, & Fianu-Jonasson, 2014). The reason for this difference is not known, but may be related to specificity and sensitivity of the analytical techniques used.

Membrane-bound enzymes degrade oxytocin released from nerves in the brain. Special enzymes open the ring structure and cleave the disulphide bond, and carboxy- and amino-peptidases clip off amino acids from the C-terminal and N-terminal sides of the oxytocin molecule, respectively (Adan et al., 1995; Burbach & Lebouille, 1983; Burbach et al., 2006; Stancampiano & Argiolas, 1993; Stancampiano, Melis, & Argiolas, 1991). Some of the fragments formed during the degradation process are biologically active (de Wied, Gaffori, Burbach, Kovacs, & van Ree, 1987; Gaffori & De Wied, 1988; Stancampiano et al., 1991). The half-life of oxytocin in cerebrospinal fluid (CSF) of guinea pigs is around 28 minutes—considerably longer than the half-life in the circulation of rats (Jones & Robinson, 1982).

Oxytocin Receptors

Oxytocin acts by binding to specific oxytocin receptors. The mammary glands and the uterus are richly provided with oxytocin receptors. Oxytocin receptors are found in many peripheral organs, e.g., in the kidneys, stomach, heart, and blood vessels. Oxytocin receptors are also widely distributed in the brain. These receptors have the same characteristics as the uterine receptors (Burbach et al., 2006; Cao & Gimpl, 2001; Freund-Mercier et al., 1987; Gimpl & Fahrenholz, 2001; Gimpl, Reitz, Brauer, & Trossen, 2008; Tribollet, Barberis, Dreifuss, & Jard, 1988).

The classical oxytocin receptor is a seven transmembrane domain G-protein coupled receptor (a G-protein linked type of receptor). When oxytocin binds to the receptor, phospholipase C is activated, thereby initiating the inositol triphosphate (IP3) and the diacylglycerol (DAG) second messenger cascade. Oxytocin increases intracellular CA2+ via IP3 and via activation of CA2+ channels in the membranes (Gimpl & Fahrenholz, 2001; Gimpl et al., 2008; Strunecka, Hynie, & Klenerova, 2009; Vrachnis, Malamas, Sifakis, Deligeoroglou, & Iliodromiti, 2011).

Oxytocin and vasopressin may to a certain extent bind to each other's receptors. The effect of vasopressin on uterine oxytocin receptors is tenfold lower than that of oxytocin, and oxytocin binds with more than ten times higher affinity to oxytocin receptors than to vasopressin receptors (Gimpl & Fahrenholz, 2001).

Antagonists directed towards the classical uterine type of oxytocin receptor do not block all effects induced by oxytocin. Therefore, other types of oxytocin receptors may exist, as is the case for many other peptides. For example, vasopressin may bind to and exert differential effects via the

V1a, V1b, and V2 types of receptors. As mentioned above, oxytocin is degraded into several fragments that induce specific effects. Such fragments may induce effects that may be mediated by other not yet fully characterized types of oxytocin receptors.

Other types of second messenger cascades may be activated when oxytocin binds to its receptors under different environmental conditions. Oxytocin, e.g., activates an intracellular pathway involving cyclic AMP when inhibiting the growth of certain cancer line cells (Cassoni, Sapino, Marrocco, Chini, & Bussolati, 2004). The phenomenon of activation of different intracellular mechanisms is referred to as "receptor promiscuity" (Strunecka et al., 2009).

The Same Oxytocin System in Females and Males

The distribution of oxytocinergic nerves and oxytocin receptors are similar in females and males (Richard et al., 1991; Sawchenko & Swanson, 1983; Swanson & Sawchenko, 1980, 1983). The effects of oxytocin may differ between males and females owing to the effects of sex hormones. Estrogens may increase the release of oxytocin and the responsiveness and/or number of oxytocin receptors (Burbach et al., 2006; Gimpl et al., 2008; Schumacher et al., 1993).

<h1 style="text-align:center">Chapter 5</h1>

Oxytocin: Effects of Administration of Oxytocin

In addition to exerting the well-known contractile effects on uterine muscles and the myoepithelial cells in the mammary glands during labor and breastfeeding, administration of oxytocin has been demonstrated to induce a multitude of other effects. Effects of oxytocin may depend on the dose of oxytocin given, the duration of treatment, and the route by which it is administered. Levels of other hormones, as well as cues from the environment, may influence the effect pattern caused by administration of oxytocin.

In this chapter, a brief summary of the effects of oxytocin that are observed following administration of oxytocin will be given. In the next chapter, the role of oxytocin when released in various physiological situations will be described. Only oxytocin-related effects relevant for this book will be described.

Ways of Administration of Oxytocin

It is difficult to induce oxytocin effects via oral administration (unless administered in extremely high amounts), since oxytocin is broken down more or less immediately in the gastrointestinal tract. If some oxytocin did survive the low pH and the degrading enzymes in the stomach and small intestine, very little oxytocin would be absorbed from the intestine. Peptides like oxytocin are electrically charged, and such substances do not easily pass biological membranes, such as the gastrointestinal mucosa. Therefore, it is preferable to inject oxytocin intravenously (IV), subcutaneously (SC), or intraperitoneally (IP) in order to obtain elevated levels of oxytocin in the circulation. Only 1% or less of oxytocin in the circulation will pass the blood brain barrier and reach the brain. In order to induce effects in the brain, it is sometimes necessary to administer oxytocin directly into the brain, e.g., intracerebroventricularly (ICV), or even by more local types of administration. In humans oxytocin may be given as a nasal spray. By this route of administration, more than 90% of the oxytocin administered passes into the brain because the blood brain barrier is weak in the nasal mucosa.

Effects of Oxytocin

Effects on Social Interaction

Oxytocin increases several types of social interactive behaviors. Oxytocin administered ICV induces maternal behavior in virgin rats after priming with estrogen (Pedersen, Caldwell, Johnson, Fort, & Prange, 1985; Pedersen, Caldwell, Peterson, Walker, & Mason, 1992; Pedersen & Prange, 1979). In sheep, endogenous oxytocin released in connection with labor, by vaginal stimulation, or by administration of exogenous oxytocin, increases maternal care and interaction with and bonding to the lamb. In contrast, blockade of oxytocin release during labor by peridural analgesia or administration of oxytocin antagonists inhibits these behaviors. As will be described more in detail later in this book, oxytocin coordinates the various aspects of maternal care. It also facilitates bonding in several ways: oxytocin increases the sensitivity to odors, facilitates some types of learning and recognition, and stimulates dopaminergic functions in the Nucleus Accumbens linked to reward (Kendrick, Keverne, & Baldwin, 1987; Keverne & Kendrick, 1992, 1994; Levy, Kendrick, Keverne, Piketty, & Poindron, 1992).

Oxytocin also stimulates pair bonding in some species, such as the monogamous prairie voles. An oxytocin-mediated release of dopamine in the NA is of importance in the formation of bonding in this species (Carter, 1998; Insel, 2003).

If oxytocin is administered to groups of rats, the rats will interact in a more friendly way. They often spend time sitting close to the other animals and may even groom each other. They don't form bonds to individual rats, but will remember each other and continue to interact in a friendly way upon renewed contact (Argiolas & Gessa, 1991; Witt, Winslow, & Insel, 1992).

Anxiolytic-Like and Calming Effect

Administration of low doses of oxytocin into the brain induces an anxiolytic-like effect in rats and mice; the animals become less fearful, more explorative, and more socially interactive. These effects are, at least in part, exerted in the amygdala (Uvnäs-Moberg, Alster, Hillegaart, & Ahlenius, 1992; Neumann, 2008; Terenzi & Ingram, 2005; Uvnäs-Moberg, Ahlenius, Hillegaart, & Alster, 1994). Knock-out mice lacking the oxytocin receptor are more anxious and more sensitive to stressors than normal mice (Amico, Mantella, Vollmer, & Li, 2004).

In response to higher doses of oxytocin, a calming or sedative effect, as expressed by decreased locomotor behavior, is induced. This effect may in part be mediated by a decrease of the activity in the LC via stimulation of alpha-2 adrenoceptors, which leads to reduced stress reactivity, wakefulness, and aggression (Petersson, Lundeberg, & Uvnäs-Moberg, 1999a; Uvnäs-Moberg et al., 1994).

Reward and Wellbeing

As mentioned above, oxytocin is linked to release of

dopamine in the NA and, therefore, to experiences of reward and wellbeing. The ability of oxytocin to induce wellbeing is an important aspect of the effect of oxytocin in different kinds of relationships, as it will make the interaction with others pleasurable. Consequently, bonding and approach towards those other individuals who are associated with oxytocin release will be promoted.

Pain Threshold and Inflammation

Oxytocin increases pain (nociceptive) thresholds, as rats treated with oxytocin react with a longer latency to heat in the tail-flick test. The effects may be exerted in the PAG and the spinal cord by an influence of the activity in endogenous opioidergic systems (Lundeberg, Uvnäs-Moberg, Agren, & Bruzelius, 1994; Petersson, Alster, Lundeberg, & Uvnäs-Moberg, 1996a). Oxytocin also exerts potent anti-inflammatory effects via central mechanisms (Clodi et al., 2008; Nation et al., 2010; Petersson, Wiberg, Lundeberg, & Uvnäs-Moberg, 2001; Szeto et al., 2008).

The HPA Axis

Cortisol or corticosterone (rats) levels fall in response to administration of oxytocin, sometimes after a short initial rise (Petersson, Hulting, & Uvnäs-Moberg, K., 1999). Oxytocin counteracts the activity of the HPA axis at several different levels in order to decrease cortisol levels: it decreases the secretion of CRF from the parvocellular neurons in the PVN (Lightman & Young, 1989; Neumann, Wigger, Torner, Holsboer, & Landgraf, 2000), it decreases the secretion of ACTH in the anterior pituitary (Legros, Chiodera, & Geenen, 1988), and it decreases cortisol secretion by a direct mechanism in the adrenal cortex (Stachowiak, Macchi, Nussdorfer, & Malendowicz, 1995). In addition, the effect of hippocampal glucocorticoid receptors is changed following administration of oxytocin (Petersson & Uvnäs-Moberg, 2003). In conclusion, oxytocin counteracts the activity of the HPA axis at many different levels.

In mice that lack the genes related to oxytocin production, stress gives rise to an increased release of corticosterone and increased levels of anxiety-like behavior, further supporting the role of oxytocin as an important anxiolytic and anti-stress agent (Amico, Miedlar, Cai, & Vollmer, 2008).

Cardiovascular Effects

Administration of oxytocin may, depending on experimental and environmental circumstances, give rise to an increase or a decrease of blood pressure (Dreifuss, Raggenbass, Charpak, Dubois-Dauphin, & Tribollet, 1988; Matsuguchi, Sharabi, Gordon, Johnson, & Schmid, 1982; Petersson, Diaz-Cabiale, Angel Narvaez, Fuxe, & Uvnäs-Moberg, 2005; Petersson, Lundeberg, & Uvnäs-Moberg, 1999b; Yamashita, Kannan, Kasai, & Osaka, 1987). After ICV administration of oxytocin, blood pressure is decreased for several hours after an initial rise. This decrease of blood pressure most likely is exerted in the rostro-ventral-lateral

medulla (RVLM) and NTS, and also in adjacent areas in the brainstem involved in the control of the autonomic nervous system. The effect may be mediated by a decreased activity in the sympathetic nerves involved in the regulation of cardiovascular tone and may involve activation of alpha-2 adrenoceptors, which exert inhibitory actions on central noradrenergic transmission (Petersson, Alster, Lundeberg, & Uvnäs-Moberg, 1996b; Petersson, Lundeberg, et al., 1999a; 1999b). Oxytocin may also decrease pulse rate by activation of parasympathetic cholinergic neurons originating in the vagas motor nucleus (DMX; Dreifuss et al., 1988).

Digestion, Metabolism, and Growth

Oxytocin influences the function in some aspects of the parasympathetic/vagal nervous system controlling the function in the endocrine system of the gastrointestinal tract via effects exerted in the dorsal vagal motor nucleus (DMX) and the nucleus tractus solitarius (NTS). Basal levels of insulin, somatostatin, gastrin, and cholecystokinin can be increased or decreased following administration of oxytocin, whereas the feeding-induced release is increased. In this way, oxytocin will contribute to a more efficient digestive function and the use of nutrients for storing, growth, and restoration will be facilitated (Bjorkstrand, Ahlenius, Smedh, & Uvnäs-Moberg, 1996; Bjorkstrand, Eriksson, & Uvnäs-Moberg, 1996; Petersson, Hulting, Andersson, & Uvnäs-Moberg, 1999).

Oxytocin in the circulation may increase glucagon release by activation of oxytocin receptors on the glucagon-producing alpha-cells in the pancreas. Glucose levels increase as a consequence of the elevation of glucagon levels and by direct effects in the liver. In this way, nutrients are recruited from its deposits, which allow transfer of nutrients, for example, to the mammary gland for milk production (Bjorkstrand, Eriksson, et al., 1996; Stock, Fastbom, Bjorkstrand, Ungerstedt, & Uvnäs-Moberg, 1990). Central administration of oxytocin may also stimulate the release of growth hormone (Björkstrand, Hulting, & Uvnäs-Moberg, 1997; Petersson, Lundeberg, Sohlström, Wiberg, & Uvnäs-Moberg, 1998; Uvnäs-Moberg & Petersson, 2005).

Oxytocin Induces Effects via Activation of Other Transmitter Systems

When oxytocin induces uterine contractions and milk ejection, it activates oxytocin receptors located in the muscular tissue. Oxytocin often exerts effects in a more indirect way by influencing the function of other classical transmitter substances, such as serotonin, dopamine, acetylcholine, noradrenaline, and opioids. In this way, oxytocin may, for example, increase the sense of wellbeing by influencing the serotonin neurons in the raphe nuclei, induce feelings of happiness or reward by stimulating the dopaminergic system in the Nucleus Accumbens (NA), decrease the sensation of pain by influencing opioidergic neurons in the Periaqueductal Grey (PAG) and in the spinal cord, decrease blood pressure and stress levels, as well as exerting stress-buffering effects, by decreasing the function in the noradrenergic system, e.g., in the LC and NTS, and increase gastrointestinal function by increasing the function of cholinergic neurons in the dorsal vagal motor nucleus (DMX).

Long-Term Effects

When oxytocin is administered repeatedly, e.g., once a day for a week, long-term effects may be induced. Blood pressure is decreased and pain thresholds increased for weeks after the last treatment. Cortisol levels, but not adrenocorticotrophic hormone (ACTH) levels, are decreased. Repeated administration of oxytocin influences the levels of gastrointestinal hormones, increases weight gain, shortens the time for wound healing, and decreases inflammation. Further, it improves learning by conditioning. Wound healing may be increased, both in response to systemic and local administration of oxytocin, and vaginal atrophy may be counteracted by intravaginal treatment with oxytocin (Bjorkstrand & Uvnäs-Moberg, 1996; Diaz-Cabiale, Petersson, Narváez, Uvnäs-Moberg, & Fuxe, 2000; Petersson, et al., 1996b; Petersson, et al. 1996a; Petersson, Diaz-Cabiale, et al., 2005; Petersson, Hulting, & Uvnäs-Moberg, 1999; Petersson, Hulting, Andersson, & Uvnäs-Moberg, 1999; Petersson, Lundeberg, et al., 1998; Petersson, Wiberg, Lundeberg & Uvnäs-Moberg, 2001; Uvnäs-Moberg, Bjorkstrand, Hillegaart, & Ahlenius, 1999; Uvnäs-Moberg, Eklund, Hillegaart, & Ahlenius, 2000).

Link Between Oxytocin and the Alpha-2 Adrenoceptor System

The long-term effects of oxytocin are linked to functional changes in release mechanisms or receptors of other signaling systems. For example, if oxytocin is administered repeatedly to rats, the sensitivity to the alpha-2 receptor agonist clonidine in noradrenergic cells of the Locus Coeruleus (LC) is increased, i.e., much less clonidine is needed to decrease the electrical activity in the noradrenergic neurons. In addition, the alpha-2 adrenoceptor function in several brain regions, such as the amygdala, the NTS, and the LC as measured by autoradiography and electrophysiology, is increased in response to repeated administration of oxytocin. Oxytocin-containing nerves emanating from the paraventricular nucleus (PVN) have been demonstrated to project to these areas in the brain.

Stimulation of the function of alpha-2 adrenoceptors underlies some of the long-term oxytocin-induced anti-stress effects, e.g., sedation and lowering of blood pressure, and the enhanced levels of insulin and gastrointestinal hormones in connection with food intake (Diaz-Cabiale, et al., 2000; Petersson et al., 1996a, 1996b; Petersson, Diaz-Cabiale, et al., 2005; Petersson, Hulting, & Uvnäs-Moberg, 1999; Petersson, Hulting, Andersson, et al., 1999; Petersson, Lundeberg, et al., 1999a; Petersson & Uvnäs-Moberg, 2003).

Oxytocin may also, in an analogous function, influence cholinergic, serotonergic, dopaminergic, and opioidergic transmission in a more permanent way to induce the long-term changes in gastrointestinal function, mood, wellbeing, and pain threshold.

The Alpha-2 Receptor System or the Energy-Conservation System

The alpha-2 receptor system has been labeled the energy-conservation system. The effects induced by activation of alpha-2 receptors are linked to behavioral and physiological changes which facilitate saving of energy. This includes increased food intake, use of energy for storing purposes, decreased energy expenditure, e.g., by decreased blood pressure and lowered stress levels, and behavioral calming. The activity of some aspects of the parasympathetic nervous system is increased, and the activity of the HPA axis and some aspects of the sympathetic nervous system are decreased.

Oxytocin Influences the Function of Alpha-2 Receptors Via Different Kind of Receptor

As mentioned previously, most effects induced by oxytocin are mediated by the classical, uterine type of oxytocin receptor. Interestingly, some of the oxytocin-mediated effects consistent with energy saving, e.g., sedation, lowering of blood pressure, and storing of nutrients, are not as easily blocked by substances that block the activity of the uterine type of oxytocin receptor. Relatively high doses are needed to induce these oxytocin-mediated effects, and the effects are not blocked by the oxytocin antagonists directed towards the uterine type of receptor, suggesting that a different kind of oxytocin receptor may be involved. When oxytocin increases the function of the alpha-2 adrenoceptor-linked energy conservation system, i.e., causes lowering of blood pressure and enhanced secretion of gastrointestinal hormones that promote storing of nutrients, and induces a calming effect, it may do so by activation of an oxytocin receptor that is different from the uterine type of oxytocin receptor.

Oxytocin Induced Activation of the Alpha-2 Adrenoceptor-Linked Energy Conservation During Female Reproduction

The oxytocin-induced activation of the alpha-2 adrenoceptor system is of extreme importance during female reproduction, i.e., during pregnancy and breastfeeding. During these periods an efficient handling of maternal energy is important not only for the individual mothers, but for survival of the human species, as it facilitates growth of the fetus and maternal milk production.

Does Oxytocin Stimulate the Release of Growth Factors?

The long-term effects induced by oxytocin are mediated

by an increased function in other classical transmitter systems. The synthesis of transmitter substances and/or their receptors is augmented by repeated exposure to oxytocin. The mechanism by which oxytocin induces these prolonged oxytocin-mediated effect is not known, but as mentioned above does not seem to be linked to activation of the classical uterine-type oxytocin receptor. It is therefore possible that the effects are induced via another type of oxytocin receptor.

Oxytocin, like the related peptide vasopressin, is metabolized to different metabolites and fragments, which are biologically active. One of the vasopressin fragments (containing amino acids number 4-8) has been shown to stimulate the production of growth factors, such as brain-derived nerve growth factor (BDNF) (Du, Yan, & Qiao, 1998; Zhou, Li, Guo, & Du, 1997). As the oxytocin molecule contains a similar fragment, it is probable that fragments or metabolites of oxytocin also stimulate the production of growth factors. In support of this, an increased release of nerve growth factor (NGF) has been demonstrated in pregnant women (Luppi et al., 1993). The increased synthesis of transmitter substances and/or their receptors and thereby the long-term effects of oxytocin may be caused by oxytocin fragments which activate growth via a receptor that differs from the uterine type of receptor. Oxytocin-mediated effects via stimulation of growth factors may be of great importance, not only in the brain, but also in peripheral organs.

Effects of Administration of Oxytocin in Humans

As mentioned above, synthetic oxytocin has been available and used clinically for many years. Oxytocin infusions are used to initiate labor and augment uterine contractions in laboring women. Oxytocin-containing spray has been and is still available in some countries and used to promote milk ejection during breastfeeding. Normally, a dose (one puff), which corresponds to 5 IU or 6.7 micrograms of oxytocin, is given. The reason for using oxytocin spray is that peptides, such as oxytocin, don't easily penetrate biological membranes, such as the gastrointestinal mucosa or the blood-brain barrier. However, if administered as a nasal spray, oxytocin enters the brain because the blood-brain barrier is relatively weak, and, therefore, permeable in the nasal mucosa (Graff & Pollack, 2005; Veronesi, Kubek, & Kubek, 2011; Wu, Hu, & Jiang, 2008).

Recently, oxytocin has been administered as a nasal spray to men and to women who are not breastfeeding in order to study possible effects of oxytocin on behavioral and physiological functions. In response to four puffs (20 IU or 26.8 microgram), several of the effects previously demonstrated to occur after administration of oxytocin to animals have now been demonstrated to occur in humans.

Effects on Social Interaction, Anxiety, Stress, Trust, and Generosity

Oxytocin administered as a spray increases social skills, e.g., the ability to read and evaluate the emotional valence of faces or voice. The latter effect lasted for several weeks in both healthy and autistic men (Domes, Heinrichs, Michel, Berger, & Herpertz, 2007; Hollander et al., 2007). The duration and frequency of gaze directed towards the eye region is also increased (Guastella, Mitchell, & Dadds, 2008).

Oxytocin spray has been demonstrated to reduce fear and to dampen activity in the amygdala. It also reduces activity in the HPA axis, as evidenced by decreased cortisol levels in response to stress (Domes, Heinrichs, Glascher, et al., 2007; Heinrichs, Baumgartner, Kirschbaum, & Ehlert, 2003; Heinrichs & Domes, 2008; Kirsch et al., 2005).

Recently, it has been observed that oxytocin spray does not always induce anxiolytic, stress-reducing, and calming effects. In some individuals, an opposite effect pattern is induced. This effect may be related to the protective, oxytocin-related effects seen in lactating mothers, which will be described later in this book (Bartz et al., 2011).

In other studies, the administration of oxytocin spray has been demonstrated to increase trust and generosity in men and to reduce abdominal pain and depression in women (Kosfeld, Heinrichs, Zak, Fischbacher, & Fehr, 2005; Ohlsson et al., 2005).

Oxytocin administered as an intravenous infusion to women during labor reduces anxiety and increases social skills. The effects last for several days after birth (Jonas, Nissen, Ransjo-Arvidson, Matthiesen, & Uvnäs-Moberg, K., 2008). The clinical effects of administration of oxytocin infusions in connection with labor will be discussed in much greater detail later.

Oxytocin, a Mammalian Pattern for Social Interaction and Stress Reduction

The fact that the effect pattern induced by administration of oxytocin spray in humans is very similar to that induced by administration of oxytocin in animals, supports the role of oxytocin as an important mammalian system for regulation of social interactive behavior and reduction of fear and stress.

As will be discussed in the next chapter, similar effect patterns are induced in response to release of endogenous oxytocin during breastfeeding and in situations involving close, tactile contact.

Administration of oxytocin as a nasal spray does not seem to give rise to the effect pattern linked to activation of alpha-2 adrenoceptors. The doses may be too low, or as will be described later, these effects are more efficiently induced when oxytocin is released in response to sensory stimulation of the skin. As will be discussed in the next chapter, the oxytocin-effect pattern differs in different physiological situations.

Disturbed Function in the Oxytocin System

Deficient Oxytocin Receptors

Several studies have implicated that the function of the oxytocin system may be deranged in individuals with social anxiety disorder, autism, and schizophrenia because they have either too high or too low oxytocin levels (Goldman, Marlow-O'Connor, Torres, & Carter, 2008; Hoge, Pollack, Kaufman, Zak, & Simon, 2008; Modahl et al., 1998) or a large fraction of precursor oxytocin molecules in plasma (Modahl et al., 1998). Recently, it has been found that some individuals with autism may have a disturbance in the function of the oxytocin receptor, based on aberrations in the structure of the gene for the oxytocin receptor. The differences in the structure of the oxytocin receptor gene may be genetic. In addition, epigenetic changes in the structure of the gene for the receptor have been demonstrated (Gregory et al., 2009).

Low Secretion of Oxytocin

Some individuals have lower oxytocin levels than others. For example, individuals with insecure attachment styles have lower levels than those with secure attachment (Gordon et al., 2008, Tops, van Peer, Korf, Wijers, & Tucker, 2007). Also, women with borderline disease have lower levels of oxytocin, and in some studies, depression and schizophrenia are linked to low oxytocin levels (Bertsch, Schmidinger, Neumann, & Herpetz, 2013; Kim et al., 2013). In addition, exposure to trauma, particularly early in life, is associated with low levels of oxytocin (Pierrehumbert et al., 2009). Low levels of oxytocin in the cerebrospinal fluid (CSF) are linked to an increased risk for suicide (Jokinen et al., 2012).

Individuals with some pain syndromes, such as fibromyalgia and recurrent abdominal pain, also have lower oxytocin levels (Alfvén, de la Torre, & Uvnäs-Moberg, 1994; Anderberg & Uvnäs-Moberg, 2000). Whether these aberrations are due to inborn genetic differences in the function of the oxytocin gene, inadequate stimulation of the oxytocin system early in life, or an acquired stress-related inhibition of oxytocin release is not yet known. Variations in the structure of the oxytocin gene have been demonstrated and are possibly linked to some clinical states (Skuse et al., 2014).

Treatment with Oxytocin

Since an impaired oxytocin function may lie behind some types of disturbances in social interaction and communication, it might be assumed that treatment with oxytocin might solve the problem. Some studies have found that administration of oxytocin increases the social competence in individuals with autistic disorders. Oxytocin infusions (in amounts normally given during labor) were found to enhance the ability to interpret the valence of voice in autistic individuals, and intranasal administration of oxytocin increased the ability to read facial expressions in young males (Guastella et al., 2010; Guastella, Howard, Dadds, Mitchell, & Carson, 2009; Hollander et al., 2007). In individuals with social phobia, intranasal administration of oxytocin seems to have some positive effects. Today, controlled clinical studies are being performed to test the effect of oxytocin against some symptoms in schizophrenic patients. Studies are being performed in which oxytocin is given together with anti-depressants to speed up the anxiolytic and anti-depressive effect of such treatment. According to the list of ongoing clinical trials published by the National Institute of Health, oxytocin treatment is also being tried to alleviate various stress disorders, drug and alcohol abuse, and as an adjunct to psychotherapy.

Oxytocin Part of Existing Pharmacological Treatments

Oxytocin is linked to the function of other neurotransmitter systems in many ways. Oxytocin is released by certain dopamine and serotonin agonists, such as 5HT1a-agonists (Uvnäs-Moberg, Alster, Hillegaart, & Ahlenius, 1995; Uvnäs-Moberg, Hillegaart, Alster, & Ahlenius, 1996). Oxytocin influences the release and production of several classical neurotransmitters, such as noradrenaline, serotonin, dopamine, acetylcholine, and opioids. Some anti-psychotic and anti-depressive drugs induce oxytocin release. It is possible that some of the effects induced by certain neuroleptics and some anxiolytic and anti-depressant drugs, e.g., serotonin uptake inhibitors (SSRI), may involve oxytocinergic mechanisms (Uvnäs-Moberg, Alster, & Svensson, 1992; Uvnäs-Moberg, Bjorkstrand, Hillegaart, & Ahlenius, 1999). Also, the positive effect of SSRIs in the treatment of obsessive-compulsive disorder was linked to increased levels of oxytocin (Humble, Uvnäs-Moberg, Engström, & Bejerot, 2013).

Chapter 6

Oxytocin: Release and Effects of Oxytocin in Response to Stimulation of Sensory Nerves

Control of Oxytocin Release

The release of oxytocin from the PVN and SON is under the influence of neural input from many parts of the brain and from substances in the circulation, e.g., hormones. Information from the environment and from different parts of the body reaches the brain via the different senses and via sensory nerves to influence the release of oxytocin.

Nervous Pathways and Signaling Substances Within the Brain

The oxytocin-producing neurons in the SON and PVN are reached by innervation from many parts of the central nervous system; therefore, the activity of the oxytocin neurons can be modulated by impulses from both newer and older parts of the brain. Nervous projections from the dorsal vagal complex (DVC), the Nucleus tractus solitarius (NTS), the Locus Coeruleus (LC), nucleus parabrachialis, BNST, amygdala, hippocampus, the raphe nuclei, and other cell groups within the hypothalamus innervate the PVN.

Many different signaling substances are involved in the control of release of oxytocin from the PVN and SON (acetylcholine, serotonin, dopamine, noradrenaline, glutamate, GABA, angiotensin II, vasoactive intestinal peptide (VIP), corticotrophin-releasing factor (CRF), prolactin, endogenous opioids, estrogens, cholecystokinin (CCK), thyrotrophin-releasing hormone (TRH), and melatonin are examples of substances that influence the release of oxytocin. Most of them stimulate the release, but GABA and endogenous opioids inhibit oxytocin release (Argiolas & Gessa, 1991; Burbach et al., 2006; Richard et al., 1991).

Feed Forward

Oxytocin also has the capacity to stimulate its own release in several ways, e.g., by activation of receptors on the dendrites of the oxytocin-producing neurons in the SON and PVN, which triggers oxytocin release. Therefore, as oxytocin is released from the dendrites, more oxytocin is released from the dendrites; a local feed-forward system is activated (Burbach et al., 2006; Ludwig & Leng, 2006).

There is also increasing evidence that circulating oxytocin may stimulate oxytocin release by activation of receptors on sensory nerves, such as the pelvic and hypogastric nerves. In addition, oxytocin released from the oxytocinergic fibers projecting to the NTS may facilitate the action of incoming sensory nerves involved in, e.g., oxytocin release.

Feed-Back Inhibition

However, oxytocin may, by other mechanisms, inhibit its own release. This effect may be exerted by oxytocin itself or by metabolites or fragments of oxytocin, since administration of a fragment of oxytocin has been demonstrated to inhibit oxytocin release (Petersson & Uvnäs-Moberg, 2004).

Estrogen

The female sex hormones, in particular estrogen, promote the secretion of oxytocin in several ways. Estrogen exerts its stimulatory effects on oxytocin release via activation of a subtype of the estrogen receptors, the estrogen receptor-beta (Shughrue, Komm, & Merchenthaler, 1996). This stimulatory effect of estrogen becomes apparent during pregnancy, when estrogen levels increase dramatically. This rise of estrogen is followed by a more moderate rise of maternal oxytocin levels (Silber, Larsson, & Uvnäs-Moberg, 1991). Estrogen may promote the effects of oxytocin in some areas of the brain by facilitating the binding of oxytocin to its receptors (Schumacher et al., 1992). For example, the binding of oxytocin to its receptors in the amygdala is reinforced by estrogen via the estrogen receptor-alpha. Some oxytocinergic nerves projecting from the PVN to the brainstem are provided with estrogen receptors, and their function is promoted by estrogen.

Release of Oxytocin in Response to Activation of Sensory Nerves

It is well known that oxytocin is released during labor and lactation to promote labor and breastfeeding by stimulation of contractions of the uterus and of myoepithelial cells. In addition, stimulation of a vast number of sensory nerves, e.g., emanating from the uterus, the genital tract, the gastrointestinal tract, the nipple, the skin, and the oral mucosa, result in oxytocin release. The role of oxytocin during labor and breastfeeding will be described in great detail later on in this book and only a short summary will be given here.

Labor

The onset of labor is induced by largely unknown central mechanisms, and during the first and second phases of labor, short oxytocin pulses occur. Each pulse is associated with a contraction of the uterus. In addition, oxytocin contributes to relaxation of the cervix and thereby to the opening of the birth canal. The frequency of the pulses increases as labor progresses. Towards the end of labor, the pulses of oxytocin and thereby the uterine contractions may occur at 90-second intervals (Fuchs et al., 1991). The release of oxytocin is enhanced via activation of the Ferguson reflex, i.e., the pressure of the fetus against the cervix of the uterus stimulates afferent fibers in the pelvic and the hypogastric nerves, which via the spinal cord and the NTS influence the oxytocin-producing cells to release oxytocin (Burbach et al., 2006; Ferguson, 1941). A subpopulation of noradrenergic neurons transmits the information from the NTS to the PVN and SON.

The autonomic nervous system participates in the control of uterine contractions and opening of the cervix. In the non-pregnant uterus, parasympathetic nervous activity increases the uterine contractions and the uterine blood flow. In contrast, the sympathetic nerves induce more long-lasting uterine contractions and a decrease of uterine blood flow (Sato, Hotta, Nakayama, & Suzuki, 1996). Oxytocin fibers projecting from the PVN project all the way down to the sacral plexa, from which the parasympathetic innervation of the uterus originates.

A subpopulation of sensory nerve afferents project from the genital organs directly to the NTS in the medulla oblongata, i.e., these fibers bypass the spinal cord.

Suckling

During lactation, the offspring's suckling leads to activation of somato-sensory nerves emanating in the nipple and the breast, which via the NTS in the brainstem leads to release of oxytocin from the SON and PVN. Nerves containing b-inhibin have been implicated in the mediation of the nervous impulses from the NTS to the SON and PVN. A sub-population of sensory nerves, which bypass the spinal cord and travel along the vagal nerves, is activated by suckling. These "afferent vagal nerves" and other cutaneous sensory nerves contribute to the release of oxytocin caused by suckling (Burbach et al., 2006; Eriksson, Lindh, Uvnäs-Moberg, et al., 1996). The release of oxytocin during suckling occurs in pulses. The myoepithelial cells surrounding the alveoli of the mammary gland contract in response to such pulses of oxytocin in the circulation, and oxytocin, together with neurogenic mechanisms, relaxes the sphincters of the milk ducts; therefore, oxytocin promotes milk ejection. Just after the start of suckling, the pulses occur at 90-second intervals (Jonas et al., 2009).

Sexual Activity

Large amounts of oxytocin are released in response to sexual activity in both male and female rats. The release of oxytocin is caused by activation of sensory nerves in the mucosa of the genital region and the skin surrounding this region, and is mediated by the pudendal, pelvic, and hypogastric nerves. Similar findings have been documented in male rabbits and humans (Burbach et al., 2006; Carmichael et al., 1987; Todd & Lightman, 1986).

The effects of stimulation of the sensory nerves emanating in the vaginal wall have been extensively studied by Komisaruk and Sansone (2003). Not only is oxytocin released into the circulation and into the spinal cord, it is connected to an increased pain threshold by actions in the spinal cord and to dilatation of the pupils. Other fibers of oxytocin are also activated, which contribute to calm and relaxation, and wellbeing and pleasure. These links may involve serotonin and dopamine released in response to oxytocin. In addition, oxytocin-mediated nerves involved in attachment are stimulated.

Food Intake

Oxytocin is released in response to feeding. Elevated oxytocin levels in the circulation have been demonstrated in cows, sows, dogs, and humans (Ohlsson, Truedsson, Djerf, & Sundler, 2006). The release of oxytocin occurring during a meal is induced by two different mechanisms, one immediate and one more protracted.

Release of Oxytocin in Response to Touch of the Oral Mucosa

A peak-shaped transient increase of oxytocin levels is induced immediately after onset of food intake in calves that suckle their mothers, but not if they drink milk from a bucket (Lupoli, Johansson, Uvnäs-Moberg, & Svennersten-Sjaunja, 2001). These immediate effects by feeding are induced by activation of touch fibers in the oral cavity. The nervous impulses, which result in release of oxytocin, reach the SON and PVN via the NTS (Svennersten, Nelson, & Uvnäs-Moberg, 1990).

Cholecystokinin and the Vagal Nerve

Oxytocin is also released in response to food intake by a second mechanism. When food is ingested and reaches the small intestine, cholecystokinin (CCK), a gastrointestinal hormone, is released. CCK not only influences digestive and metabolic processes, it also influences brain function, e.g., the release of oxytocin via activation of afferent vagal nerves. In support of this, both afferent electrical stimulation of the vagal nerves and administration of CCK lead to a rise of oxytocin levels into the circulation (Ohlsson, Forsling, Rehfeld, & Sjölund, 2002; Svennersten, Nelson, & Uvnäs-Moberg, 1990; Uvnäs-Moberg, 1989, 1994). The afferent vagal fibers connect with a subset of noradrenergic fibers in the NTS, which project to the SON and PVN.

Tactile Stimulation

Release of Oxytocin

Oxytocin is released in response to stimulation of sensory nerves originating in the skin. In anesthetized rats, oxytocin levels rise in response to electrical stimulation of the sciatic nerve and stroking of the skin (Stock & Uvnäs-Moberg, 1988). In addition, oxytocin levels rise both in plasma and cerebrospinal fluid in response to vibration, warm temperature, and acupuncture, like electrical stimulation, in anesthetized male rats (Uvnäs-Moberg, Bruzelius, Alster, & Lundeberg, 1993). In experiments performed on conscious rats (the rats were treated very gently and were not afraid), stroking, in particular of the ventral side at a rate of 40 strokes per minutes, results in a rise of oxytocin levels (Lund et al., 2002). The oxytocin observed in the circulation emanates from the magnocellular neurons, which project to the posterior pituitary. At the same time, oxytocin is released within the brain to induce oxytocin-mediated effects.

Effects of Stroking, Warmth, and Touch (Non-Noxious Sensory Stimulation)

In anesthetized rats, weak electrical stimulation and brushing or stroking of the skin lowers the levels of corticosterone and adrenaline in the circulation (Araki, Ito, Kurosawa, & Sato, 1984; Kurosawa, Suzuki, Utsugi, & Araki, 1982; Tsuchiya, Nakayama, & Sato, 1991) and blood pressure is reduced (Kurosawa, Lundeberg, Agren, Lund, & Uvnäs-Moberg, 1995; Uvnäs-Moberg, Posloncec, & Ahlberg, 1986), showing that the activity of the HPA axis and some aspects of the sympathetic nervous system are reduced by non-noxious stimulation. Furthermore, the levels of gastrointestinal hormones, such as gastrin, cholecystokinin, and insulin, are influenced as a result of activation of vagal nerve fibers that exert a regulatory effect on the release of these hormones (Uvnäs-Moberg, Lundeberg, Bruzelius, & Alster, 1992; Uvnäs-Moberg et al., 1986). Pain sensitivity is reduced as a response to application of warm temperature on the chest (Uvnäs-Moberg, Bruzelius, et al., 1993).

In conscious rats, stroking of the chest reduces blood pressure (particularly if applied to the front side), decreases sensitivity to pain, and induces a sedative effect (Agren, Lundeberg, Uvnäs-Moberg, & Sato, 1995; Lund, Lundeberg, Kurosawa, & Uvnäs-Moberg, 1999; Uvnäs-Moberg, Alster, Lund, et al., 1996). In response to repeated treatments, the pain-relieving effect is reinforced (Lund et al., 2002). In addition, the levels of gastrointestinal hormones are influenced and weight gain is promoted (Holst, Lund, Petersson, & Uvnäs-Moberg, 2005). Stroking in conscious rats also influences behavior and induces calming effects (Uvnäs-Moberg, Alster, Lund, et al., 1996).

Taken together, these data indicate that mild or non-noxious sensory stimulation exerts anti-stress effects by inhibiting the activity in the HPA axis and certain aspects of the sympathetic nervous system. Further, it stimulates the function of the parasympathetic/vagal system and the endocrine system of the gastrointestinal tract, and thereby anabolic metabolism and growth. In addition, behavioral calm is induced. In this way, anti-stress effects are exerted, and growth and development are promoted (Uvnäs-Moberg & Petersson, 2011).

Whether the effects induced by somatosensory stimulation summarized above are mediated by the CT fibers or by other types of sensory fibers remains to be established.

Role of Oxytocin in the Effects Mediated by Sensory Stimulation

The effects induced by administration of oxytocin were described in chapter 5. It is obvious that the effect pattern induced by non-noxious sensory stimulation, which was described above, very much resembles that of administration of oxytocin. Given the fact that oxytocin is released by non-noxious sensory stimulation, it is likely that oxytocin participates in the mediation of the effects described above that are induced in response to non-noxious sensory stimulation.

The connection between release of oxytocin and the effects induced by sensory stimulation of the skin is supported by some experimental findings. For example, the elevation of pain threshold caused by warm temperature and stroking of the front side of rats is blocked if the animals are given an oxytocin antagonist before treatment with sensory stimulation (Agren et al., 1995; Uvnäs-Moberg, Bruzelius, et al., 1993).

Mechanisms Involved in the OT-Related Effects Caused by Sensory Stimulation

The effects of oxytocin released in response to sensory stimulation may be induced by several different mechanisms. The sensory information by stimulation of somatosensory nerves is relayed to the PVN via the NTS. Then oxytocin is released from oxytocinergic fibers originating in parvocellular neurons from the PVN, which project to specific areas within the brain. The oxytocin released may exert local effects at the site of release in the brain by itself. It may also act in conjunction with other signaling substances, such as serotonin, opioids or dopamine.

The elevation of pain threshold and the anxiolytic and calming effects may be exerted by oxytocin released in the periaqueductal gray (PAG), amygdala, and Locus Coeruleus (LC). In fact, increased oxytocin levels have been demonstrated in the periaqueductal grey, an area in the brain that is of central importance for nociception in response to repeated stroking (Lund et al., 2002).

Somatosensory stimulation may influence, e.g., pulse rate, blood pressure, and the levels of gastrointestinal hormones by local reflexes in the brain stem, e.g., in the LC, RVLM, DMX, and NTS. The effect on pulse rate, blood pressure, and the levels of gastrointestinal hormones in response to stroking and other types of sensory stimulation may also involve an effect of oxytocin released from oxytocinergic nerves, emanating from parvocellular neurons in the PVN.

Oxytocin released from the nerve fibers projecting to the centers in the brainstem controlling autonomic nervous function may facilitate the effects of shorter and more direct effects "brain stem reflexes" in this area (Sato, Sato, & Schmidt, 1997).

The oxytocinergic nerve fibers projecting to the NTS may also act by modulation (facilitation or inhibition) of the activity of incoming sensory information in the NTS, as a kind of gating system (Burbach et al., 2006).

NTS – An Important Relay Station for Oxytocin Release via Sensory Stimulation

The NTS seems to be a very important relay station for all the afferent nervous impulses, irrespective of being triggered by suckling, labor, feeding (CCK), or tactile stimulation, which result in the release of oxytocin.

Many different transmitter substances participate in the signaling between the NTS and the oxytocin-producing cells in the SON and PVN. Noradrenergic neurons emanating from a specific cell group in the NTS seems to play a major role during labor and in response to food intake, whereas fibers containing B-inhibin seem to be more important for the release of oxytocin during suckling (Burbach et al., 2006).

It is important to note that the different sensory inputs to the NTS, which result in oxytocin release, are not necessarily linked to the same oxytocin-effect patterns. The oxytocin-effect patterns related to labor, breastfeeding, food intake, and tactile stimulation are to a certain extent similar, but are not completely identical, since the response patterns are adapted to the situations in which they are involved. This will be described in more detail in subsequent chapters.

Oxytocin Release via Other Senses

Pheromones and Olfaction

Pheromones may trigger oxytocin release. Rats that have received oxytocin may influence untreated neighboring animals via airborne substances. Not only does the oxytocin level rise in the recipient animal, they also develop some of the classical oxytocin-mediated effects, such as elevation of pain threshold and anti-stress effects. These substances influence the recipient animal via the olfactory organ, since local anesthesia applied in the nasal cavity abolishes the oxytocin-mediated effects on oxytocin release, pain threshold, and stress reactivity (Agren, Olsson, Uvnäs-Moberg, & Lundeberg, 1997; Uvnäs Moberg, Bystrova, et al., 2014).

Visual and Auditory Stimuli

Oxytocin may also be released via visual and auditory stimuli. Mothers may release oxytocin when they see pictures of their infant (Strathearn, Iyengar, Fonagy, & Kim, 2012). Infants may release oxytocin not only in response to touch, but also in response to their mothers' voice. Mothers' oxytocin release may increase in response to their infants' cries (McNeilly, Robinson, Houston, & Howie, 1983; Seltzer, Ziegler, & Pollak, 2010).

Mental Representations and Conditioning

Oxytocin is released in the mother and milk is ejected when the baby suckles, but as mentioned above, it is also released when she sees her baby or hears the baby cry. These effects may be triggered directly by the sound or sight of the baby, but they may also be developed into conditioned, Pavlovian reflexes that are activated by sight or sound. It is well known that the milk ejection reflex can be conditioned. These effects will be described in more detail in the next chapters.

Coordinating Effects of Oxytocin

Parallel Release of Oxytocin into the Circulation and the Brain

Oxytocin is sometimes, but not always, released in parallel into the circulation and the brain. A subpopulation of magnocellular neurons from the PVN project to the posterior pituitary and to several areas in the brain, including the amygdala and the hippocampus via axon collaterals. When these neurons are activated, a parallel secretion of oxytocin in the brain and the circulation occurs (Knobloch et al., 2012).

In addition, magnocellular and parvocellular neurons may be activated at the same time. A parallel secretion of oxytocin into both the brain and the circulation has been shown during suckling, feeding, parturition, and vaginocervical stimulation (Kendrick, Keverne, Baldwin, & Sharman, 1986; Kendrick, Levy, & Keverne, 1991). In rats, electroacupuncture, vibration, and thermal stimuli significantly increase oxytocin levels in the cerebrospinal fluid (Uvnäs-Moberg, Bruzelius, et al., 1993).

Oxytocin Coordinates Different Effect Patterns

Oxytocin is released into the circulation and into the brain in response to labor and suckling, and both behavioral and physiological effects are induced. By integrating different combinations of effects, oxytocin may create effect patterns, which are adaptive in different situations. For example, different patterns of oxytocin-related effects are activated in connection with labor and breastfeeding. During labor, the HPA axis is activated and blood pressure is increased, whereas breastfeeding and skin-to-skin contact are linked to inhibition of HPA axis and the sympathetic nervous system (Risberg, Olsson, Lyrenas, & Sjöquist, 2009; Jonas, Nissen, Ransjo-Arvidson, Wiklund, et al., 2008). On the other hand, oxytocin, e.g., promotes social interaction, decreases levels of anxiety, and increases pain thresholds in both situations. The release of oxytocin and the different effect profiles induced by oxytocin during labor and breastfeeding will be discussed in more detail later in this book.

Oxytocin Antagonizes Stress Reactions

The different components of the stress system were described in great detail in chapter 3.

As will be demonstrated below, oxytocin inhibits the stress system by influencing the activity of almost all mechanisms involved in stress regulation.

Oxytocin Inhibits Activity in the HPA Axis

Oxytocin counteracts the activity of the HPA axis in several ways. It decreases the release of CRF within the PVN, it inhibits adrenocorticotrophic hormone (ACTH) secretion from the anterior pituitary, and it inhibits the release of cortisol in the adrenal cortex. Oxytocin also influences the function of pathways in the hippocampus, which are involved in the regulation of the HPA axis.

Oxytocin Released in the Amygdala and LC Decreases Reactions to Stress

Oxytocin released from oxytocinergic nerves originating from parvocellular neurons in the PVN antagonizes stress reactions by counteracting the inputs to the HPA axis from other areas in the brain.

As described in detail in chapter 3, fear induces stress reactions by activating the amygdala, which, in turn, activates noradrenergic neurons in the LC, stimulating the secretion of CRF in the hypothalamus. Oxytocin released within the amygdala reduces the activity in the amygdala-LC pathway by dampening the reaction to fear in the amygdala.

In addition, oxytocin released into the LC reduces the activity of the noradrenergic neurons of the LC, since oxytocin activates alpha-2 adrenoceptors, which decrease the function of noradrenergic neurons. As activity of the HPA axis is activated by NA, activity in the HPA axis is further counteracted by the oxytocin-mediated decrease of noradrenergic activity.

Oxytocin Decreases Sympathetic Tone and Increases Parasympathetic Tone

Oxytocin released from parvocellular neurons projecting from the PVN to the brainstem decreases blood pressure and cardiovascular function and increases the function in the gastrointestinal tract by actions in the RVLM, NTS, and DMX, or in other terms, by decreasing the function of the sympathetic and increasing the parasympathetic innervation of the brain.

Oxytocin Inhibits Stress Reactions by Noxious Sensory Stimulation by Actions in the NTS

Finally, oxytocin dampens the effects of noxious or painful stimulation transmitted to the NTS via somatosensory nerves. Non-noxious sensory stimulation increases oxytocin release from the SON and PVN. When oxytocin is released from parvocellular neurons in the PVN, which project to the NTS, alpha-2 adrenoceptors are activated on the noradrenergic neurons originating in the NTS. Since activation of alpha-2 adrenoceptors decreases the activity in noradrenergic neurons projecting to the CRF neurons in the PVN, the effects of noxious somatosensory stimulation resulting in stimulation of noradrenergic neurons are dampened.

In contrast, as described above, low intensity somatosensory stimulation facilitates oxytocin release. In this way, non-noxious sensory stimulation acts as a kind of feed-forward system for oxytocin release, in addition to inhibiting the transmission of noxious stimulation (Burbach et al., 2006).

Reciprocal Facilitating Effects by Oxytocin and Non-Noxious Sensory Stimulation

Oxytocin is released in response to non-noxious somatosensory stimulation in a dose-dependent way, i.e. the more sensory stimulation the more oxytocin is released.

In addition, oxytocin released into the NTS from neurons originating in the PVN facilitate the function of the sensory nerve fibers, which are involved in oxytocin release. This means that the effects of sensory stimulation on oxytocin release will be subject to a feed-forward stimulation, and further oxytocin will be released in response to the stimulation.

As oxytocin facilitates the transmission of non-noxious sensory stimulation in the NTS, the effects of sensory stimulation can also be increased by oxytocin released by other types of stimuli, which increase the activity of the oxytocinergic system. Therefore, if the oxytocin levels in the NTS are high because oxytocin release has been stimulated by, e.g., visual stimuli or by labor, more oxytocin will be released by somatosensory stimulation. This means that the higher the oxytocin levels are in the NTS, the more efficient the effects of non-noxious sensory stimulation become.

No Oxytocin, No Release of Oxytocin in Response to Somatosensory Stimulation

However, this also means that in the absence of oxytocin release in the NTS, somatosensory stimulation is not going to result in oxytocin release. This may e.g., occur if the individual is frightened or in other situations when oxytocin release is shut down, e.g., in mothers having had a Cesarean section and in mothers and babies who have high levels of marcaine in their circulation. This relationship between oxytocin release and sensory stimulation will be discussed further later in the book.

Approach Versus Interaction

Some aspects of the oxytocin-release profile are activated in various kinds of interaction by visual, olfactory, and auditory stimuli. For example, oxytocin released by seeing a beloved person/dog. When oxytocin is released into the amygdala, it facilitates social-approach reactions and reduces anxiety. If social interaction results in closeness or touch, oxytocin is additionally released in response to activation of sensory nerves. No such prolonged release of oxytocin occurs in the absence of closeness and touch.

In response to close contact, the anti-stress effects of oxytocin are particularly pronounced, as oxytocin from parvocellular neurons projecting to the NTS is released. The effect of touch and stroking on short brainstem reflexes involved in the regulation of autonomic nervous tone is potentiated. In addition, alpha-2 adrenoceptors are also stimulated, which results in a decreased activation of noradrenergic fibers, which stimulate the CRF neurons in the HPA axis and the sympathetic nervous system, thereby resulting in a facilitation of oxytocin-induced effects of an anti-stress and relaxing nature.

Internal and External Cues May Shift the Oxytocin Effect Pattern From Anti-stress to Stress Patterns

Sometimes oxytocin may give rise to aggression and stress reactions. Which type of oxytocin pattern will be induced is dependent on the levels of other hormones, e.g., estrogen and cortisol levels, and on other internal and environmental factors. In principle, the calming aspects of oxytocin are induced in a familiar environment in response to soft, tactile stimulation and warmth. In contrast, stress-related oxytocin effects may be induced in a hostile and unfamiliar environment. These differences will be described in more detail later on in this book.

Psycho-Physiological Reaction Patterns

The Fight or Flight Response and the Relaxation and Growth Response or Calm and Connection Reaction

From an evolutionary point of view, mammals and humans share some very old psycho-physiological reaction patterns, which are protective and have survival value. These reaction patterns involve both behavioral and physiological effects, and are mediated by nervous and hormonal effects. They involve activation of the autonomic nervous system and hormones from the HPA axis. The gastrointestinal tract may also play an important role in the expression of these reaction patterns.

It is well known that *defense or stress reactions* are activated by danger, physical damage/pain, and fear. The *fight or flight reaction* described by Cannon (1929) is an example of an integrated stress response involving mental and physiological adaptations. Fear, anger, and arousal are part of this response pattern. In addition, more blood reaches the muscles to provide them with nutrients and

oxygen; cardiovascular activity is increased, as is the lung function. The function in the gastrointestinal tract is reduced, and nutrients are recruited from the liver and used as fuel for activity. Sensitivity to touch is low, as is social competence and ability for compassion. The *fight or flight reaction* is characterized by high activity in the HPA axis and sympathetic nervous system, and low activity in the parasympathetic nervous system (Cannon, 1929; Selye, 1976; Uvnäs-Moberg, Arn, & Magnusson, 2005).

An almost opposite reaction pattern exists in which social skills are promoted, stress levels are decreased, and nutrients are used for growth and restoration. This reaction pattern has been named the *growth and relaxation response* or the *calm and connection reaction response*. It is activated by touch, warmth, and light pressure on the skin, and also in situations perceived as friendly, safe, and calm, for example, being in the presence of liked and trusted persons. In this situation, calm, wellbeing, and relaxation prevail. The sensitivity to pleasant and innocuous sensory stimuli is high, as is the capacity for compassion and social interaction. The activity in the HPA axis and the sympathetic nervous system is low, and the activity in the parasympathetic nervous system is high. Nutrients are used for growth and restorative processes (Uvnäs-Moberg et al., 2005; Uvnäs-Moberg, 1997, 1998a, 2003).

Influence of Hormones, Sensory Interaction, and Genes

It is well established that CRF and vasopressin produced in the PVN of the hypothalamus (and in the amygdala) together with NA from the Locus Coeruleus (LC) in the brainstem regulate behavioral and endocrine aspects of defense and stress reactions.

In contrast, oxytocin produced in the PVN integrates important aspects of the *relaxation and growth response/calm and connection reactions*.

The tendency to react with defense reactions or the calm and connection type of reaction patterns differs between individuals and may also differ within the same individual over time. There may be genetic differences between individuals, and hormonal, sensory, and emotional experiences may influence the level of expression of these reaction patterns in a short- or long-term perspective. The tendency to react with aggression may be promoted by testosterone, and also by frightening, painful, and stressful events. By analogy, the expression of the calm and connection type of reaction patterns may be strengthened by exposure to female sex hormones, such as estrogen and progesterone, and also by emotional and sensory experiences of a non-noxious, pleasant, and calming type. As a rule, the effect of hormonal, emotional, and sensory stimuli give rise to more powerful and sustained effects if experienced early in life, even in utero (Bystrova et al., 2009; Cameron et al., 2008; Glover, O'Connor, & O'Donnell, 2010).

Chapter 7

Milk Production: Role of Prolactin and Oxytocin

As mentioned in the preface, one of the main aims of this book is to describe the role of oxytocin during breastfeeding. The following four chapters are dedicated to this topic. The first important aspect to be dealt with is the role of oxytocin in milk production. The main hormone for stimulation of milk production is prolactin, but oxytocin exerts an important regulatory influence. How these interactions occur will be described in this chapter.

The following two chapters (8 and 9) will be devoted to the role of oxytocin in milk ejection and giving of warmth. In chapter 10, the role of oxytocin and prolactin in breastfeeding mothers will be described.

The Mammary Glands

Mammalian females most often give birth to live offspring, and they feed their young with milk produced in their mammary glands. The term mammal is actually derived from the Latin word for mammary glands, mammae.

The gross anatomy of the mammary glands in which the milk is produced differs between mammalian species. Some have udders with several teats, some have many nipples along the entire front side, from the axillar region down to the groins, and others have just two nipples. In some species, large amounts of milk are stored in big cisterns, allowing the offspring to ingest large amounts of milk at one time. In other species with a smaller storing capacity, the offspring must suckle more frequently.

Structure of the Mammary Glands

The milk-producing mammary glands are of cutaneous origin and have a relatively simple arrangement, which resembles that of the sweat glands (Long, 1969). In the mammary glandular tissue, milk is produced and secreted from a specialized type of epithelial cells, the lactocytes, which cover the inside of the small alveoli. From the alveoli, the milk is drained into small and then larger milk ducts, which open on the nipple. The alveoli and the smaller milk ducts, but not the larger milk ducts, are surrounded by myoepithelial cells, which cause milk ejection when they contract.

In humans, the glandular tissue of the mammary gland is composed of 15-20 lobes, each comprised of smaller lobules that contain 10-100 smaller alveoli. The alveoli are drained by small ducts, which coalesce into larger ducts that converge into five to nine main milk ducts, which open on the nipple. The nipple pores are 0.4-0.7 mm in diameter, and these openings are surrounded by circular muscle fibers (Geddes, 2007).

The Nipple

The nipple is the specialized part of the mammary gland to which offspring attach while suckling. It consists of connective tissue with elastic fibers and smooth muscle, in which blood vessels, nerves, and milk ducts are embedded (Giacometti & Montagna, 1962).

Milk Production

The composition of the milk may vary. Some species, for example, whales and rabbits, produce extremely high fat milk, which keeps the young satisfied for a long time. Other species, for example, rats, produce milk with a low concentration of fat, and rat pups must suckle very often in order to ingest larger volumes. These variations reflect adaptations to the extremely varying lifestyles of different mammals.

The alveoli and milk ducts in the mammary glands are prepared for milk production during pregnancy. During this period, the mammary epithelial cells are transformed into mammary secretory cells, the lactocytes, which synthesize milk. The high levels of estrogen, progesterone, and placental lactogens (the chemical structure resembles that of growth hormone and prolactin) are responsible for the development of the mammary glands.

Milk Production in Human Mothers

In human mothers, like in other mammals, milk production starts during pregnancy, but the secretion of milk is under inhibitory control by the high levels of estrogen and progesterone until after birth. As soon as the placenta is expelled, the levels of the pregnancy hormones drop and milk secretion starts.

Immediately after birth, small amounts of protein-rich colostrum are secreted. The composition of milk undergoes a gradual change after birth, and within days, the "mature milk" containing 7% lactose, 0.8% protein, and 4.1% fat is produced. Most of the constituents in milk are synthesized in the mammary glands, the exception being certain types of fat, which need to be transferred to the lactocytes from maternal stores (Czank, Henderson, Kent, Tat Lai, & Hartmann, 2007). The average volume of milk produced per day by mothers that are exclusively breastfeeding approaches around 250 ml after one week and 750-800 ml per day after one month (Bystrova, Matthiesen, et al., 2007; Hartmann, 2007).

Regulation of Milk Production

Prolactin

Prolactin is the main hormone involved in milk production during the lactation period. It is a peptide hormone produced in a special type of hormone-producing cell in the anterior pituitary, the lactotrophs. The chemical structure of prolactin differs between different mammalian species. Growth hormone, which from a chemical point of view is related to prolactin, seems to be the major stimulant for milk production in cows (Cowie, Forsyth, & Hart, 1980; Czank et al., 2007).

Prolactin Stimulates Milk Synthesis from the Lactocytes

Prolactin stimulates milk synthesis in the mammary glands by binding to specific prolactin receptors on the milk-producing cells, the lactocytes (Rosen, Wyszomiersky, & Hadsell, 1999; Tucker, 2000). Intense exposure to prolactin may not only increase the capacity of milk production of the individual lactocytes, it may even increase the amount of lactocytes, and thereby the milk-secreting capacity of the mammary gland. Prolactin has been suggested to be of greater importance for milk production in the beginning of lactation, when the amount of milk production is increasing, than later on during established lactation (Czank et al., 2007).

Link Between Intensity and Frequency of Suckling, Prolactin Release, and Milk Production

As suckling stimulates milk production via a release of prolactin, the production of milk is linked to the intensity and frequency of suckling. The more suckling, the more prolactin is released, and the more milk is produced from the milk-producing lactocytes in the mammary gland, since the activity of the cellular mechanisms involved in milk production is promoted by prolactin (Czank et al., 2007).

Regulation of Prolactin Release

Inhibitory Effect of Dopamine

Suckling stimulates the secretion of prolactin into the circulation from the anterior pituitary. The release of prolactin from the anterior pituitary is under inhibitory control of dopamine, which is secreted from the tuberoinfundibular system in the hypothalamus. As the levels of dopamine are reduced in response to suckling, prolactin is released into the circulation from the anterior pituitary and milk secretion is stimulated (Freeman, Kanyicska, Lerant, & Nagy, 2000).

Administration of substances that bind to dopamine receptors and have dopamine-like effects (dopamine agonists) decrease milk production. In contrast, substances that reduce the activity of dopamine, dopamine antagonists, increase milk production. Such substances may be used to increase milk production, particularly during the early phase of breastfeeding when prolactin is considered to be of greater importance for milk production than later on during established lactation. The ability of dopamine antagonists to increase milk production is why treatment with some anti-psychotic drugs, which have dopamine-antagonistic properties, gives rise to milk production as a side effect (Cowie, 1974; Cowie et al., 1980; Czank et al., 2007; Ostrom, 1990).

Stimulatory Effect of Oxytocin

Oxytocin is of prime importance for prolactin release from the anterior pituitary. Oxytocin receptors have been demonstrated on a sub-population of the lactotrophs, and administration of antibodies that block the effect of oxytocin inhibit suckling-induced release of prolactin. These data show that oxytocin released locally in the anterior pituitary reinforces the release of prolactin from the lactotrophs in response to suckling (Helena et al., 2011; Kennett, Poletini, Fitch, & Freeman, 2009; McKee, Poletini, Bertram, & Freeman, 2007; Mori et al., 1990; Samson, Lumpkin, & McCann, 1986; Samson & Schell, 1995; Sarkar & Gibbs, 1984). Oxytocin may be secreted into the hypothalamohypophysial-portal system to the anterior pituitary from axon swellings of the magnocellular and parvocellular neurons. Oxytocin-containing nerve fibers may reach the anterior pituitary directly from the paraventricular nucleus. Finally some magnocellular oxytocinergic neurons that project to the posterior pituitary, where oxytocin is released into the circulation, also send collaterals or branches to the anterior pituitary (Buma & Nieuwenhuys, 1988; Burbach et al., 2006; Sheward, Coombes, Bicknell, Fink, & Russell, 1990; Pittman, Blume, & Renaud, 1981; Swanson & Sawchenko, 1983; Zimmerman et al., 1984).

The Inhibitory Factor FIL

Milk production is, however, not only controlled by the prolactin-related stimulation of milk secretion, it is also dependent on the presence of an inhibitory factor (FIL), which is produced from the alveolar epithelium and is secreted into milk. The inhibitory effect exerted by FIL is removed as soon as the milk is emptied from the mammary glands (Czank et al., 2007; Wilde, Addey, Boddy, & Peaker, 1995). By inducing efficient milk ejection and removing the inhibitory factor, FIL, oxytocin indirectly acts in concert with prolactin to stimulate milk production (Wilde et al., 1998). The inhibitory mechanism exerted by FIL does not operate during the first days of lactation, but becomes increasingly important during the period of established lactation.

The chemical identity of FIL has not been established. It

has been suggested to correspond to a protein component in the milk. Another possibility is that the inhibitory effect is simply caused by local neurogenic mechanisms activated when the pressure increases in the alveoli.

Oxytocin Receptors on the Lactocytes

Oxytocin receptors have recently been demonstrated on the milk-producing cells, the lactocytes, suggesting that oxytocin may also contribute to milk production by direct action in the mammary gland (Kimura et al., 1998).

Oxytocin receptors are also present on all epithelial cells in alveoli and milk ducts in the mammary glands. Oxytocin has been suggested to be involved in the regulation of growth of the mammary gland epithelium via these receptors (Ito et al., 1996; Gimpl et al., 2008).

Stimulation of Milk Production by Neurogenic Mechanisms

Stimulation of local neurogenic mechanisms in the udder or spinal reflexes may also influence milk production. If quarters of cows' udders are provided with extra sensory stimulation by hand-milking, this quarter may produce milk with a higher fat content than other udder quarters receiving less stimulation (Geddes, 2007; Uvnäs-Moberg, Johansson, Lupoli, & Svennersten-Sjaunja, 2001).

Activation of local neurogenic mechanisms may also explain why the kangaroo may produce milk of different composition from different udders for their younger and older offspring, respectively, at the same time.

In both examples, the circulating levels of prolactin and oxytocin reaching the mammary glands are identical; therefore, the differential effects induced on milk composition are not induced by hormonal effects, but must be induced by local neurogenic mechanisms. In the first case, the quantity of stimulation applied to the different quarters of the cow's udder was varied. In the second case, the quality and quantity of the suckling performed by the younger and older kangaroo offspring differed. Activation of local axon reflexes and nervous reflexes at the spinal level may be involved in these effects on milk production. The role of nervous mechanisms in the control of milk production and milk ejection, in particular, will be discussed in more detail in the next chapter.

- An inhibitory substance, FIL, produced in milk inhibits milk secretion from the lactocytes. The effect of FIL disappears as soon as milk is removed from the mammary gland.

- Oxytocin may contribute to stimulation of milk production by activation of oxytocin receptors on the lactocytes.

Summary

- Prolactin is the main stimulator of milk production at the level of the lactocytes, where it binds to specific prolactin receptors.

- Prolactin release from the lactotrophs in the anterior pituitary is under inhibitory control of dopamine from the hypothalamus. Oxytocin released via nervous mechanisms into the anterior pituitary stimulate prolactin release from the lactotrophs.

Chapter 8

Milk Ejection and Giving of Warmth: Role of Oxytocin

As described in the previous chapter, prolactin produced in the lactotrophs of the anterior pituitary is the main stimulator of milk production, even if oxytocin exerts a positive regulatory input. In contrast, oxytocin released from the posterior pituitary into the circulation is the main stimulatory factor behind milk ejection.

Oxytocin released in response to suckling induces an additional effect as it dilates the blood vessels in the skin of the mammary glands and the chest, thereby allowing "giving of warmth," in addition to giving of milk.

Milk Ejection

Milk ejection is the process whereby milk is expressed from the alveoli and the ducts of the mammary glands to the opening of the ducts on the nipple. It is induced by suckling, but the pathways in the spinal cord and the brain, as well as the hormonal mechanisms involved, differ from those of milk production.

Milk Ejection in Breastfeeding Women

In connection with milk ejection induced by the suckling stimulus during breastfeeding, milk that has already been produced becomes available to the infant in connection with milk ejection. In lactating women, most of the milk stored in the alveolar portion of the gland is expressed into the milk ducts and ejected from the nipples during milk ejection.

The occurrence of the milk-ejection reflex during breastfeeding can be established by a sensation of tingling or pressure in the mother's breast. Not all women sense this reflex. Alternatively, an observed flow of milk from the contra-lateral nipple or swallowing sounds from the infant can be used to establish the milk-ejection reflex. By using these types of observations, milk ejection was found to occur within 60-90 minutes after the start of breastfeeding (Widstrom et al., 1984).

Recently, an ultrasound technique has been developed which allows milk ejection to be visualized as opening of the pores on the nipple. The opening of the pores was shown to parallel ejection of milk in experiments in which milk flow was studied in the contra-lateral breast during milk pumping. The first milk ejection occurred after 120 seconds and was then followed by several others at 90-120-second intervals (Geddes, 2007; Prime et al., 2009; Prime, Geddes, Hepworth, Trengove, & Hartmann, 2011; Prime, Kent, Hepworth, Trengove, & Hartmann, 2012; Ramsay, Kent, Owens, & Hartmann, 2004; Ramsay et al., 2006).

Role of Oxytocin

A pituitary extract was found to increase milk flow in the beginning of the 20th century. Later on, this unknown substance was found to correspond to oxytocin (Ott & Scott, 1910). As described in detail in a previous chapter, oxytocin is produced in nerve cells in the SON and PVN in the hypothalamus. Oxytocin produced in the magnocellular neurons of the SON and PVN is transported down to the posterior pituitary by long nerve endings to be released into the blood stream, e.g., in response to suckling.

Interestingly, an oxytocin-like peptide is released into the circulation in connection with egg laying in birds, suggesting that milk ejection in mammals is functionally related to behaviors, such as egg laying in birds, and perhaps to other even more primitive animals (Burbach et al., 2006)

Oxytocin is necessary for milk letdown. Female animals lacking oxytocin fail to give milk to their young, and the offspring die of starvation (Nishimori et al., 1996; Young et al., 1996).

Oxytocin Induces Contraction of Myoepithelial Cells

During suckling, milk ejection occurs when oxytocin released into the circulation reaches the mammary glands. After binding to specific receptors, oxytocin contracts the myoepithelial cells that surround the alveoli, thereby raising the intra-alveolar pressure. Milk is consequently expelled into the smaller milk ducts. Since the myoepithelial cells lining the small milk ducts are disposed longitudinally, the ducts shorten and widen in response to oxytocin, thereby expelling the milk into the larger ducts, which lack myoepithelial cells (Ely & Petersen, 1941; Gaines, 1915; Kimura et al., 1998; Ott & Scott, 1910; Petersen & Ludwick, 1942; Prime et al., 2009; Prime et al., 2011).

Oxytocin Opens the Sphincters of the Larger Milk Ducts

Oxytocin may also widen the larger milk ducts and dilate the circular muscles surrounding the openings of the larger milk ducts on the nipple, "opening the doors" for the milk to be ejected. These effects may be mediated by oxytocin receptors on the milk ducts and in smooth muscles located in the connective tissue surrounding the ducts, as well on circular muscles surrounding the sphincters, as oxytocin receptors are not only present on the myoepithelial cells surrounding the alveoli (Kimura et al., 1998). These effects may be indirectly mediated via an oxytocin-induced release of locally produced peptides that relax smooth muscles. As will be described later in this chapter, the sensory nerves innervating the nipple and the mammary glands contain peptides, such as calcitonin gene-related peptide (CGRP), SP, and VIP, which may relax smooth muscle (Holzer, Taché, & Rosenfeldt, 1992; Pernow, 1983; Said & Mutt, 1970). In support of this assumption, oxytocin has been demonstrated to release VIP (Stock & Uvnäs-Moberg, 1985).

Giving of Warmth

In addition to stimulating milk production and milk ejection, suckling also increases the temperature in the skin overlying the mammary glands and adjacent areas on the front side of the chest. In women, this phenomenon is called flushing and can be visualized by cameras sensitive to heat.

Functions of Increased Skin Temperature

The increase of maternal skin temperature helps the mother warm her offspring and prevent hypothermia, which may be lifesaving, particularly immediately after birth (Kimura & Matsuoka, 2007).

The maternal capacity to give warmth to newborns has other important functions for the offspring. Newborns are extremely sensitive to small changes in temperature. Since they are attracted by warmth, it may help them find the nipple and start suckling. Newborn piglets, for example, move towards the udder, because the temperature of its base is increased by 0.5 degrees Celsius (Algers & Uvnäs-Moberg, 2007).

The warm temperature makes the newborns feel well and calm, and their stress levels are reduced when they are close to their mothers. Together with touch and stroking, it also stimulates processes related to growth and maturation in the newborn. In this way, the mother continues to regulate metabolic and physiologic processes in the newborn after birth (Hofer, 1994). In fact, by transferring warmth to the offspring, the mother gives a more basic form of "calories or energy" than when she gives milk. All these effects will be described in more depth in the chapters describing the effects of skin-to-skin contact.

Giving of Warmth in Birds

Perhaps the ability to give warmth to mammalian offspring is related to the process by which birds warm their eggs and offspring before hatching. Some birds have a network of superficial blood vessels on their "chest," and some species pick their feathers on the "chest" before they are going to lie on their eggs to increase the contact between their skin and the egg. In this way, the parents give warmth to the eggs when they lie on them. It is by transferring warmth to their eggs that birds make their unborn chicks grow and develop inside the egg. They also warm newborns by lying on them in the nest.

It is as if mammals have retained the capacity to give warmth to their offspring, and in this way, contribute to growth and development of the offspring.

Role of Oxytocin

The increased skin temperature in the skin overlying the mammary glands is due to an increased circulation in the thoracic arteries and to dilation of the blood vessels of the skin. When the blood vessels in the skin dilate, the circulation in the skin increases, which leads to increased temperature (Kimura & Matsuoka, 2007).

Circulating oxytocin plays an important role in the increase of skin temperature. In fact, the mechanisms involved are not so different from those involved in milk ejection. As described above, circulating oxytocin does not only contract the myoepithelial cells in the alveoli in connection with milk ejection, it also dilates the larger milk ducts to allow expression of milk. In parallel, blood vessels in the skin are dilated.

Experiments

The role of oxytocin on skin temperature was studied by Eriksson and collaborators in a series of experiments performed on lactating rats (Eriksson, Lundeberg, & Uvnäs-Moberg, 1996). The experiments showed that:

- The temperature of the skin overlying the mammary glands increased in connection with milk letdown when the pups suckled.

- Injections of oxytocin in amounts that gave rise to the same circulating oxytocin levels as observed in response to suckling induced a similar rise of skin temperature as observed during suckling.

- Injections of CGRP, SP, and VIP into the circulation of the mammary gland increased the temperature in the skin overlying the mammary glands to the same extent as suckling and injections of oxytocin.

- Injections of NPY into the circulation of the mammary glands decreased the temperature of the skin overlying the mammary glands.

These data show that oxytocin released by suckling not only induces milk ejection, it also increases the circulation and the temperature in the skin overlying the mammary glands. Peptides, such as CGRP, SP and VIP, are produced in or close to blood vessels and increase skin temperature, so the effect of oxytocin may be secondary to a release of locally produced peptides (Eriksson, Lundeberg, et al., 1996). The results do not exclude the possibility that circulating oxytocin also dilates the blood vessels in the skin by a more direct action via oxytocin receptors in the blood vessels (Kimura et al., 1998).

Stimulation of Milk Ejection and Increase of Skin Temperature in Response to Other Sensory Cues or Mental Stimuli

As will be discussed in more detail later in this book, maternal oxytocin is not only released into the circulation by suckling and skin-to-skin contact, but may be released when the mother sees and hears her newborn or simply thinks of him or her, as oxytocin release can be conditioned to other stimuli. Therefore, milk ejection may occur and the skin temperature may rise (flushing), in response to increased levels of circulating levels of oxytocin before the onset of, or even in the absence of, suckling (Tancin, Kraetzl, Schams, & Bruckmaier, 2001).

Summary

- Milk ejection is the process whereby milk is expressed from the alveoli and the ducts of the mammary glands.

- Oxytocin stimulates milk ejection by contracting the myoepithelial cells in the alveoli and smaller milk ducts, and facilitates milk ejection by dilating the larger milk ducts.

- Oxytocin increases chest and breast skin temperature by dilating the blood vessels in the skin. The relaxation of the milk ducts and the blood vessels in the skin may be induced by direct effects of oxytocin on the smooth muscles or indirectly by a local release of vasoactive peptides.

• Oxytocin: The Biological Guide To Motherhood

Chapter 9

Milk Ejection and Giving of Warmth: Role of Nervous Mechanisms

As described in the previous chapters, both prolactin and oxytocin are released in response to suckling. In this way, milk production and milk ejection are stimulated by hormonal actions of prolactin and oxytocin, respectively. In addition, the temperature of the skin on the chest is increased in response to the elevated levels of oxytocin.

Milk ejection and the increased temperature of the skin are not only regulated by hormonal actions, but also by local nervous mechanisms induced by axon reflexes from the somatosensory nerves and by the sympathetic nervous system in the mammary glands. These effects will be described in this chapter.

Innervation of the Mammary Gland

The mammary gland receives its innervation via the intercostal nerves. When the different parts of the mammary glands are studied, somatosensory nerves have been associated with the major duct system, but not with the smaller ducts (Findlay & Grosvenor, 1969; Linzell, 1971). The areola and the nipple are sparsely innervated by sensory nerve fibers (Geddes, 2007). The mammary glands are reached by sympathetic efferent or motor nerves from the paravertebral sympathetic ganglia, which innervate blood vessels and contractile muscles in the nipple and the areola, and there is also a sparse innervation of the large ducts (Cowie, 1974). In contrast, no parasympathetic motor fibers have been demonstrated in the mammary gland (Findlay & Grosvenor, 1969; Linzell, 1971).

Peptides as Co-Transmitters in Mammary Gland Innervation

Nerves originating in the skin, e.g., somatosensory nerves, and nerves belonging to the autonomic nervous system often contain co-transmitters of a peptidergic nature. When present in sensory nerves such peptides often exert local actions at the site of origin of the nerves by being released in a backwards direction via axon-reflexes. The nerves in the mammary gland are no exception.

Experiment

An extensive study of the presence of such peptides in nerves within the nipple and the mammary gland in both rats and humans has been performed by Eriksson and collaborators (Eriksson, Lindh, et al., 1996). More specifically, the localization of calcitonin gene-related peptide (CGRP), substance P (SP), and vasoactive polypeptide (VIP) previously demonstrated to coexist with other transmitters in somatosensory nerves, e.g., originating from the skin (Gibson et al., 1984; Hokfelt et al., 1975; Shehab & Atkinson, 1986), and of neuropeptide Y (NPY), previously demonstrated to occur in motor neurons of the sympathetic nervous system (Lundberg et al., 1983), were studied. CGRP, SP, and VIP are all peptides that exert relaxing effects on smooth muscle, e.g., blood vessels and milk ducts, whereas NPY is a peptide which contracts smooth muscles (Edvinsson, Ekblad, Hakånson, & Wahlestedt, 1984; Holzer et al., 1992; Pernow, 1983; Said & Mutt, 1970).

In the study by Eriksson, Lindh, et al. (1996), a rich distribution of immuno-reactive nerve fibers containing CGRP, SP, VIP, and NPY was demonstrated in structures of the mammary gland related to milk ejection and production, such as epidermis, blood vessels, smooth muscle, and connective tissue surrounding the alveoli and the milk ducts. Similar findings were obtained in mammary tissue from both humans (non-lactating) and lactating rats. Since these peptides are of functional importance during lactation or breastfeeding and are linked to the effects exerted by oxytocin, a more detailed description of their localization and function in the mammary gland will be given below.

The peptides studied were demonstrated in three different types of nerves:

1. CGRP and SP immuno-reactivity was demonstrated in cell bodies in the dorsal root ganglia close to the spinal cord, where sensory nerves have their cell bodies. CGRP and SP immuno-reactivity was also present in the epidermis of the nipple and the areola, demonstrating that the sensory nerves have their origin in the skin. In addition, these peptides were present in axon collaterals surrounding non-vascular smooth muscle, blood vessels, and milk ducts in the nipple and mammary gland tissue. These peptides, which most often exert relaxing effects on smooth muscles, may therefore be released in a retrograde direction (via axon reflexes) when the somato-sensory nerves are activated in response to suckling to induce nipple erection and to stimulate blood and milk flow.

2. The VIP-containing fibers had their cell bodies in the nodose ganglia, which contains the cell bodies from sensory nerves in the parasympathetic vagal

nerve, suggesting that these fibers represent a special type of sensory nerves or "vagal afferents." Fibers containing VIP were also found in axon collaterals in the muscular tissue of the nipple and in the muscles surrounding blood vessels and milk ducts in both the nipple and the breast tissue. Since VIP also has a relaxing effect on smooth muscle, VIP released locally from axon reflexes in response to suckling may contribute to nipple erection and increased blood and milk flow during suckling.

3. By contrast, the nerve fibers containing NPY had their origin in the stellate ganglia, the site of the cell bodies of motor fibers of the sympathetic nervous system. Both NA, the main transmitter in the sympathetic motor nerves, and NPY may contract smooth muscle. Since fibers containing NA and NPY were present in both non-vascular smooth muscle in the nipple, as well as in smooth muscle surrounding blood vessels and milk ducts, NA and NPY may exert a contractile effect on non-vascular muscles in the nipple and contract blood vessels and milk ducts, thereby inhibiting blood and milk flow in response to activation of the sympathetic nerves.

Taken together, the sensory nerves of the mammary glands contain peptides, such as CGRP, SP and VIP, which relax blood vessels and milk ducts, thereby facilitating the circulation and flow of milk. The sympathetic nerves innervating the mammary glands and the nipple contain the substances NA and NPY, which act in an opposite direction, i.e., they constrict blood vessels and the milk ducts, thereby inhibiting blood flow and milk ejection (Eriksson, Lindh, et al., 1996; Uvnäs-Moberg & Eriksson, 1996).

Role of Axon Reflexes in Milk Ejection and "Giving of Warmth"

As presented in detail above, sensory nerves originating in the nipple, areola, and mammary gland tissue contain peptides, such as CGRP, SP, and VIP. These peptides are also present in axon collaterals, which terminate close to the origin of the somatosensory nerves in the mammary gland. Since suckling induces stimulation of sensory nerves, these peptides are released locally in the mammary gland in response to the suckling stimulus.

Nipple Erection

A suckling-related local release of these peptides may contribute to nipple erection, which occurs at the onset of suckling to make it easier for the offspring to attach to the nipple (Eriksson, Lindh, et al., 1996).

Opening of Milk Ducts and Increased Circulation in Blood Vessels

The local release of SP, CGRP, and VIP relaxes the circular muscles surrounding the milk ducts, thereby widening the openings to facilitate milk flow. Such neurogenic effects may explain why touching a cow's udder may cause milk secretion, the tapping reflex. In addition, the locally released peptides increase the circulation in the mammary gland and in the skin overlying the mammary gland, thereby increasing skin temperature.

Facilitation of Hormonal Effects

The local neurogenic effects induced by suckling facilitate milk ejection and vasodilation in skin induced by circulating oxytocin. As an immediate response to suckling, locally released CGRP, SP, and VIP start to relax muscles in blood vessels and milk ducts in the nipple. In a second step and after a small delay, these effects are reinforced when circulating oxytocin released by suckling reaches the mammary gland to induce contraction of myoepithelial cells and dilation of blood vessels and milk ducts.

Pre-stimulation in Cows

The need for pre-stimulation when cows are milked by milking machines is an expression of the need for activation of neurogenic mechanisms in order to obtain optimal milk ejection. The mechanism involved in milk ejection induced by milking machines is mainly based on vacuum extraction of the milk. This may not provide sufficient sensory stimulation, and, therefore, needs to be supplemented by manual sensory stimulation (Uvnäs-Moberg et al., 2001).

Delayed Milk Ejection After Breast Pumping in Women

Interestingly, the milk ejection observed after breast pumping in women was slightly delayed when compared to milk ejection induced by breastfeeding (120 versus 90 seconds; Geddes, 2007; Widstrom et al., 1984). This difference may be due to the fact that breast pumps may not induce the same quality of stimulation of the sensory nerves emanating in the nipple as does suckling. As described above, the suckling stimulus not only induces a release of oxytocin into the circulation, it also gives rise to activation of axon reflexes and a local release of peptides, which facilitate milk ejection by opening the milk ducts in the nipple. Since breast pumping is to a large extent based on milk extraction caused by vacuum, the local relaxing effect may not be induced, and, consequently, milk ejection occurs with a short delay (Geddes, 2007; Prime et al., 2009; Prime et al., 2011).

Role of the Sympathetic Nervous System

The mammary glands are innervated by the sympathetic nervous system (but not by the parasympathetic nervous system). As shown by Eriksson et al. (Eriksson, Lindh, et al., 1996), the sympathetic nerve fibers in the mammary gland contain NA and NPY (as a co-transmitter). NA, as well as NPY, may contract the milk ducts and blood vessels in the mammary gland and in the skin overlying the mammary gland, which results in an inhibition of milk ejection and a decrease in skin temperature (Bruckmaier, Wellnitz, & Blum, 1997; Bruckmaier, Schams, & Blum, 1993; Eriksson, Lundeberg, et al., 1996).

Stress Activates the Sympathetic Nervous System

The sympathetic nervous system and the HPA axis are important components of the stress system as described in chapter 3. As the mammary glands are innervated by the sympathetic nervous system, stress may influence the function of the mammary glands via the sympathetic nervous system.

Stress Inhibits Milk Ejection and Giving of Warmth

Stress may inhibit the letdown of milk in two different ways:

1. The milk ducts may contract in response to activation of the sympathetic nervous system, inhibiting milk ejection.

2. The release of oxytocin and, thereby, the hormonal aspect of the letdown reflex is easily inhibited by stress.

Stress Contracts the Milk Ducts and Blood Vessels in the Mammary Gland

During stress, increased amounts of NA and NPY are released from the sympathetic fibers within the mammary gland. As these substances exert contractile effects on smooth muscles in milk ducts and blood vessels, milk ejection and blood flow is inhibited (Bruckmaier et al., 1997). As demonstrated in the results presented in the previous chapter from the study by Erikson et al. (1996), infusions of NPY decrease blood flow in the skin overlying the mammary gland and decrease skin temperature.

Stress Inhibits Oxytocin Release

Stress may also inhibit milk ejection by inhibition of the hormonal aspect of the milk ejection reflex, i.e., by inhibition of oxytocin release. Relatively subtle stimuli, such as being in an unfamiliar environment, may inhibit oxytocin release in connection with being milked by a milking machine and, thereby, milk ejection in cows until the situation is again considered normal (Bruckmaier, Pfeilsticker, & Blum, 1996; Bruckmaier et al., 1997).

Newton demonstrated that stress also inhibits oxytocin secretion and the milk ejection reflex, albeit temporarily, in women (Newton, 1992). Oxytocin release and, thereby, the milk ejection reflex can be inhibited by quite subtle factors, such as being in an unfamiliar environment or feeling unsafe. In fact, oxytocin has been called the shy hormone (Odent, 2012). The inhibition of oxytocin release taking place when mothers feel unsafe will be discussed further in the chapter on maternal protective strategies.

Prevention of Stress-Induced Inhibition of Oxytocin Release and Milk Letdown by Suckling and Sensory Stimulation

Suckling Inhibits Activity in the Sympathetic Nervous System

Suckling promotes milk ejection in several ways. It not only stimulates oxytocin release into the circulation, it also influences milk ejection via local neurogenic mechanisms in the mammary gland, and sometimes also via spinal reflexes.

The suckling stimulus, however, exerts powerful anti-stress effects. These effects are exerted at many levels in the CNS (central nervous system), and important anti-stress effects are induced in the area in the brainstem involved in the control of the autonomic nervous system. Suckling decreases the function of the sympathetic nervous system and increases the function of the parasympathetic nervous system in this area. These generalized effects will be dealt with more extensively later on in this book. Here only the consequences of the suckling induced inhibition of sympathetic nervous tone on functions in the mammary gland will be discussed.

Pathways Involved in the Inhibition of Sympathetic Nerve Activity

The suckling stimulus leads to an activation of the NTS in the medulla oblongata (Burbach et al., 2006). This effect is induced by activation of the somatosensory nerves projecting to the spinal cord and in response to activation of the special "vagal afferents" innervating the mammary gland (Burbach et al., 2006; Eriksson, Lindh, et al., 1996). Non-noxious stimulation of sensory nerves, as induced by suckling, has been demonstrated to decrease the activity in the sympathoneural and in sympathoadrenal systems (Araki et al., 1984; Kurosawa et al., 1982; Tsuchiya et al., 1991; Uvnäs-Moberg et al., 1986). These effects are induced in areas within and close to the NTS in the brainstem involved in the control of the autonomic nerve system.

In addition to the "direct" effects in the NTS and adjacent areas in the medulla oblongata, effects induced by non-noxious sensory stimulation are exerted at the level of the hypothalamus by activation of a population of oxytocinergic nerves emanating from the paraventricular nucleus that innervate the NTS (Buijs, 1983; Buijs & Swaab, 1979; Sofroniew, 1983; Stern & Zhang, 2003). In support of this, oxytocin is released in response to non-noxious stimulation of sensory nerves, and administration of oxytocin may decrease the activity in some parts of the sympathetic nervous system (Stock & Uvnäs-Moberg, 1988).

In summary, the effects of suckling seem to involve a two-step pathway. The first effect is exerted directly in the brainstem and the second effect is exerted in the hypothalamus. The oxytocin released from the paraventricular neurons emanating in the hypothalamus into the areas involved in autonomic nervous control in the brainstem facilitate or reinforce the effects induced by the direct effects in the brainstem.

By inhibition of the activity of the sympathetic nervous fibers projecting to the mammary gland, suckling may antagonize the contraction of the muscles surrounding the milk ducts and the blood vessels in the mammary gland, and as a consequence, increase milk flow and skin temperature.

Skin-to-Skin Contact Contributes to the Relaxing Effects

Before suckling, the offspring or infants often lie close to their mothers' chest or even massage the udders. The activation of sensory nerves induced by close contact contributes to the inhibition of sympathetic nerve activity caused by suckling, and, therefore, facilitates oxytocin release and milk ejection. The effects of skin-to-skin contact will be discussed more in detail later in this book.

Application of Warmth

Application of warmth, e.g., by immersing the breasts in warm water, may induce an immediate milk flow. This is because warm temperature stimulates sensory nerves, which, in turn, decrease sympathetic nervous tone by reflex actions in the NTS and by a release of oxytocin (Uvnäs-Moberg, Bruzelius, et al., 1993).

Summary

- Local neurogenic reflexes induced by the suckling stimulus contribute to milk ejection and increased blood flow/skin temperature.

- The hormonal effects of oxytocin on milk ejection and increase in skin temperature are facilitated by nervous mechanisms induced by the suckling stimulus.

- The sympathetic nervous system, which is activated during stress, inhibits milk ejection and decreases skin temperature by contraction of smooth muscles in milk ducts and blood vessels.

- Suckling may decrease sympathetic nervous tone, thereby counteracting the inhibitory actions on milk ejection and decrease of skin temperature caused by stress. These effects are exerted at multiple sites in the brain.

Table 9.1. Suckling-Induced Mechanisms that Promote Milk Ejection and Increase Skin Temperature

Suckling	Effect
Induces release of local peptides	Relaxes opening of milk ducts and blood vessels in skin overlying mammary glands
Induces release of oxytocin into the circulation	Contracts myoepithelial cell to induce milk ejection
Induces activity in the NTS	Decreases activity in the sympathetic nervous system
Releases oxytocin from the PVN into the brain	Decreases activity in the sympathetic nervous system
Decreases fear and anxiety	Decreases activity in the sympathetic nervous system
All of the above	Act in conjunction to increase skin temperature and cause milk ejection

Chapter 10

Role of Prolactin and Oxytocin in Breastfeeding Women

In the former three chapters, the regulatory mechanisms involved in milk production and milk ejection, including the role of prolactin and oxytocin were presented. In this chapter, the levels of prolactin and oxytocin in breastfeeding women will be presented and the role of these hormones in the control of milk production and milk ejection will be described.

A substantial number of studies have been performed which demonstrate that prolactin and oxytocin levels rise in response to suckling in breastfeeding women (Drewett, Bowen-Jones, & Dogterom, 1982; Glasier, McNeilly, & Howie, 1988; Johnston & Amico, 1986; Lucas, Drewett, & Mitchell, 1980; McNeilly et al., 1983; Widstrom et al., 1984).

Prolactin and Oxytocin Levels

Clinical Studies

Three different clinical studies have provided detailed information on the release profile of prolactin and oxytocin in response to breastfeeding. Other breastfeeding variables, such as duration of suckling and breastfeeding, and the amount of milk ejected during a breastfeed were recorded, and the relationship between hormone levels and these breastfeeding variables was established. The results from these studies will be described and discussed in some detail.

1. Repeated blood samples were collected before, during, and after breastfeeding in the beginning (four days after birth) and during established breastfeeding (three to four months after birth) in 55 primiparous women. Oxytocin and prolactin levels were measured and related to other breastfeeding variables, such as milk yield, duration of suckling, duration of breastfeeding, and weaning. Oxytocin levels were measured by RIA (Uvnäs-Moberg, Widstrom, Werner, et al., 1990).

2. Twenty-four blood samples were collected in 37 primiparous women in connection with breastfeeding two days after birth. The amount of milk ejected in connection with the breastfeed and the duration of breastfeeding were recorded. Oxytocin and prolactin levels were measured and related to other breastfeeding variables. Oxytocin levels were measured with RIA (Nissen et al., 1996).

3. Blood samples were collected in 61 breastfeeding primiparous women according to the same schedule as in study II. Oxytocin and prolactin levels were measured. Oxytocin levels were measured with enzyme-linked immunoassay (EIA). Other breastfeeding variables, such as duration of suckling, were also measured (Jonas et al., 2009).

Prolactin and Oxytocin Levels

Main Results—Prolactin

The most important findings from the three clinical studies regarding prolactin levels were:

*   Basal prolactin levels were higher the first days after birth than later on during breastfeeding (Uvnäs-Moberg, Widstrom, Werner, et al., 1990).

*   Prolactin levels rose 10-20 minutes after the start of breastfeeding to reach a maximum after about 20-30 minutes when measured at two and four days after birth and at three to four months postpartum. The rise of prolactin levels persisted for at least one hour after the start of suckling (Uvnäs-Moberg, Widstrom, Werner, et al., 1990; Nissen et al., 1996; Jonas et al., 2009).

*   The longer the period of suckling, the more prolactin was released (Nissen et al., 1990; Jonas et al., 2009).

*   Basal, as well as suckling-related, prolactin levels decreased over time, as the rise of prolactin levels was higher four days after birth than at three to four months postpartum. Still, the rise of prolactin levels amounted to about 50% of basal levels at both time points (Uvnäs-Moberg, Widstrom, Werner, et al., 1990).

*   Basal prolactin levels at three to four months postpartum predicted the duration of the remaining breastfeeding period (Uvnäs-Moberg, Widstrom, Werner, et al., 1990).

*   Prolactin levels decreased significantly within 24 days of weaning (Uvnäs-Moberg, Widstrom, Werner, et al., 1990).

Main Results—Oxytocin

The most important findings from the three clinical studies

regarding oxytocin levels were:

- Basal oxytocin levels were higher the first days after birth than later on during breastfeeding (Uvnäs-Moberg, Widstrom, Werner, et al., 1990).

- The suckling-related oxytocin release occurred in pulses, which started to appear within one minute after onset of suckling on both day four and at three to four months postpartum. Up to five oxytocin pulses, with approximately 90-second intervals, were recorded during the first ten minutes of breastfeeding. Oxytocin levels during the pulses were about five-fold higher than presuckling levels. Basal oxytocin levels were reached within 20-60 minutes after onset of suckling (Uvnäs-Moberg, Widstrom, Werner, et al., 1990; Nissen et al., 1996; Jonas et al., 2009).

- The rise of oxytocin levels caused by suckling increased over time and was more pronounced at three to four months postpartum than at four days after birth. The individual peaks were difficult to discern at this stage of lactation, as they coalesced into one major peak (Uvnäs-Moberg, Widstrom, Werner, et al., 1990).

- In spite of the difference in amounts of oxytocin released four days after birth and three to four months postpartum, the amount of oxytocin released correlated strongly within individual mothers (Uvnäs-Moberg, Widstrom, Werner, et al., 1990).

- Oxytocin levels decreased after weaning, i.e., 24 hours after the last breastfeeding session (Uvnäs-Moberg, Widstrom, Werner, et al., 1990).

Prolactin

The finding of a rise of prolactin levels in response to suckling that occurred after around ten minutes and which lasted for at least 60 minutes in the studies summarized above (Uvnäs-Moberg et al., 1990; Nissen et al., 1996; Jonas et al., 2009) are in line with previous studies demonstrating a suckling-related release of prolactin (Battin, Marrs, Fleiss, & Mishell, 1985; Frantz, 1977; Johnston & Amico, 1986; McNeilly et al., 1983; Yokoyama, Ueda, Irahara, & Aono, 1994).

Prolactin Levels and Duration of Suckling

The finding of a relationship between the duration of suckling and the amount of prolactin released in response to breastfeeding supports the role of prolactin as an important stimulator of milk production, and is consistent with the fact that frequent and relatively long periods of breastfeeding are important in stimulating milk production (Houston, Howie, & McNeilly, 1983; Houston, Howie, Smart, McArdle, & McNeilly, 1983; Salariya, Easton, & Cater, 1978).

Prolactin Levels Decrease Over Time

Prolactin levels were lower when studied in response to breastfeeding three to four months after birth than after four days. A similar decrease of prolactin levels during the course of breastfeeding has been reported previously and has been attributed to a less important role for prolactin in milk production in later stages of breastfeeding (Battin et al., 1985; Johnston & Amico, 1986).

Prolactin Levels and Duration of Breastfeeding

The finding that prolactin levels recorded at four months postpartum were closely associated with the remaining period of breastfeeding in exclusively breastfeeding women, indicate that prolactin levels still play a role in milk production at later stages of breastfeeding (Uvnäs-Moberg, Widstrom, Werner, et al., 1990). Prolactin levels in these women probably reflected the frequency of suckling, as women who breastfeed often are more likely to be able to breastfeed successfully in the long term.

The finding of a fall in prolactin levels 24 hours after the last breastfeeding session, i.e., in connection with weaning, provides further evidence for a suckling-related stimulation of prolactin release at the end of lactation (Uvnäs-Moberg, Widstrom, Werner, et al., 1990).

Oxytocin

In all of the studies described above, the rise in oxytocin occurred in pulses, even if the individual peaks were difficult to discern at later stages of breastfeeding, when the amounts of oxytocin release was bigger. The findings of a pulsatile suckling-related oxytocin pattern is in line with other reports (Drewett et al., 1982; Johnston & Amico, 1986; Lucas et al., 1980; McNeilly et al., 1983; Yokoyama et al., 1994).

RIA and EIA

In order to determine blood levels of oxytocin, the use of radioimmunoassay (RIA) has been the norm. This technique is indirect and based on how much a sample containing oxytocin influences the binding between radioactive (iodinated oxytocin) and an antibody to oxytocin. The more oxytocin the sample to be analyzed contains, the more the binding between oxytocin and the oxytocin antibody is shifted. Since it is known how much standards of oxytocin (the quantity is known) influences the binding, it is possible to deduce how much oxytocin the unknown samples contain.

This equilibrium reaction can be disturbed by other substances; therefore, the samples (e.g., blood samples) need to be purified before they are analyzed. The blood samples in the studies by Uvnäs Moberg and Nissen et al. were analyzed by this technique, using RIA basal levels of oxytocin around 10-20 pg/ml.

As the RIA is relatively complicated to perform and

involves radioactive material, another type of technique based on binding between oxytocin and an oxytocin antibody has been developed. This technique, called enzyme-linked immunoassay (ELISA or EIA), gives rise to higher oxytocin values, particularly if the samples to be analyzed are not purified before analysis. If EIA is used to measure oxytocin levels without purification of the plasma samples prior to the analysis, non-specific reactions with larger plasma molecules also occur, which give rise to even higher levels (Szeto et al., 2011). If samples are purified, different values from those obtained with RIA may still be obtained, indicating that the analytical techniques do not always measure the same thing. Such differences may be linked to several differences between the techniques. One important aspect is which antibody is used, how specific it is for recognizing and binding only to oxytocin and to other related peptides, such as vasopressin. Another important aspect is whether the antibody recognizes the whole oxytocin molecule or just part if it. In the latter case, smaller metabolites or fragments of oxytocin are detected.

RIA and ELISA May Give Rise to Different Results

Oxytocin levels in the study by Jonas et al. were performed by EIA without extraction and, consequently, the basal levels of oxytocin were 10-20-fold higher than in the two previous studies in which RIA was used. As mentioned above, in spite of the very different basal levels of oxytocin obtained by RIA and EIA, breastfeeding was associated with a pulsatile release of oxytocin irrespective of the use of RIA or EIA, suggesting that the immediate oxytocin release induced by suckling is recorded by both techniques (Jonas et al., 2009, Nissen et al., 1996; Uvnäs Moberg et al., 1990).

When comparing results from different studies in which oxytocin levels have been recorded, it is important to keep in mind which analytical method has been used, as different analytical methods give rise to different basal oxytocin levels and sometimes different response patterns.

In a recent study, EIA was used to determine oxytocin levels in plasma and saliva in breastfeeding women (White-Traut et al., 2009). The patterns obtained are very different and completely opposite to the ones obtained in the studies in which RIA was used. In fact, in these studies oxytocin levels decreased in response to breastfeeding. Since so many other studies demonstrated that oxytocin levels rise in response to suckling in breastfeeding women, the results are not likely to represent oxytocin levels, but should be due to a methodological problem. To analyze oxytocin levels in saliva is also problematic, since circulating oxytocin is not likely to penetrate into saliva. As described in chapter 3, oxytocin is a peptide hormone, and it is electrically charged. Such hormones do not easily penetrate biological membranes, e.g., to reach the salivary glands.

The reason for these aberrant results is probably that EIA is a less specific technique and measures substances in plasma that do not only correspond to the nine amino acid oxytocin molecule itself, but also to other circulating substances, e.g., oxytocin fragments or metabolites or other completely unrelated substances. By contrast, RIA more selectively detects oxytocin.

Oxytocin Levels and Milk Ejection

The finding that oxytocin levels rise within 60-90 seconds after onset of suckling fits nicely with the timing of onset of the milk ejection reflex and supports the role of oxytocin for milk ejection in breastfeeding mothers. As mentioned in the previous chapter, milk ejection occurs within 60-90 seconds of breastfeeding, which coincides with the first suckling-induced peak of oxytocin (Widstrom et al., 1984; Uvnäs Moberg, Widstrom, Werner, et al., 1990; Nissen et al., 1996; Jonas et al., 2009).

In studies performed on women in which a breast pump is applied to one breast, milk can be observed to be ejected from the contralateral breast at 90-second intervals (Geddes, 2007; Prime et al., 2009; Prime et al., 2011). As mentioned above, oxytocin is released at 90-second intervals; therefore, the ejection of milk occurring at 90-second intervals is likely to be induced by individual oxytocin peaks. In other words, each pulse of oxytocin is associated with ejection of milk in human mothers.

Association Between the Number of Oxytocin Pulses, the Amount of Milk Ejected, and the Duration of the Entire Breastfeeding Period

The finding that milk is ejected in response to each individual oxytocin pulse indicates that the number of oxytocin peaks observed during suckling should be linked to the amount of milk ejected. Indeed, this assumption is supported by findings of Nissen and collaborators showing that the number of oxytocin peaks recorded during the first ten minutes of a breastfeed two days after birth correlated with the amount of milk ejected. The more oxytocin pulses induced by suckling, the more milk was ejected (Nissen, Gustavsson, Widstrom & Uvnäs-Moberg, 1998).

The number of oxytocin pulses recorded during the first ten minutes of breastfeeding two days after birth was also associated with the duration of exclusive breastfeeding, i.e., the more pulses the longer the mothers breastfed (Nissen et al., 1996). Whether the long period of breastfeeding in mothers having many oxytocin pulses during the first 10 minutes of breastfeeding is because they have a good milk production, which, of course, facilitates breastfeeding, or if the bonding between mother and infant is particularly strong is not known.

Maternal Oxytocin Levels During Pregnancy and Breastfeeding May Predict the Duration of Breastfeeding

The mothers' oxytocin levels not only during breastfeeding, but also during pregnancy, seem to predict duration of breastfeeding, as data from several studies suggest that there is an association between high maternal oxytocin levels and a long duration of breastfeeding. Oxytocin levels recorded during pregnancy and breastfeeding were demonstrated to correlate with duration of breastfeeding (Silber et al., 1991), i.e., the higher the oxytocin levels, the longer the period of breastfeeding.

Exclusive Breastfeeding Is Associated With Higher Oxytocin Levels Than Bottle Feeding

Mothers who were exclusively breastfeeding had higher oxytocin levels during breastfeeding than mothers of infants who received supplementation with formula (Uvnäs-Moberg, Widstrom, Werner, et al., 1990). The reason why women with high oxytocin levels breastfeed exclusively more often than those with lower levels is not known. Mothers with high oxytocin levels could, as suggested above, have innately high oxytocin levels, a good milk production, and a good bonding to the baby, which would, of course, make breastfeeding easier.

The high oxytocin levels in exclusively breastfeeding mothers could also be secondary to the more frequent breastfeeding and intense close contact with the baby, which is associated with breastfeeding. Not only breastfeeding, but also close contact and interaction with the babies increase oxytocin levels as will be described below. The finding that basal oxytocin levels decreased 24 hours after weaning suggests that oxytocin levels in breastfeeding is actually associated with increased basal levels of oxytocin (Uvnäs Moberg, Widstrom, Werner, et al., 1990).

Effect of Massage and Infant Cues

Both prolactin and oxytocin are released by the suckling stimulus. The release profile differs and the nervous pathways mediating suckling-related prolactin and oxytocin release are separate; however, as will be discussed below, oxytocin may promote the release of prolactin by effects in the anterior pituitary.

Oxytocin, but not prolactin, can also be released by other types of sensory stimulation. Breast massage in breastfeeding mothers is associated with oxytocin release, although the release profile differs from that seen during suckling, as it is not pulsatile (Cowie, Tindal, & Yokoyama, 1966). In addition, oxytocin release is promoted by skin-to-skin contact with the baby and when the infant massages the mother's breast (Nissen, Lilja, Widstrom, & Uvnäs-Moberg, 1995; Yokoyama et al., 1994).

None of these stimuli are directly associated with milk ejection, as they do not induce the short oxytocin peaks typical of suckling and necessary for milk ejection. Instead, more protracted elevations of oxytocin levels are induced. Still, this type of oxytocin release will influence breastfeeding in a positive way. The increased oxytocin levels will result in increased prolactin secretion from the pituitary and, thereby, increased milk production as described more in detail below. It will also, as discussed in detail in chapter 9, contribute to the relaxation of the

sphincters of the milk ducts, thus facilitating milk ejection. The effect of tactile interaction between mother and infant will be described more in detail in the chapters on skin-to-skin contact.

Maternal oxytocin can also be released by other types of infant cues, e.g., infant crying (McNeilly et al., 1983). Just looking at the infant or even a picture of it may be linked to maternal oxytocin release (Strathearn, Fonagy, Amico, & Montague, 2009). These effects may be due to direct responses to the different sensory cues mentioned above. They may also be secondary and a result of conditioning of the oxytocin release to the infant cues. This would be in analogy with the well-known conditioning of the maternal milk ejection reflex to the sight, sound, smell, or even thought of the baby. All of these different ways of increasing oxytocin levels in connection with breastfeeding should facilitate milk production and milk ejection.

Oxytocin Levels; Trait or State

The reason why women with high oxytocin levels during breastfeeding breastfeed longer than those with low oxytocin levels may either be the consequence of breastfeeding or the reason for long-term breastfeeding (Uvnäs-Moberg, Widstrom, Werner, et al.1990). Intense exposure to skin-to-skin contact and frequent suckling may create high levels of oxytocin in the mothers, *a high oxytocin state*. If the mothers naturally have high oxytocin levels, *a high oxytocin trait*, the high oxytocin levels may facilitate long-term breastfeeding. In fact, high oxytocin levels may represent both a state and a trait.

Relationship Between Oxytocin Levels Obtained on Different Occasions

An interesting feature of oxytocin levels is that mothers seem to have a certain oxytocin level, i.e., the oxytocin levels obtained on different occasions in a single mother are associated. For example, the oxytocin levels in breastfeeding mothers obtained four days after birth correlated significantly with oxytocin levels obtained at four months, even if the rise of oxytocin was much larger on the second occasion (Uvnäs-Moberg, Widstrom, Werner, et al., 1990).

Oxytocin levels obtained in individual mothers during pregnancy and during breastfeeding have also been demonstrated to correlate with each other in two different studies (Feldman, Weller, Zagoory-Sharon, & Levine, A., 2007; Levine, Zagoory-Sharon, Feldman, & Weller, 2007; Silber et al., 1991). It, therefore, seems as if oxytocin levels to a certain extent are a characteristic or a trait of each individual mother.

Are Oxytocin Levels Genetic or Learned?

The reason why some mothers have higher oxytocin levels than others is not known. Some mothers might simply have higher oxytocin levels than others due to genetic factors. Others may have high oxytocin levels as a consequence of positive experiences early in life. It is becoming more and more clear that experiences early in life may influence social interactive skills and stress reactivity for life via epigenetic mechanisms in both positive and negative directions, depending on the type of early interactions the individual is exposed to (Champagne & Meaney, 2001; Szyf, McGowan, & Meaney, 2008). In humans, the experience of early trauma is associated with lower oxytocin levels and higher stress reactivity later in life (Heim et al., 2009; Pierrehumbert et al., 2010) and, therefore, by analogy, positive experiences early in life should be related to higher oxytocin levels later in life.

Role of Estrogen for Prolactin and Oxytocin Release

Basal levels of both prolactin and oxytocin were shown to be higher the first days after birth than later on during breastfeeding. The high prolactin and oxytocin levels observed after birth are due to effects of the high estrogen levels during pregnancy, since estrogen stimulates the production and the release of both prolactin and oxytocin (Amico, Seif, & Robinson, 1981; Freeman et al., 2000). When estrogen levels fall after birth (a consequence of the expulsion of the placenta—an important site of estrogen production during pregnancy), the levels of prolactin and oxytocin also start to fall during the first days postpartum (Uvnäs-Moberg, Widstrom, Werner, et al., 1990). Still, the levels of prolactin and oxytocin remain elevated in the period; therefore, the hormonal mechanisms involved in milk production and milk ejection are active at birth.

Relationship Between Oxytocin and Prolactin Levels

Oxytocin levels correlate with prolactin levels in breastfeeding women (Jonas et al., 2009). Regulation of prolactin release is partly under the control of oxytocin released within the anterior pituitary (Samson et al., 1986). In addition to being released from the posterior pituitary into the circulation, oxytocin is also released into the anterior pituitary in response to suckling. As described in detail in a previous chapter, this release may occur as a consequence of activation of axon reflexes originating from the axons of the magnocellular neurons that project to the posterior pituitary, from a release of oxytocin into the blood vessels that connect the hypothalamus and the anterior pituitary, and from oxytocin-containing nerves that project to the anterior pituitary.

These data implicate that oxytocin has a more important role during breastfeeding than previously thought. It not only stimulates milk ejection, it also increases milk production by stimulating prolactin release. In other words, milk production to a certain extent is regulated by the activity of the oxytocin system. The release of oxytocin is influenced by many different factors, such as stress, closeness, food intake, and perceived trust. The oxytocin system may serve as a hub where inborn propensities interplay with environmental cues to regulate breastfeeding.

Summary

- Both prolactin and oxytocin are released in response to breastfeeding. The suckling-induced prolactin release occurs after a delay of 10-20 minutes and lasts for at least one hour. By contrast, oxytocin is released in short pulses that appear within minutes after onset of suckling. The rise of oxytocin levels lasts only 20-30 minutes.

- Basal and suckling-related prolactin levels decrease during the breastfeeding period, whereas the amount of oxytocin released by suckling increases over time.

- Prolactin is only released by suckling of the nipple, whereas oxytocin can be released by tactile stimulation of the breasts and by visual and auditory cues. In addition, oxytocin release can be triggered by conditioned reflexes.

- The suckling-related prolactin release is associated with the duration of each suckling period, i.e., the longer the period of suckling the more prolactin is released.

- By contrast, the number oxytocin pulses released during the first ten minutes of breastfeeding correlates with the amount of milk ejected, i.e., the more pulses, the larger the milk volume.

- Several oxytocin pulses in the beginning of a breastfeed and high oxytocin levels are predictive of long duration of breastfeeding.

- The amount of oxytocin measured on different occasions correlated strongly, suggesting that a woman has a certain level of oxytocin. No such relationship was demonstrated for prolactin.

- Oxytocin levels correlate with prolactin levels. Oxytocin facilitates prolactin secretion and, therefore, milk production.

Chapter 11

Maternal Behavior: Role of Oxytocin and Sensory Cues

In the previous chapters, the role of oxytocin as a circulating hormone that promotes milk ejection, milk production, and giving of warmth was described. In addition to giving milk to their offspring, mothers take care of and interact with them, and they protect them in many different ways. These effects also involve integrating effects of oxytocin, but are induced in the brain in response to a release of oxytocin from oxytocin-containing nerves in important regulatory areas.

In the following six chapters, different aspects of maternal caring and interactive behaviors, "maternal behavior," will be summarized, together with the effects and responses induced in the offspring. The first two chapters will deal with the different components of maternal behavior and how they are influenced by oxytocin and by visual, auditory, olfactory, and somatosensory (e.g., touch and warmth) cues. In the next two chapters, immediate and long-term effects of skin-to-skin contact in women who have just given birth will be described. The last two chapters will discuss expressions of maternal caring and protective behavior.

Maternal Behavior—How Mammalian Mothers Take Care of Their Newborns

Mammalian females are not only programmed to feed their offspring, they also have innate programs to help them take care of and protect their newborns. These inborn behaviors are often referred to as maternal behavior.

The expression of maternal behavior in mammals varies between species and depends on the environment in which a particular animal species lives and how mature or immature their offspring are at birth.

Grazing animals live in herds and give birth to relatively mature offspring. The newborns can stand up and walk immediately after birth, and they can control their temperature. The offspring are dependent on their mothers, as the mothers provide them with food and protection.

Other mammals give birth to very immature offspring. Such newborns need the mother's closeness and full attention more or less constantly for a period of time after birth to keep them warm and to help them grow and develop. Rats, for example, give rise to immature offspring. In this species, maternal behavior includes not only giving of milk and protection from potential enemies, but also licking and grooming, and keeping the pups warm by lying close to them. By lying close to the offspring, the mother acts as a regulator of their temperature and metabolism, and keeps them calm (Hofer, 1994; Numan, 2006; Numan & Woodside, 2010; Rosenblatt, 1994, 2003).

Recognition, Bonding and Attachment

It is necessary for mother and offspring to stay together after birth in order for the offspring to receive milk, care, and protection. In species that give rise to relatively mature young that can walk by themselves, the mothers rapidly learn to recognize the smell, sound, and looks of their offspring and develop a preference for it. As they become bonded to the offspring and stay close to it, they reject alien offspring and only allow their own offspring to suckle. The bonding is most efficiently established during the first 24 or 48 hours after birth (Kendrick, Da Costa, et al., 1997; Keverne & Kendrick, 1994).

The offspring learn to recognize their mother and develop a preference for her, as they become attached to her. They need to recognize their own mother in order to receive milk and protection from her, since if they approach mothers of other offspring, they will often be rejected (Nowak, Murphy, et al., 1997).

Sensory cues—visual, auditory, and olfactory—play important roles in the formation of recognition and bonds between mothers and infants. The role of olfaction is extremely important in more primitive mammals, e.g., in rodents and sheep, because the mothers learn to identify their infants' specific scents (Kendrick, Guevara-Guzman, et al., 1997). In animals with a more developed neocortex, such as monkeys and apes, the bonding process becomes more complex, and visual cues become of greater importance for recognition between individuals (Broad, Curley, & Keverne, 2006, 2009). As will be described later on, pheromones do play a significant role in the interaction between human mothers and their infants, particularly early in life.

Role of Oxytocin in Maternal Behavior and Bonding

In spite of species' differences in the expression of maternal care, the neuroendocrine organization of maternal behavior may still be very similar. In principle, hormones and nerves interact during pregnancy, birth, and lactation to induce maternal behavior. Oxytocin plays an important role in the brain by integrating the sensory inputs and by coordinating different behaviors into a specific pattern of effects—the maternal behavior—by neuroendocrine actions (Febo, Numan, & Ferris, 2005; Numan, 2006). The medial preoptic area (MPOA) plays an important coordinating role in the expression of maternal behavior.

Maternal Behavior

Experiments performed in animals support the important role of oxytocin for the development of maternal behavior. For example, intracerebroventricular (ICV) administration of oxytocin facilitates the development of maternal behavior in rats and sheep (Kendrick et al., 1987; Keverne & Kendrick, 1992, 1994; Levy et al., 1992; Pedersen, Ascher, Monroe, & Prange, 1982; Pedersen & Prange, 1979). Furthermore, administration of oxytocin antagonists, which block the effects of oxytocin, or a peridural anesthesia, which blocks the release of endogenous oxytocin into the circulation and the brain during labor and the period, inhibit the spontaneous development of maternal behavior in ewes. The maternal behavior can be restored by exogenous oxytocin administered into the brain or by stimulation of endogenous oxytocin released by mechanical vagino-cervical stimulation (Kendrick, Da Costa, et al., 1997; Keverne & Kendrick, 1992, 1994; Kendrick et al., 1986; Kendrick et al., 1991; Keverne & Kendrick, 1994; Levy et al., 1992).

Recognition and Bonding

The establishment of recognition and bonding between the mother and her young is linked to a release of oxytocin in the mother's brain during labor and in response to suckling. Administration of oxytocin into the brain facilitates bonding, and administration of oxytocin antagonists inhibits it. Peridural anesthesia, which blocks afferent nervous pathways in the spinal cord, blocks the development of maternal bonding to the young in the same way as it affects the development of maternal behavior (Kendrick et al., 1986; Kendrick et al., 1991; Keverne & Kendrick, 1994).

In addition, oxytocin increases the sensitivity to odors by effects in the olfactory bulb and learning by actions, e.g., in the hippocampus. In this way, the recognition of the newborn via its odor is facilitated. As oxytocin increases the release/effects of dopamine in the nucleus accumbens (NA), the experience of the newborn will be remembered as pleasurable.

The bonding or attachment process is reciprocal. The newborn's suckling and ingestion of colostrum trigger the development of attachment by inducing a release of oxytocin. The hormone cholecystokinin, released from the small intestine in the gastrointestinal tract, plays an important promoting role in the development of attachment in part by facilitating oxytocin release (Lupoli, et al., 2001; Nowak, Goursaud, et al., 1997; Nowak, Murphy, et al., 1997). The important role of cholecystokinin (CCK) in promoting suckling-related events in both mothers and their offspring will be described in a later chapter.

The closeness or presence of the newborn reduces stress levels in the mother and a reciprocal effect occurs in the offspring. Consequently, separation causes anxiety in both mother and offspring, which is relieved by closeness to the "other." This calming effect contributes to bonding between mother and young, and to the development of attachment between the newborn and its mother. The mechanisms involved in these effects will be discussed in more detail in the next chapter.

Communication and Interaction Between Mothers and Offspring, Role of Oxytocin

Mothers and their young communicate with each other in different ways during the lactation period to attract attention, to stimulate certain behaviors, or simply to bring information to the other individual. Several "sensory languages" are used. Vocal communication, odors and pheromones, tactile stimuli, and even closeness and skin temperature can confer information between mother and baby. Oxytocin plays an important role in the communication between mother and baby, irrespective of the type of communicative "language." Some examples will be given below.

Vocal Communication

In some species, mother and young communicate with sounds to inform each other about how they feel and where they are.

Call for Help

Rat pups that are separated from their mothers produce special distress calls to attract their mothers' attention. The distress calls stop as soon as the mother and the pups have reunited. Administration of oxytocin also stops the distress calls, suggesting that oxytocin may be involved in the anxiolytic or calming effect that closeness brings (Hofer, Brunelli, & Shair, 1993; Shair, Masmela, & Hofer, 1999). Cholecystokinin released from the gastrointestinal tract also plays an important role in calming effects during suckling and closeness in the pups.

Time to Suck and Swallow

When it is time for a sow to give milk to her piglets, she calls for them by emitting grunting sounds. When the piglets are suckling, just before milk ejection occurs, the sows change the frequency of their grunting. As a response to this change, the piglets stop suckling and start swallowing the ejected milk (Algers & Uvnäs-Moberg, 2007). As the change of grunting frequency occurs just as maternal oxytocin levels rise in plasma to induce milk ejection, it is likely that it is mediated by oxytocin released by suckling in areas that regulate the tone of the vocal cords. Oxytocin-containing nerves have been found not only in the larynx, but also in areas of the brain related to both vocalization and hearing, suggesting that adaptations occur to optimize the vocal interaction between mother and her young (Algers & Uvnäs-Moberg, 2007; Kanwal & Rao, 2002).

Odors and Pheromones

The role of olfaction in the communication between individuals is often forgotten, but it plays an important role in the interaction between mothers and offspring of many species. The process of bonding and attachment involves learning and recognition of the other's specific scent, and oxytocin released in the olfactory bulb promotes the process of bonding and attachment.

Time to Suck

Specific substances, released from the Montgomery glands located around the nipples, may attract the attention of newborns, help them find the nipples, and even stimulate suckling behavior. They also promote the process of learning (Coureaud et al., 2010; Doucet, Soussignan, Sagot, & Schaal, 2009). Oxytocin may indirectly contribute to such pheromonal effects by increasing the circulation in the skin overlying the mammary gland, thereby facilitating secretion of the odors (Eriksson, Lundeberg, et al., 1996).

Calming Effect of Mother

Pheromones secreted from the mother influence the behavior of the newborns. When rat pups, which have been separated from their mother, are reunited, they calm down. This effect is, in part, due to olfactory cues emitted from the mother (Hofer, 1994).

Lactating animals, e.g., guinea pigs, exert a profound calming effect on other individuals in their close vicinity (N. Sachser, personal communication, 1998), suggesting that an odor with calming effects is emitted from the lactating females.

Oxytocin Exerts Calming Effects on Neighboring Animals Via a Pheromonal Effect

When oxytocin is administered to a rat, it becomes more socially interactive, calm, less stressed, and less sensitive to pain. Surprisingly, a similar effect pattern is induced in other rats that are in the close vicinity of the animal that received oxytocin. If, however, the nasal mucosa of the recipient animals has been anesthetized, no effects are induced, suggesting that the effects in the recipient animals are mediated by a pheromone secreted from the animal given oxytocin (Agren et al., 1995; Agren, Olsson, et al., 1997). Interestingly, the levels of oxytocin rise in the recipient animals, suggesting that the other effects observed in these animals are mediated by a release of endogenous oxytocin (Uvnäs-Moberg, Bystrova, et al., 2014). In this way, a chain reaction is induced. When oxytocin levels are high in one animal, the neighboring animals will be influenced by pheromones to raise their oxytocin levels, and so on. These types of reactions synchronize behaviors within groups of animals.

Calming Effect of Mother; Role of Oxytocin

The pheromone that induces oxytocin release and oxytocin-linked effects in neighboring animals may be identical to the one ejected from lactating animals, which exerts a similar calming-effect profile. The secretion of this calming substance from lactating animals may be induced or facilitated by oxytocin released in response to the suckling stimulus. Lactating mothers may eject such odors not only to keep their offspring calm and content, but also to "pacify" possible intruders that may threaten the offspring.

Summary

- Mammals have inborn programs for taking care of their offspring. Maternal behaviors consist of feeding, caring for, and protecting their young.

- Environmental sensory cues and oxytocin are important regulators of these innate behaviors. An oxytocin-mediated decrease of anxiety and stimulation of social-interactive behaviors by actions in the amygdala, as well as oxytocin-mediated integration of behavioral effects take place in the MPOA.

- Oxytocin facilitates bonding between mother and newborns, and attachment between newborns and their mothers by increasing the sensitivity to smell in the olfactory bulb, as well as by formation of memories in the hippocampus. Oxytocin-related stimulation of dopaminergic reward mechanisms in the NA and of mechanisms involved in calming and relaxation within the hypothalamus and the brainstem also contribute to the development of bonding and attachment.

- Mother and newborns communicate in several "sensory languages," e.g., by auditory and olfactory signals. Oxytocin facilitates this communication by increasing receptivity to auditory and olfactory signals in the brain, stimulating vocal interaction, and facilitating the release of pheromones.

Chapter 12

Maternal Behavior: Role of Tactile Stimulation and Closeness

As mentioned in the previous chapter, maternal behavior not only consists of feeding and protection of their young, it also involves communication and interaction via other senses, e.g., visual, auditory, olfactory, and tactile cues. In some species in which the offspring are born very immature (precocious), mothers interact by licking their offspring and staying close to them, not only during suckling, but most of the time. In addition to the tactile interaction, warmth plays an important role in this kind of interaction.

During closeness, the boundaries between mother and infant are more or less eradicated. It is, in fact, a continuation of pregnancy, but the umbilical cord is substituted by the close skin-to-skin contact. The effects of closeness are bi-directional, and mother and young influence each other.

Role of Closeness, Tactile Stimulation, and Warmth

Closeness is Active

Closeness between mother and offspring from an external perspective is completely passive, but from an internal perspective, closeness is extremely active. By lying close to the offspring, the mother acts as a regulator of the physiology of her offspring. She regulates temperature, metabolism, growth rate, cardiovascular function, and stress levels. She keeps them calm (Hofer, 1994). The offspring are not in the womb any longer, but the mother transfers warmth and other types of tactile information to them by activation of multiple types of sensory nerves in the skin.

Tactile Stimulation Reduces Stress Levels

In some species, e.g., rats, the mothers lick their offspring as a part of their care. The positive effects induced by maternal tactile interaction have often been studied in the context of stress and the ability of these interactions to reverse stress levels. Extra tactile stimulation of pups can counteract stress reactivity by a decrease in the activity in the hypothalamo-pituitary axis (HPA axis). It may also reverse other negative consequences of exposure to stress, such as decreased growth and development caused by prenatal stress or separation between mother and offspring (Wakshlak & Weinstock, 1990; Levine, Alpert, & Lewis, 1957; Pauk, Kuhn, Field, & Schanberg, 1986; van Oers, de Kloet, Whelan, & Levine, 1998). Licking of the anogenital region of the rat pups is particularly frequent and important in rats. It reduces stress levels and increases growth and development (Fleming et al.,

2002).

Effects of Warmth

The mother does not only give milk to its offspring, it also actively gives warmth to them as a consequence of dilation of blood vessels in the mucosa of the skin on the chest. The mechanisms, including the role of oxytocin, involved in giving of warmth were described in chapters 8 and 9. When the mother stays close to the newborn, the warmth from her skin temperature influences the physiology and behavior of the newborn. The warmer the mother, the more content and relaxed the offspring, and its sensitivity to pain is reduced (Uvnäs-Moberg, Bruzelius, et al., 1993).

Warm teats direct the newborns to the teats to start suckling. This effect may be reinforced by pheromones released from the teats or mammary glands. Oxytocin is, as mentioned above, involved in the increase of skin temperature, as it helps dilate blood vessels in the skin. The increased circulation in teats and mammary glands also promotes the release of maternal pheromones, which will help the newborn find its way and also to feel calm and safe.

The Effects of Closeness are Bi-directional

The consequences of closeness are bidirectional, as the mother is also influenced by close contact with the offspring. In experiments performed on lactating rats, closeness with the offspring (in the absence of suckling) calmed the mothers. The anxiolytic effect, however, only lasts for a few hours after separation from the pups, but is re-instituted after reunion with them (Bonetto et al., 1999; Lonstein, 2005). Also, the presence of the pups increases the maternal chest skin temperature (Erikson, Lindh, et al., 1996)

Long-Term Effects of Sensory Stimulation in the Newborn Period

Closeness between mother and offspring not only induces calm, reduces stress levels, and stimulates growth during the actual period of closeness, repeated exposure to tactile stimuli tends to develop all these variables into more sustained effects. If induced during the first week of life, the effects may become lifelong.

Closeness to Mother Necessary for Normal Development

The detrimental effects of maternal deprivation and the importance of closeness or "skin-to-skin contact" were described by Harry Harlow in the 1950s. He showed that close contact with the mother (and siblings) was necessary for young rhesus monkeys to develop normal interactive behaviors as adults. Rhesus monkeys that were brought up separated from their mothers became not only socially incompetent, they also became extremely anxious and had difficulties handling stress.

To a certain extent, an artificial "surrogate mother" could compensate for deprivation from the real mother. To be brought up with a furry surrogate mother almost normalized the behavior of the monkeys, which was not the case if the surrogate mother was made of steel wire. Monkey babies that were allowed the soft, tactile contact of the furry surrogate mother had almost normalized behavioral and physiological reaction patterns as adults (Harlow, 1959; Harlow & Seay, 1964; Harlow & Zimmermann, 1959; Seay & Harlow, 1965).

Newborns Have a Specific Skin Hunger, Not Only Food Hunger

Harlow's results suggest that in addition to having a hunger for food, newborns also have a hunger for skin. They need contact with something that feels soft and warm in order to feel satisfied and to develop normally. Although Harlow clearly pointed to an important role of the skin in early development, he did not discuss the role of somatosensory nerves originating in the skin as mediators of these effects.

Intense Tactile Stimulation and Closeness in the Newborn Period Increases Social Interaction and Reduces Stress Levels in Adulthood

High and Low Licking Mothers

In rat studies, some strains of rat mothers licked and groomed their newborn pups more than other rat mothers during the first week of life. The rat pups of highly interacting mothers received more tactile stimulation during the first week of life. These rats became more socially interactive, less anxious, and had a better ability to cope with stress as adults. The female rat pups receiving extra sensory stimulation became better mothers, in the sense that they interacted more with their own newborns. The interactive pattern was thus transferred to the next generation, as these pups, when they became mothers, displayed the same highly interactive maternal behavioral pattern as their mothers (Champagne & Meaney, 2001; Champagne, Curley, Keverne, & Bateson, 2007; Champagne & Meaney, 2007).

Epigenetic Programming

These effects were, at least in part, not genetic, since the effects were not expressed if rat pups born to highly interactive mothers were moved to a less interactive mother after birth and they received less tactile interaction. The results of these studies indicate that the stimulation of social interactive skills, the decreased levels of anxiety, and the ability to better cope with stress were instead due to epigenetic programming, i.e., tactile stimuli applied during the first week of life, which may have activated or deactivated certain genes (Cameron et al., 2008; Francis, Champagne, Liu, & Meaney, 1999; Szyf, Weaver, Champagne, Diorio, & Meaney, 2005).

Administration of Extra Sensory Stimulation

Another way to show the important role and effects of sensory stimulation in the newborn period is to supply the newborn with repeated periods of extra sensory stimulation by brushing during the first week of life. By using this technique, an effect pattern that resembles the one induced by high licking mothers in their offspring is induced. For example, blood pressure is decreased in adulthood in rats having received extra sensory stimulation as pups (Holst, Uvnäs-Moberg, & Petersson, 2002). Increased stress levels and retarded growth caused by separation in early life could be restored by extra tactile stimulation (Pauk et al., 1986; van Oers et al., 1998). The amount of dopamine-2 receptors was also increased by extra sensory stimulation (Holst, Uvnäs-Moberg, & Petersson, 2000).

Effect of Handling

Handling of newborn rats, i.e., separation of rat pups from their mothers for various periods of time during the first period of life, has been shown to influence the behavior of the newborns and their mothers in a long-term way. In some experiments, rats exposed to handling as pups have been shown to be calmer and more stress tolerant in adulthood. This paradoxical effect has been attributed to increased maternal interaction when mother and pups are reunited after a period of separation. In other words, these pups are exposed to more sensory stimulation than non-handled rats as compensation for what was lost during the periods of separation. It should be noted that not all studies demonstrated similar results in the physiology and behavior of rats that were exposed to early handling. These data suggest that the long-term effects of early handling are highly influenced by other factors, e.g., epigenetic, genetic, and environmental factors (Eklund, Johansson, Uvnäs-Moberg, & Arborelius, 2009).

Mechanisms Involved in the Effects Induced by Tactile Stimulation and Closeness

The effects induced by closeness in both mother and offspring are to a great extent mediated via activation of sensory nerves originating in the skin. Oxytocin, released into important regulatory areas in the brain from parvocellular neurons originating in the PVN, plays an important role in these effects. Oxytocin also contributes to the effects pattern induced by non-noxious sensory stimulation in a more indirect way by reinforcing the effects of sensory stimulation in the NTS and other areas in the brainstem that are involved in the control of autonomic nervous tone. This is the reason why the anti-stress and growth-promoting effects of oxytocin are so prominent when induced by stimulation of some types of somatosensory nerves, e.g., from the skin.

The animal experimental data, which support the important role of non-noxious stimulation in the control of anxiety levels, pain threshold, stress levels, cardiovascular and gastrointestinal function, as well as the role played by oxytocin in these effects were to a large extent described in earlier chapters. Since these basal mechanisms are of such fundamental importance in understanding the effects caused by closeness and skin-to-skin contact, a summary will be given here.

Nervous Mechanisms Involved in Somatosensory Stimulation and Oxytocin Release

Different Types of Nerve Fibers May Mediate Non-Noxious Information

Touch, stroking, light and strong pressure, and warmth can activate sensory nerve fibers that transmit non-noxious information from the skin. The nerve fibers transmitting these types of sensory information may belong to the group of myelinated fibers or could correspond to C fiber afferents. The latter are, from a phylogenetic perspective, older than the myelinated fibers, and they transmit nerve impulses at a slower pace. In addition, vagal afferents of cutaneous origin may mediate effects from the skin of the chest (Eriksson, Lindh, et al., 1996).

Effects Induced by Non-Noxious Sensory Stimulation

The activity of the HPA axis and some aspects of the sympathetic nervous system are reduced by non-noxious stimulation in anesthetized animals (Araki et al., 1984; Kurosawa et al., 1982; Tsuchiya et al., 1991) and blood pressure is reduced (Kurosawa et al., 1995; Uvnäs-Moberg et al., 1986). The levels of gastrointestinal hormones are influenced as a result of activation of efferent (outgoing) vagal nerve fibers that exert a regulatory effect on the release of these hormones (Uvnäs-Moberg, Lundeberg, et al., 1992; Uvnäs-Moberg et al., 1986). Pain sensitivity is reduced as a response to application of warm temperature on the chest (Uvnäs-Moberg, Bruzelius, et al., 1993).

In conscious rats, stroking of the chest reduces blood pressure, decreases sensitivity to pain, and induces a sedative effect (Agren et al., 1995; Lund et al., 1999; Uvnäs-Moberg, Alster, Lund, et al., 1996). In response to repeated treatments, the pain-relieving effect is reinforced, the levels of gastrointestinal hormones are influenced, and weight gain is promoted (Holst et al., 2005; Lund et al., 2002).

Taken together, these data indicate that mild or non-noxious sensory stimulation exerts anti-stress effects by inhibiting activity in the HPA axis and certain aspects of the sympathetic nervous system. Further, it stimulates the function of the parasympathetic/vagal system and the endocrine system of the gastrointestinal tract, and thereby anabolic metabolism and growth. Calm is also promoted.

Noxious Stimuli Induce an Opposite Effect Pattern

Noxious, painful stimulation, on the other hand, causes an opposite effect pattern characterized by anxiety, aggression, and increased activity in the HPA axis and the sympathetic nervous system, as well as a decrease in the activity of the parasympathetic nervous system, i.e., *a fight or flight response pattern* (Uvnäs-Moberg & Petersson, 2011).

Oxytocinergic Pathways in the Brain

Oxytocin is produced in the SON and PVN of the hypothalamus. Oxytocin is released into the circulation from magnocellular neurons in the SON and PVN, which terminate in the posterior pituitary. Oxytocin, however, is also produced in oxytocinergic nerves that project from the parvocellular neurons in the PVN to many important regulatory areas in the brain, e.g., the amygdala, other areas in the hypothalamus, as well as brainstem areas, such as the LC, the RVLM, the NTS, and the vagal motor nucleus (DMX).

Effects of Oxytocin

Administration of oxytocin results in a multitude of behavioral and physiological effects. It results in decreased anxiety via an effect in the amygdala. It may decrease the activity of the HPA axis by reducing the release of CRF in the PVN. It may decrease cardiovascular function by actions in the LC, RVLM, NTS, DMX, and other areas involved in the control of sympathetic nervous tone. And, it may increase the function of the gastrointestinal tract via actions in the DMX.

Release of Oxytocin in Response to Non-Noxious Stimulation

Oxytocin is released into the circulation and into the brain in response to non-noxious stimulation of sensory nerves originating in the skin (Lund et al., 2002; Stock & Uvnäs-Moberg, 1988; Uvnäs-Moberg, Bruzelius, et al., 1993; Uvnäs Moberg et al., 1993) and in the brain.

Oxytocin is not only released into the circulation from magnocellular neurons in the SON and PVN, but also from parvocellular neurons originating in the PVN, which project to important regulatory areas in the brain.

Similarity Between the Effect Profile Induced by Non-Noxious Sensory Stimulation and Oxytocin

Interestingly, administration of oxytocin induces an effect pattern that resembles that of non-noxious sensory nerve stimulation. As oxytocin is released from parvocellular neurons projecting to many important regulatory areas in the brain in response to non-noxious sensory stimulation, some of the effects observed by non-noxious stimulation could, to a certain extent, be mediated by a release from oxytocinergic neurons. Some effects induced by non-noxious sensory stimulation, e.g., the increased pain threshold, can be blocked by oxytocin antagonists.

Neural Pathways Involved in the Release of Oxytocin

Several types of sensory stimuli stimulate oxytocin release. Nerve impulses from the genitourinary tract (in connection with labor and sex) and from the breast and nipple (in connection with suckling), as well as vagally mediated information from the gastrointestinal tract (and the skin on the chest) result in oxytocin release from both magno- and parvocellular neurons in the SON and PVN. Sucking in the offspring is related to an activation of vagal nerve afferents in the oral mucosa, which project to the oxytocin-producing neurons in the SON and PVN. In a similar way, nerve impulses from somatosensory nerves originating in the skin may trigger oxytocin release from the SON and PVN.

The NTS—An Important Relay Station

Some of these sensory pathways project directly to the NTS (vagal afferents from the gastrointestinal tract, urogenital tract, and oral cavity). Other fibers, e.g., from the urogenital tract, the mammary glands, and the skin, project indirectly to the NTS via the spinal cord.

Connections Between the NTS, SON, and PVN

Within the NTS, neurons are activated which connect the NTS with the SON and PVN. For example, discrete bundles of noradrenergic fibers originating in the NTS innervate magno- and parvocellular neurons in the SON and PVN, which produce oxytocin, vasopressin, or CRF (PVN).

Oxytocinergic Projections Between the PVN and Brainstem Areas

As mentioned above, oxytocin is released from the magnocellular neurons in response to the various types of somatosensory stimuli listed above via the NTS. The oxytocinergic fibers projecting from the PVN to the areas in the brain stem in which the function of the HPA axis and the autonomic nervous system is controlled, e.g., the LC, the RVLM, the NTS, and the DMX, are of particular importance for the functions described in this summary, as this is the site where input from sensory nerves and oxytocinergic nerves converge to potentiate its other effects.

Reflexes Induced From the Gastrointestinal Tract are Facilitated by Oxytocin

When the vagal afferent nerves originating in the gastrointestinal tract are activated, e.g., in response to food intake, local "brainstem" reflexes are induced. Nervous connections between the NTS and the DMX influence the function of the gastrointestinal tract, e.g., motility and secretion.

As mentioned above, afferent vagal nerve activity also releases oxytocin from parvocellular neurons into the DMX and the NTS. Oxytocin released from the parvocellular neurons in these areas plays an important role in the control of gastrointestinal function, as it modulates the function of the local reflex arcs between the NTS and the DMX.

Reflexes Induced From the Skin Are Facilitated by Oxytocin

Just as in the case of activation of afferent vagal nerves from the gastrointestinal tract, activation of the somatosensory nerves emanating in the skin induce actions in a two-step way. First, actions are induced in the brainstem via neural pathways projecting from the NTS to other brainstem centers involved in the control of autonomic nervous tone. As mentioned in the paragraph on the effects induced by non-noxious sensory stimulation, blood pressure is decreased as a result of decreased sympathetic nervous tone and the levels of gastrointestinal hormones are influenced as a result of increased parasympathetic nervous activity.

In a second step, oxytocin, released from parvocellular neurons emanating in the PVN into the brainstem, e.g., the LC, the RVLM, the NTS, and the DMX, modulates the activity of the more local reflex arcs. The oxytocinergic hypothalamic pathway potentiates or facilitates the activity of the brainstem reflexes, and in this way, the anti-stress pattern induced by non-noxious sensory stimulation from the skin is strengthened (Sato et al., 1997).

Simultaneous Increase of Oxytocin Levels and Sensory Stimulation of the Skin Facilitates Anti-stress Effects and Growth

An important consequence of the cooperation between the activity of local brainstem reflexes and oxytocin released from nerves originating in the PVN of the hypothalamus is that the anti-stress-effect pattern induced by non-noxious stimulation of sensory nerves from the skin becomes very prominent.

Oxytocin Stimulates Alpha-2 Adrenoceptors

Repeated administration of oxytocin has been demonstrated to increase the number of alpha-2 adrenoceptors in the noradrenergic neurons in many areas in the brain, such as the amygdala, the hypothalamus, the LC, and the NTS. Since alpha-2 adrenoceptors exert an inhibitory action on the transmission in some noradrenergic neurons, oxytocin will counteract noradrenergic transmission.

Oxytocin Counteracts Noxious and Facilitates Non-Noxious Stimulation

Oxytocin released by non-noxious stimulation into the NTS may act as a gating system by which the transmission of non-noxious information is promoted and noxious information is counteracted. When oxytocin is released in the NTS from parvocellular neurons originating in the PVN, the function of alpha-2 adrenoceptors on the noradrenergic neurons, emanating in the NTS and which project to the CRF neurons in the hypothalamus, is increased. As the alpha-2 adrenoceptors inhibit the release of noradrenaline, the function of the noradrenergic neurons that connect the NTS with the PVN and which stimulate the activity of the CRF neurons in the HPA axis is reduced. Consequently, the function of the HPA axis is decreased, as its function is highly dependent on the intensity of afferent noradrenergic input.

The ability of oxytocin to act like a gating mechanism in the NTS has important functional consequences, since it may indirectly influence "downstream" many other functions in the brain, e.g., stress reactivity, without acting directly on oxytocin receptors in this area.

Oxytocin may facilitate the effect of non-noxious somatosensory stimulation in yet another way. Oxytocin nerve fibers originating in the PVN that project to the NTS have been demonstrated to increase the activity in the afferent nerve fibers that project to the NTS and are linked to oxytocin release. In this way, even more oxytocin is released in response to sensory stimulation, a kind of feed-forward mechanism.

Role of Oxytocin in Effects Induced by Tactile Interaction and Closeness

Role of Oxytocin During Interaction Between Mother and Offspring

As oxytocin is released from the SON and PVN by sensory stimulation, the immediate effects induced during interaction between mother and offspring must involve a release of oxytocin from parvocellular neurons at the sites in the brain discussed above. As discussed in detail above, oxytocin released into the NTS acts by facilitating direct effects caused by sensory stimulation at regulatory centers in the brainstem area, by promoting effects of non-noxious sensory and inhibiting effects of noxious stimulation, and

finally by facilitating the effect of sensory neurons that promote oxytocin release. In this way, oxytocin released in the brain will stimulate social interaction between mother and offspring, and reduce pain and stress levels.

It is highly probable that oxytocin also plays an integrative role in the long-term adaptations caused by non-noxious stimulation. As presented above, some rat mothers interact more with their offspring during the first week of life than others.

Rats born to highly interacting mothers, who therefore received extra sensory stimulation during the first week of life, had more oxytocin receptors in the amygdala, an important area for the control of social interactive behavior and fear as adults, than those who received less stimulation (Francis, Young, Meaney, & Insel, 2002).

The lifelong reduction of the activity in the HPA axis induced by intense maternal tactile interaction of newborn rats has convincingly been demonstrated to be linked to change in the activity of serotonin receptors in the PVN, which regulate the release of CRF. However, these results do not rule out a role for oxytocin in the anti-stress pattern. In this case, oxytocin may act downstream, i.e., in the brainstem, to change sensory information reaching the hypothalamus.

Interestingly, one effect of repeated exposure to oxytocin is an increased amount of alpha-2 adrenoceptors in the NTS and some other areas in the brain. Therefore, the decreased stress reactivity seen in the pups exposed to increased maternal care may also be related to an increased release of oxytocin in response to tactile contact, increased amounts of alpha-2 adrenoceptors, and decreased sensitivity to stress. The decreased stress reactivity could be associated with decreased activity in the noradrenergic fibers innervating aspects of the CRF neurons in the hypothalamus. Indeed, the number of alpha-2 adrenoceptors in the NTS of rats is associated with the amount of tactile stimulation they received during the first week of life, when the levels of CRF are also decreased (Caldji, Diori, & Meaney, 2000).

Administration of Oxytocin to Newborns Causes Life-Long Effects

In further support of a role for oxytocin in these maternally induced adaptations, are findings that show that administration of oxytocin to rat pups during the first week of life stimulates growth, makes the animals more resistant to pain, and reduces cortisol levels and blood pressure in adulthood (Holst et al., 2002; Olausson, Uvnäs-Moberg, & Solstrum, 2003; Petersson & Uvnäs-Moberg, 2008; Sohlstrom, Carlsson, & uvnas-wallensten; Uvnäs-Moberg, Alster, Petersson, Sohlstrom, & Bjorkstrand, 1998).

The integrative effects of oxytocin may become permanent as the effects of the stimuli applied during this early period of life turns into long-lasting effects by epigenetic mechanisms as described above. Oxytocin may act by influencing the production and function of many other transmitter systems.

Summary

- Closeness and other forms of tactile interaction are important aspects of maternal behavior in mammals giving birth to immature offspring.

- Warmth, light pressure, and stroking/licking activate sensory nerves in the skin, which stimulate social interactive behaviors, calm, anti-stress effects and stimulation of growth.

- These effects are immediate consequences of closeness and tactile interaction, but if induced during the first week after birth, they may be transformed into life-long effects. The long-term effects are "dose dependent," i.e., the more sensory stimulation the offspring receives, the stronger the long-term effects become. The long-term effects are induced by epigenetic mechanisms.

- Oxytocin released into the brain from oxytocinergic neurons emanating in the PVN in response to the somatosensory stimulation, takes part in the regulation of the above-mentioned effects.

- The increased social interactive behavior and reduced levels of anxiety are exerted in the amygdala. The long-term effects are linked to an increased production of oxytocin receptors in the amygdala.

- Oxytocin released into brainstem areas induces anti-stress effects by reinforcing direct effects caused by somatosensory nerves in areas involved in the regulation of autonomic nervous tone in the brainstem.

- The long-term anti-stress and growth-promoting effects may involve an oxytocin-induced stimulation of alpha-2 adrenoceptors, which decreases the activity in noradrenergic neurons.

- Oxytocin may also stimulate the function of other transmitter systems by increasing the production of transmitters or the function of receptors in many other signaling systems.

Table 12.1. Neurogenic Pathways Involved in Oxytocin Release and Effects in Response to Closeness

Neurogenic Pathways	Effects in Response to Closeness
Myelinated sensory nerve fibers or unmyelinated C fiber afferents in skin project to or connect with the NTS when stimulated by touch, warmth, stroking, and pressure	Mediate effects of non-noxious (pleasant) stimulation
Nerve fibers from NTS connect with brainstem areas involved in control of the sympathetic and the parasympathetic nervous system	Influence the function of the gastrointestinal tract and some aspects of cardiovascular function
Nerve fibers from NTS connect with SON and PVN	Cause release of oxytocin from magno- and parvocellular neurons
Oxytocinergic fibers originating in PVN project to brainstem areas involved in control of the sympathetic and parasympathetic nervous systems	Decrease function of stress axis and sympathetic nervous system; increase function of parasympathetic nervous system
Oxytocin released from parvocellular neurons in the NTS	Facilitates direct effects induced by non-noxious stimuli in brainstem
Oxytocin released from parvocellular neurons in the NTS	Increase activity of non-noxious sensory fibers projecting to the NTS from, e.g., the skin; increased release of oxytocin
Oxytocin released from parvocellular neurons in the NTS	Increase activity of alpha-2 adrenoceptors; decrease function of noradrenergic neurons in PVN; decrease function of HPA axis

Chapter 13

Skin-to-Skin Contact Between Mother and Infant Postpartum: Immediate Effects

In the two previous chapters, different aspects of maternal behavior and how hormones and different types of sensory cues take part in the control of these behaviors were described. Closeness, giving of warmth, and tactile stimulation are important aspects of maternal behavior, particularly in species in which the newborns are born immature.

In this chapter, we will highlight the effects of skin-to-skin contact, i.e., effects of somatosensory stimulation—touch, stroking, light pressure, and warmth, during the first hours postpartum in women and their newborns. Both behavioral and physiological adaptations are induced in both the mother and the newborn, and oxytocin plays an important regulatory role in these innate and basic expressions of a human "maternal behavior and mother/infant interaction"

as shown in Figure 13.1.

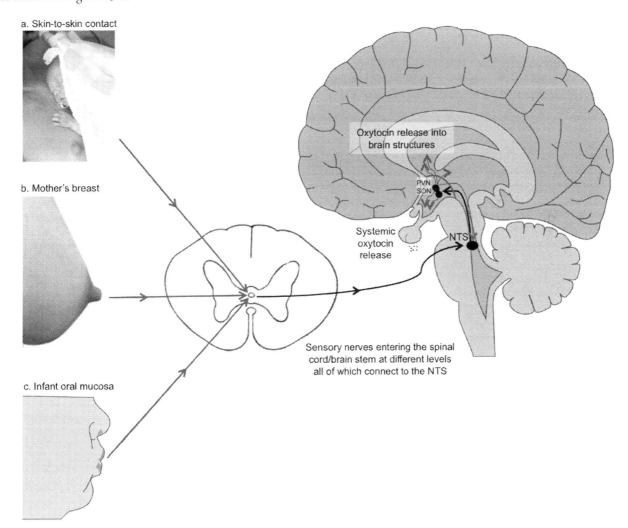

Figure 13.1. Mother and Baby, Suckling and Skin-to-Skin Contact, Connections with the Brain

Source: Uvnäs-Moberg & Prime, 2013. Reprinted with permission.

The First Meeting of Mother and Infant

From the beginning of the existence of the human species, human mothers, perhaps after a brief period of inspection, have brought their newborns to their chest to hold, breastfeed, and protect them after birth. When the mother holds her newborn in skin-to-skin contact, several maternal caring and protective behaviors and some adaptive physiological reactions are automatically induced. Corresponding behavioral changes are induced in the newborn baby, which approaches the mother not only to receive food, but also care and support. Nature facilitates the first meeting between mother and newborn by making it a pleasurable experience. For the mother, it is a joyful experience, and the stress of being born is reduced in both mother and infant. In this way, the bonding between mother and infant starts to develop immediately after birth.

This early close contact between mother and infant was not possible any longer when births were moved to hospitals, as mothers and infants were separated from each other after birth. A renewed insight as to the importance of closeness between mother and infant immediately after birth has emerged based on the pioneering studies by Klaus and Kennel. Their studies showed that early skin-to-skin contact between mother and infant promoted future mother and infant interaction, not only immediately after birth, but also in a long-term perspective.

Clinical Studies

A number of clinical studies have been performed in order to extend the knowledge regarding various aspects of the effect of skin-to-skin contact between mothers and their newborns. Both behavioral observations and physiological measurements were obtained in both mothers and their newborns immediately after birth. In two of the studies (2 and 6), data was also collected at a later time point. The immediate effects of skin-to-skin contact after birth will be presented in this chapter. The more long-term effects will be presented and discussed in the next chapter.

1. Twenty-one newborn infants were placed on their mothers' chests immediately after birth and the interaction between mothers and infants was videotaped for a 120-minute period. Detailed observations of mothers' and infants' behaviors were recorded from the videotapes. Some of the infants were subjected to gastric suction, and the effect of this procedure was studied and recorded (Widstrom et al., 1987).

2. Fifty mother-infant dyads were randomized to either skin-to-skin contact alone or to skin-to-skin contact in addition to suckling of the breast immediately after birth. Four days after birth, the mothers were observed during a breastfeeding session and their interaction with their children was recorded. Milk production was measured and blood samples were analyzed for prolactin and gastrin before and after a breastfeed. The mothers were asked to describe how anxious they were and how close they felt to their children. In addition, the mothers were asked to fill in a diary regarding the amount of time they spent with their infants four days after birth. At this time, the infants were kept in a nursery in the maternity ward, and the mothers fetched them when they were supposed to breastfeed or just when they wanted to be with them (Widström et al., 1990).

3. Right after birth, 44 infants were either placed in skin-to-skin contact with the mother or in a cot and thereafter in skin-to-skin contact with the mother. The newborns' cries were recorded by a tape recorder for 90 minutes after birth (Christensson, Cabrera, Christensson, Uvnäs-Moberg, & Winberg, 1995).

4. Eighteen healthy women were allowed skin-to-skin contact after birth. Ten blood samples were collected at 15-minute intervals. Oxytocin levels were measured with RIA (Nissen, Lilja, Widstrom, et al., 1995).

5. The behavior of 28 mother-infant dyads were video recorded during a two-hour period of skin-to-skin contact after birth. A detailed study of the infants' hand movements and sucking activity was performed based on the video recordings. Ten of the mothers had not received any analgesia during labor, whereas 18 mothers had received one or two types of analgesia in connection with labor. Ten blood samples were collected at 15-minute intervals for a two-hour period after birth. Plasma levels of oxytocin were analyzed by RIA. Finally, the amount of hand massage and suckling were related to oxytocin levels (Matthiesen, Ransjo-Arvidson, Nissen, & Uvnäs-Moberg, 2001a).

6. In the St. Petersburg study, 176 mother-infant dyads were randomized to either have skin-to-skin contact with their infants (group 1), to hold their dressed infants (group 2), or to be separated from their infants, who were placed in a cot in a nursery (groups 3 and 4). Half of the group of infants that were separated immediately after birth were reunited with their mothers two hours after birth and were allowed rooming in at the maternity ward, whereas the others were placed in a nursery at the maternity ward. The mothers who had skin-to-skin contact or who held their dressed children immediately after birth were allowed rooming-in at the maternity ward. These infants were allowed to breastfeed if they wanted to. Maternal breast temperature and the infants' axillar, scapular, thigh, and foot skin temperatures were recorded at 15-minute intervals from 30 minutes until two

hours after birth. The skin temperatures recorded in the different treatment groups were compared.

When the children were one year old, behavioral observations were performed on both mother and infant. The interaction between mothers and infants were studied in two different situations, during free play, i.e., the mothers and children played with whatever they wanted, or during a structured play, when the mothers and infants played after receiving certain instructions. Both interactions were recorded on videotapes, and the tapes were analyzed by psychologists according to a standardized schedule (the PCERA). According to this method, certain aspects of the interaction between mother and infant and the behavior of mothers and infants were studied (Bystrova et al., 2009; Bystrova, Matthiesen, Vorontsov, et al., 2007; Bystrova et al., 2003).

7. Forty-two infants born by Cesarean section were randomized to have skin-to-skin contact with either their mothers or fathers for a 25-minute period after birth. The interaction between parents and their infants during the first two hours after birth was observed and recorded on videotape, allowing recording of sounds. Detailed observations of motor behavior, tactile interaction, and vocal communication were performed from the video recordings. Differences between mothers and fathers, and between boys and girls were noted. The amount of oxytocin the mothers had received postpartum was recorded. Seventeen blood samples were collected in five- or 15-minute intervals in both mothers and fathers during the 90-minute period, and oxytocin levels were analyzed by RIA. Behavior and oxytocin levels in mothers and fathers who had skin-to-skin contact were compared with those who hadn't. The influence of infusion of exogenous oxytocin on endogenous oxytocin levels was explored (Velandia, Matthiesen, Uvnäs-Moberg, & Nissen, 2010; Velandia, Uvnäs-Moberg, & Nissen, 2011).

Main Results

- Newborn babies perform a spontaneous breast-seeking behavior (Widström et al., 1987).

- The maternal interaction with the newborn increases during skin-to-skin contact and the vocal interaction between mother and infant becomes more synchronized (Velandia et al., 2010).

- Maternal oxytocin levels increase in response to skin-to-skin contact with the newborn (Nissen, Lilja, Widström, et al., 1995).

- Infants' breast massage stimulates maternal oxytocin release (Matthiesen et al., 2001a).

- Maternal breast skin temperature starts to pulse when mother and infant are in skin-to-skin or close contact (Bystrova, Matthiesen, Vorontsov, et al., 2007).

- The infant's skin temperature, in particular at peripheral sites, such as the feet, increase during skin-to-skin contact (Bystrova et al., 2003).

- Maternal and infant skin-to-skin contact synchronizes (Bystrova et al., 2003).

- Newborn babies cry less if placed in skin-to-skin contact (Christensson et al., 1995).

Interactive Behaviors

Infants in Skin-to-Skin Contact Express an Approach and Breastfeeding Behavior

When the newborn infant was placed in skin-to-skin contact on the mother's chest immediately after birth and the mother was told not to interfere, the infant displayed a very regular, spontaneous breast-seeking behavior. The infant was lying on the mother's chest without moving, and then the activity increased gradually. The infants tried to move towards the breast by crawling and pushing with their feet. They put their hands to their mouth and from there to the nipple. They performed rooting movements and massaged their mothers' breasts with their hands, very much like kittens do before suckling. Finally, the infants managed to move up to the breast by pushing with their feet and lifting their heads, then reaching for and attaching to the nipple. The infants started to breastfeed within approximately 60 minutes (Widstrom et al., 1987). The hand movements and the sucking was coordinated in such a way that the massage-like hand movements stopped when the infants were sucking, but reappeared when they stopped sucking (Matthiesen et al., 2001a). After breastfeeding, the infants fell asleep.

Mammalian Heritage

The approach or breast-seeking behavior described above is not an entirely normal sequence of events, since unless instructed not to interfere, most mothers will spontaneously reach for, touch, and hold their infants during these first moments. Still, any behavior that occurs during the period immediately after birth is of particular interest, since any behaviors or reactions that occur during this period must be innate and not learned, as this is the first time the mother and infant have met. Therefore, the infant's active inborn breast-seeking behavior may represent an important mammalian heritage, which in ancient times and under some circumstances, e.g., if the mothers were extremely exhausted, might have been lifesaving.

Skin-to-Skin Contact Stimulates Vocal and Tactile Interaction Between Parents and Infants

When infants born by Cesarean section were put in skin-to-skin contact immediately after birth with either their father or mother, the parents touched, looked at, and smiled more at their infants in comparison to when they were not in skin-to-skin contact (Velandia et al., 2010). The parents increased their vocal interaction by soliciting sounds and verbal communication compared to when they were not in skin-to-skin contact with their infant. Parents and infants synchronized or mirrored each others' vocalizations during skin-to-skin contact (Velandia et al., 2010).

Sex Differences

Some sex differences were observed. Mothers touched their infants more than fathers, and they used more finger-tipping touch than fathers when they touched their infants. Mothers touched their newborn boys more than their newborn girls. Fathers talked more to their newborn boys than to their newborn girls (Velandia et al., 2011). These data suggest, but, of course, do not prove, that mothers and fathers may have an innate preference for the other sex!

Maternal Oxytocin Release Postpartum

Maternal oxytocin levels are increased during the first hour after birth (Nissen, Lilja, Widstrom, et al., 1995). The rise coincides with expulsion of the placenta and may represent an inborn release of oxytocin aimed at causing contractions of the uterus to deliver the placenta. Suckling also plays an important role (Uvnäs-Moberg & Prime, 2013).

It is also a consequence of the close contact between mother and infant. Maternal oxytocin levels were raised when the infants were sucking or massaging the mothers' breasts, and also by the effects of the skin-to-skin contact itself during the first hours postpartum. When maternal oxytocin levels were related to the observations of mother-infant interaction from the video recordings, it was found that oxytocin levels rose when the infants were massaging the breasts of the mothers, in addition to when they were sucking the breasts. Periods of increased hand massage or sucking were both accompanied by higher oxytocin levels (Matthiesen et al., 2001a). These data are supported by the findings showing that breast massage is associated with oxytocin release in breastfeeding women (Yukoyama et al., 1994).

Increased Sensitivity to Touch, An Effect of Oxytocin Released During Birth?

The release of oxytocin in the period may be facilitated by an increase in tactile sensitivity of the areola and skin of the breast around birth (Robinson & Short, 1977). It is tempting to suggest that this increased sensitivity is, in fact, due to the high amounts of oxytocin being released during birth. As has been described in the previous chapters, oxytocin released from oxytocin-producing neurons projecting to the nucleus tractus solitarius (NTS) facilitates the transmission in the incoming sensory nerve fibers involved in oxytocin release. As will be discussed in greater detail in the chapter on Cesarean section, oxytocin release in response to the infant's hand massage and suckling is practically absent in mothers having given birth via an elective Cesarean section. The effect was, however, restored in those mothers who had received infusions of exogenous oxytocin (Velandia, Uvnäs-Moberg, & Nissen, 2014a).

Oxytocin Also Released by Other Sensory Cues

Maternal oxytocin is not only released by the infant's sucking, hand massage, and warmth during skin-to-skin contact, but also by visual, auditory, and olfactory cues. Indeed, oxytocin has been demonstrated to be released in response to an infant's crying or other expressions of being needed (McNeilly et al., 1983). The activity in areas of the brain which are rich in oxytocin receptors and are associated with the brain's reward system are activated when mothers viewed pictures of their infants (Bartels & Zeki, 2004; Strathearn et al., 2009). In fact, the rise in circulating oxytocin levels is associated with the oxytocin-induced activation of areas in the brain linked to the reward system. It is also well known that maternal oxytocin release can develop into a conditioned reflex, and after a while, not only the sight, sound, and smell of the baby can trigger maternal oxytocin release and milk ejection, but also the thought of the baby.

Maternal Skin Temperature

Maternal breast skin temperature increased in mothers who were close to their infants after birth. Maternal breast skin temperature displayed different patterns depending on how close they were to their children. The breast skin temperature of mothers having their infants close to them, particularly if they had them in skin-to-skin contact, started to pulse. In contrast, the temperature curve of the mothers of infants that stayed in the nursery was absolutely flat (Bystrova, Matthiesen, Vorontsov, et al., 2007).

As described in previous chapters, mothers give warmth to their infants as the breast and chest temperatures rise, particularly if this is associated with a pulsative pattern. The warmth gives rise to many positive effects. As the infants like warmth, they will move towards it. The warm temperature is perceived as pleasant and relaxes the infant.

Infant Temperature

Newborns' skin temperatures normally rise after birth. This rise is reinforced if the children are in skin-to-skin contact with their mothers (Christensson et al., 1992).

In the St. Petersburg study, the skin temperature increased the most in infants in skin-to-skin contact with their mothers. There was a moderate increase in the foot temperature of the infants close to their mothers, but dressed in clothes. In contrast, the foot temperature of the infants in the nursery decreased during the two hours after birth.

The rise in skin temperature was most clearly expressed in the infants' feet, and this rise amounted to several degrees Celsius during the first two hours after birth. The temperature of the skin in the axilla, the back, and the thigh showed a similar, but less clear temperature pattern. These data show that it is not just closeness, but skin-to-skin contact per se, which is the best trigger for the rise of the infant's skin temperature (Bystrova et al., 2003).

It took two days for the skin temperature of infants that were separated from their mother to reach the same skin temperature as the infants that had been allowed skin-to-skin after birth (Bystrova et al., 2003).

Association Between Maternal and Infant Temperature

The maternal temperature was strongly related to the infant's temperature (Bystrova, Matthiesen, Vorontsov, et al., 2007; Bystrova et al., 2003). The higher the maternal skin temperature, the higher the infant's skin temperature was.

The synchronization of maternal and infant skin temperature may be interpreted from an evolutionary, physiological, and psychological point of view. The warmer the mother is, the more energy she can afford to give to the infant. When the infant receives warmth, it relaxes and physiological systems related to growth are activated.

The Language of Temperature

The results from the St. Petersburg study show that the mother and infant interact and communicate with each other not only by visual, auditory, olfactory, and tactile stimuli, but also by the language of skin temperature. In a sense, this synchronization of maternal and infant temperature can be regarded as a primitive kind of mirroring.

Infants in Skin-to-Skin Contact Cry Less

Infants placed in skin-to-skin contact during the first hours after birth displayed very little crying in comparison to infants put in a cot. Infants that were first placed in a cot, but then reunited with their mothers by being placed in skin-to-skin contact reduced their crying (Christensson et al., 1995).

The crying of the separated infants, e.g., after birth, has been suggested to be a human representation of the distress calls seen in mammalian young when separated from their mothers, which is relieved upon reunion with the mother (Christensson et al., 1995).

Other Expressions of Anti-stress Effects in Response to Skin-to-Skin Contact After Birth

As will be described below, labor is an extremely stressful event for both mother and infant. Nature has created a way by which the stress reaction caused by labor is dampened. A series of studies by Bergman and collaborators has demonstrated how the cardiac reactivity becomes more regular in infants receiving skin-to-skin after birth and how their chance of survival increases (Bergman, 2005; Bergman, Linley, & Fawcus, 2004; Moore, Anderson, Bergman, & Dowswell, 2012). Also, cortisol levels decrease in response to skin-to-skin contact after birth as an expression of decreased activity in the HPA axis (Takahashi, Tamakoshi, Matsushima, & Kawabe, 2011).

When premature infants are placed in skin-to-skin contact with their mothers, their basal levels of CCK decrease, and at the same time, the rise of CCK in response to bolus feeding increases (Tornhage, Serenius, Uvnäs-Moberg, & Lindberg, 1998). In this way, the premature infant's digestive function and use of energy will be optimized.

Approach, Interaction, Anti-stress, and Growth in Response to Skin-to-Skin Contact Represents Different Kinds of Oxytocin-Mediated Effects

All the different effects caused by skin-to-skin contact in mothers and their infants to some extent involve oxytocinergic mechanisms. As described in the previous chapter, oxytocin is released into the maternal circulation in response to skin-to-skin contact. At the same time, oxytocin is released into the brain. Different oxytocinergic pathways are involved in the different effects described. In real life, the effects described as separate entities above, do, in fact, occur at the same time and could therefore be induced in different brain areas simultaneously in response to activation of the oxytocin system.

Oxytocin release induced by somatosensory stimulation, i.e., warmth, touch, stroking, and light pressure, is not always revealed by elevated circulating oxytocin levels. In response to this kind of stimulation, some of the oxytocinergic pathways in the brain are preferentially activated. Whether oxytocin levels are increased in the circulation of the newborn infants in response to skin-to-skin contact is not known. It would not be possible for practical and ethical reasons to collect several blood samples from a newborn infant. However, the finding of elevated levels of oxytocin after vaginal birth, as well as effect profiles induced by skin to skin, strongly suggest that oxytocin is released in both mother and infant during birth and in response to skin-to-skin contact postpartum. This is why they synchronize and mirror each others' reactions, both regarding social interaction, e.g., vocal interaction, and also the anti-stress effects, e.g., skin temperature.

Oxytocin Contributes to Increased Maternal Breast Skin Temperature

As described above, maternal breast skin temperature increased when the mother was in skin-to-skin contact or very close to the infant (Bystrova, Matthiesen, Vorontsov, et al., 2007). The flushing of skin of the chest is due to two different effects of oxytocin. Oxytocin released into the circulation dilates the blood vessels in the skin of the chest via activation of oxytocin receptors in the muscles surrounding the blood vessels. In addition, the effect is caused by a decrease of sympathetic nervous activity, due to oxytocin being released in areas involved in the regulation of the autonomic nervous system, in combination with activation of local neurogenic effects in the chest area.

Oxytocin and Approach or Breast-Seeking Behavior

As described above, infants express a breast-seeking behavior when put skin-to-skin after birth. Oxytocin release triggered by the skin-to-skin contact most likely facilitates the spontaneous approach behavior, as oxytocin has been demonstrated to stimulate several types of social approach. It is also possible that pheromones, small air-born substances that influence the receiver by actions in the brain, are released from the glands and blood vessels on the nipple and areola when the blood vessels dilate in response to skin-to-skin contact. Such substances attract the infant to the breast and stimulate the approach and breast-seeking behavior (Varendi, Porter, & Winberg, 1994). In addition, pheromones and other odors may help the infant learn to recognize the mother's smell outside the womb and contribute to the development of attachment to the mother (Winberg, 2005).

Oxytocin Released in, e.g., the Amygdala Increases Tactile and Vocal Interaction

As described in the previous chapters, oxytocin plays an important role in regulation of maternal interactions with their offspring. The high hormone levels during pregnancy prepare the mother for motherhood. Elevated levels of oxytocin released into the brain in connection with labor triggers maternal behavior and stimulates the process of bonding, effects which involve activation of parvocellular oxytocin-producing neurons originating in the PVN (Kendrick et al., 1986; Keverne & Kendrick, 1994).

By analogy, the observed release of oxytocin into the circulation in the mothers after birth is probably linked to a parallel increase of oxytocin levels in the brain, which facilitates maternal caring behaviors and bonding. The increased tactile and vocal interaction between mothers and their newborn infants is likely to reflect one aspect of such an oxytocin-mediated maternal behavior. This assumption is supported by the fact that administration of oxytocin to humans does increase social interaction and reduce anxiety as described in detail in chapter 5.

Increased Skin Temperature in the Infant

When sensory nerves in the infant's skin are activated by touch, light pressure, stroking, and warm temperature, the activity of the sympathetic nervous system is decreased. The blood vessels in the skin dilate, and since more blood is transported in the vessels, the skin gets warmer. The effect is more pronounced in peripheral parts of the body, such as the feet, since the basal sympathetic tone is stronger in these areas.

The decreased activity in the sympathetic nervous system caused by skin-to-skin contact is exerted in the area in the brainstem, where autonomic nervous tone is controlled, e.g., the NTS. The effect is induced in two steps. First, activation of sensory nerves in the skin decreases the sympathetic tone by a direct action in the NTS and adjacent areas involved in the control of sympathetic nervous tone. Second, oxytocin released from neurons that project from the PVN to the NTS reinforce the decrease of sympathetic nerve activity caused by the direct action.

Increased Skin Temperature, Part of Generalized Pattern of Anti-stress and Growth-Promoting Effects

Sensory stimulation of the breast by touch and warmth reduces sympathetic tone and facilitates the milk ejection reflex and the stress-reducing effects of breastfeeding. The mechanisms behind the effects of skin-to-skin contact in both mothers and infants are from a mechanistic view very similar. Sensory stimulation induced by touch, warmth, and light pressure from the entire body influence the activity in the autonomic nervous system. It reduces the activity in the HPA axis, decreases sympathetic tone, and increases parasympathetic tone. Central nervous mechanisms contributing to stress and arousal are blocked, whereas systems related to restoration and growth are activated by a release of growth factors. Oxytocin plays an important role in orchestrating these effects. From a physiological perspective, skin-to-skin contact decreases the activity in the fight-flight system and increases the activity in the calm and connection system (Uvnäs-Moberg et al., 2005).

Skin-to-Skin Contact Counteracts the Stress of Being Born

During normal labor, the infant is exposed to enormous stress, in part caused by uterine contractions. Consequently, stress levels are high when the baby is born. The levels of NA and cortisol are higher after birth in infants born by vaginal delivery than in those born by Cesarean section. The high levels of noradrenalineand adrenaline are important components of an acute stress reaction. The elevated levels of cortisol contribute to the maturation of many physiological functions, e.g., lung function in the infant (Lagercrantz & Slotkin, 1986).

Even if the infant profits from the high stress levels in

connection with birth, a longstanding stress reaction may delay further development and growth. The original and natural way to counteract the stress of being born may be skin-to-skin contact with the mother. The increased skin temperature (particularly in the feet of the infants) in connection with skin-to-skin contact suggests that the infants' sympathetic nervous tone is decreased. Also, the regularization of pulse rate indicates that sympathetic nervous tone is decreased. The lower levels of cortisol show that the activity of the HPA axis is reduced. The decreased crying indicates that pain and anxiety is relieved.

After labor, maternal stress levels are likely relieved in a corresponding way.

Summary

Skin-to-skin contact between mother and infant is associated with behavioral and physiological effects in both mothers and infants:

- The newborn infant performs a spontaneous breast-seeking behavior.

- Mothers and infants interact more and their vocal communication is more synchronized.

- Maternal oxytocin levels are increased in response to the infant's suckling and hand massage.

- Maternal breast temperature increases and pulses.

- The infant's skin temperature increases.

- Maternal and infant skin temperature are synchronized.

- In addition to the rise of skin temperature, other anti-stress effects, such as lowering of cortisol levels and pulse rate, occur in the infant.

- The skin-to-skin contact calms the infant, as it cries less.

- The rise of oxytocin levels during birth sensitizes the skin to non-noxious stimuli, such as touch, stroking, and warmth.

All of the above effects are promoted by oxytocin released in response to sensory stimulation of the skin in both mothers and infants. Effects of oxytocin are exerted via the circulation in the mother and via oxytocinergic pathways in the brain, which project to different regulatory centers in the brain in both mothers and infants.

Chapter 14

Skin-to-Skin Contact Between Mother and Infant Postpartum: Long-Term Effects

In the former chapter, the immediate effects induced by skin-to-skin contact immediately after birth were described and discussed. The immediate effects induced by skin-to-skin contact after birth may be converted into long-term effects, which will be described in this chapter.

The Concept of the Early Sensitive Period in Humans

Some studies demonstrate that skin-to-skin contact immediately after birth may induce not only acute, but also long-lasting positive effects. This period has been named the early sensitive period by Klaus and Kennel, who observed that even a very short period of skin-to-skin contact between mother and infant after birth increased the likelihood of long-term breastfeeding and a better relationship between mothers and infants. Several studies show that both mothers and babies smile and communicate more with each other three months later if they are allowed skin-to-skin contact after birth (De Chateau & Wiberg, 1977a, 1977b, 1984; Kennell, Trause, & Klaus, 1975; Klaus et al., 1972; Wiberg, Humble, & de Chateau, 1989).

Clinical Studies

In two of the clinical studies described in the previous chapter in which the effects of extra stimulation of the breast or skin-to-skin contact after birth were investigated, observations were also performed later, at four days after birth or at one year. The experiments were described in the previous chapter.

Extra Stimulation of the Breast After Birth Increases Maternal Interaction and Bonding with the Infant Four Days Later

In the study in which the mother-infant dyads were allowed either skin-to-skin contact only (the control group) or skin-to-skin contact and breastfeeding (the case group) immediately after birth, some behavioral differences emerged at day four, even though most of the infants allowed to suckle after birth failed to do so. Instead of suckling, the infants touched and licked the nipple. In this way, the mothers in the case group received more breast stimulation than the mothers in the control group (Widstrom et al., 1990).

Increased Interaction

When the mothers were observed during a breastfeed at day four, the mothers who had received extra sensory stimulation in connection of the breast after birth were more interactive during a breastfeeding session four days later. They talked more with their infants and smiled more at them than did the mothers in the control group (Widstrom et al., 1990).

Increased Bonding

At the time the study was performed, the infants were routinely placed in a nursery. The mothers having received extra sensory stimulation of the breast after birth spent significantly more time with their infants during the four-day stay at the maternity ward, i.e., they fetched them more often from the nursery.

The increased interaction between mother and infant during the breastfeeding session, along with the increased wish or need to be with the infant, suggests that extra sensory stimulation received by the infant's suckling or attempts at suckling in the postnatal period increased the bonding between the mother and the infant (Widstrom et al., 1990).

Extra Stimulation of the Breast After Birth Decreases Maternal Gastrin Levels Four Days Later

Both gastrin and prolactin levels were measured before and after suckling four days after birth in the mothers who had been exposed to just skin-to-skin contact or to both skin-to-skin contact and suckling (licking of the breast) immediately after birth.

Prolactin levels did not differ between the groups, but the levels of the gastrointestinal hormone gastrin were decreased in connection with a breastfeed four days after birth in the group of women who had had both skin-to-skin contact and suckling after birth. The lowered gastrin levels suggest that vagal nerve activity had been enhanced by the short period of nipple touching postpartum to influence the activity of the endocrine system of the gastrointestinal tract (Widstrom et al., 1990).

Association Between the Duration of Time Spent With the Infants and Low Gastrin Levels

There was an association between gastrin levels and the amount of time the mothers spent with their infants during the stay in the maternity ward. The more time the mothers spent with their children, the lower their gastrin levels were, indicating a link between low gastrin levels and maternal bonding to the infant (Widstrom et al., 1990). The association between low gastrin levels and the time spent with the infants may be due to an effect on both these variables induced during the early sensitive period after birth or it could be secondary to the more frequent interaction between mothers and infants.

Skin-to-Skin Contact After Birth Increases Maternal Interaction and Bonding with the Infant a Year Later

In the study performed by Bystrova and collaborators in which mother-infant interaction was studied one year after birth, the quality of the interaction differed between mothers and infants who had been exposed to the different treatments immediately after birth. The mothers and infants allowed to have skin-to-skin contact after birth interacted better with each other and in a more intuitive and sensitive way according to the PCERA scale one year later than did the mother-infant dyads of the other groups. Second best were the mothers and infants in the group in which the infants were held by their mother, but dressed in clothes. The nursery group, i.e., mothers and infants who were separated from each other in the labor and maternity wards, did not do as well as the other groups (Bystrova et al., 2009).

Skin-to-Skin Contact After Birth Increases the Infant's Ability to Handle Stress One Year Later

When the infants' abilities to regulate stress were compared between the groups, it followed the same pattern as the interaction between mother and infant. Infants having had skin-to-skin contact after birth were better at handling stress than those having been close to their mothers, but with clothes on. The infants separated from their mothers after birth did not do as well as the infants that had been close to their mothers after birth (Bystrova et al., 2009).

Role of Sensory Stimulation in the Development of Social Interaction and Ability to Handle Stress

The mothers and infants that were close, but the infants were dressed, did not do as well according to the PCERA scores as to interaction and handling of stress than did mothers and infants belonging to the skin-to-skin group. If the mother-infant dyads in the dressed group were separated into those that were suckled or not, a difference emerged. In the dyads in which the infants had been suckled, the results were as good as in the skin-to-skin group. This means that the extra sensory stimulation received by suckling compensated for the loss of skin-to-skin contact caused by the clothes. On the other hand, there was no difference in the skin-to-skin group in the dyads who suckled and those who did not, suggesting that the sensory stimulation caused by skin-to-skin contact in the immediate period is sufficient to trigger the long-term effects on social interaction and stress reactivity (Bystrova et al., 2009).

The Early Sensitive Period

The crucial importance of skin-to-skin contact immediately after birth was demonstrated by the finding that a two-hour separation period immediately after birth inhibited the development of positive effects on social interaction and stress buffering. The mother-infant dyads reunited after a two-hour separation period after birth, behaved like those that were separated not only in the labor ward, but also during the four-day stay at the maternity ward. These results point to a particular role of skin-to-skin contact during the first two hours after birth, "the early sensitive period." More surprisingly, the group in which the babies wore clothes differed from the skin-to-skin group, suggesting that clothes act like an insulator from real skin-to-skin contact (Bystrova et al., 2009).

Long-Term Increase in Social Interaction, Ability to Handle Stress, and Facilitated Digestion as a Result of Sensory Stimulation After Birth—A Link to Oxytocin?

Facilitated Interaction Between Mother and Child

The results of the two studies described above demonstrate the interaction between mother and infant is strengthened at four days (increased interaction with the child during breastfeeding and increased bonding as the mother spent more time with the infant otherwise placed in a nursery) and at one year (increased and more intuitive and sensitive interaction between mother and infant according to the PCERA scores) in mother-infant dyads who have been allowed extra suckling, extra stimulation of the breast, or skin-to-skin contact after birth. These studies support the results of previous studies showing that increased skin-to-skin contact after birth promotes interaction between mothers and their infants long after birth (De Chateau & Wiberg, 1977a, 1977b, 1984; Kennell et al., 1975; Klaus et al., 1972; Wiberg et al., 1989).

Skin-to-Skin Contact Facilitates Mother Infant Interaction After Birth

Both maternal tactile and vocal interaction was increased during the period of skin-to-skin contact after birth. The infants' vocal interactions were increased and synchronized with that of the parents' (Velandia et al., 2010; Velandia et al., 2011) suggesting a link between the immediate and the more long-term facilitation of interaction or continued synchronization between mother and infant.

Role of Oxytocin in the Brain

Administration of oxytocin increases social interaction in humans. A reciprocal release of oxytocin in response to the sensory stimuli caused by skin-to-skin contact (light pressure, stroking, touch, and warmth), as well as other sensory cues, may have triggered the effect on social interaction in mothers and children. The infant's hand massage and sucking during the breast-seeking behavior may have contributed to the effects by a further release of oxytocin in the mothers (Matthiesen et al., 2001a).

It is important to keep in mind that the effects of oxytocin on social interaction are exerted within the brain via parvocellular oxytocinergic fibers emanating in the PVN, which project to areas involved in social interaction, e.g., the amygdala. Therefore, rising oxytocin levels in the circulation may not necessarily occur. If they do, they represent a parallel release of oxytocin from magnocellular neurons into the circulation and from parvocellular neurons into the brain.

It is plausible that oxytocin released in both mother and infants are involved in the long-term effects induced by skin-to-skin contact immediately after birth. The mechanisms involved in these effects will be discussed later in this chapter.

Link Between Temperature Patterns After Birth and Behavioral Observations One Year Later

The skin temperature variations recorded during skin-to-skin contact express some interesting associations with the effects observed one year later. The mothers' chest temperatures increased by skin-to-skin contact as oxytocin levels rose (Bystrova, Matthiesen, Vorontsov, et al., 2007; Matthiesen et al., 2001a; Nissen, Lilja, Widstrom, et al., 1995). It is particularly interesting that maternal breast temperature and infant skin temperature observed after birth were related to the outcome in the behavioral studies performed one year later. The more the maternal breast skin temperature increased and pulsed, the more the infant's skin temperature (in particular foot skin temperature) increased (Bystrova, Matthiesen, Vorontsov, et al., 2007; Bystrova et al., 2003). The more pulsatile the mother's breast temperature and the higher the infant's foot temperature were after birth, the higher the maternal and infant interaction scores were, as well as the score of calm in the infants, according to the PCERA one year later (Bystrova et al., 2009).

Link Between High Skin Temperature and Low Sympathetic Nervous Tone

A warm skin temperature to a certain extent reflects a low sympathetic nervous tone, as more blood reaches the blood vessels in the skin when the sympathetically driven constriction of blood vessels is decreased. One of the immediate effects of skin-to-skin contact is a decrease in skin temperature in infants (Bystrova et al., 2003). Perhaps the feeling of warmth in the period is converted into a warm behavior, or the warm skin just reflects a high oxytocinergic tone, as parvocellular neurons project from the PVN to areas involved in the control of the sympathetic nervous system in the NTS and RVLM. Perhaps it is the effects of the high oxytocinergic tone, which becomes permanent. Warm temperature is linked to oxytocin release (Uvnäs Moberg, Bruzelius, et al., 1993).

Decreased Stress Levels

The increased skin temperature in the newborn is an expression of a decreased tone in the sympathetic nervous system. Cortisol levels and pulse rate fell more in infants allowed skin-to-skin contact than in those separated from their mothers (Takahashi et al., 2011). Whether the activity in the sympathetic nervous system and in the HPA axis remains lower in infants allowed skin-to-skin contact postpartum in a longer time perspective is not known. However, the infants of the St. Petersburg study that had been randomized to skin-to-skin contact with their mothers were better at handling stressful situations one year later according to the PCERA scores. These results indicate that skin-to-skin treatment after birth reduces stress reactivity in a more long-term perspective. The finding of an inverse association between oxytocin and cortisol levels in blood samples collected four days after birth in the infants from the skin-to-skin group, but not in the other groups, suggests that oxytocin may give rise to sustained effects on the activity of the HPA axis after birth (Agren, Lundeberg, & Uvnäs-Moberg, 1997).

Increased Vagal Nerve Activity

The lower gastrin levels observed in the mothers exposed to both suckling and skin-to-skin contact than to skin-to-skin contact alone, i.e., mothers who had received more sensory stimulation, was likely due to activation of the vagal nerves.

Stimuli of low intensity, such as touch or stroking, decrease basal levels of digestive hormones, such as gastrin, CCK, and insulin, whereas the release of these hormones is enhanced in connection with the stronger stimulation caused by suckling during breastfeeding. In studies performed during skin-to-skin contact in premature infants receiving kangaroo care, a decrease in the levels of CCK was observed. In contrast, the feeding-induced rise was enhanced (Tornhage et al., 1998). By the initial lowering of the levels of gastrointestinal hormones, the set point for the suckling-related release becomes more favorable, and the digestive process is optimized. These results indicate that the maternal digestive capacity is activated by extra sensory stimulation immediately after birth.

Skin-to-skin contact triggers maternal oxytocin release, which stimulates maternal interaction and bonding. Administration of oxytocin into the brain lowers gastrin levels via activation of the vagal nerves (Bjorkstrand, Ahlenius, et al., 1996). Therefore, the low gastrin levels observed in the mothers having received extra sensory stimulation after birth may be caused, in part, by oxytocin released from parvocellular neurons projecting to the areas in the brain where vagal functions are controlled (vagas motor nucleus—DMX). The lowered gastrin levels may parallel an oxytocin-related enhancement of maternal bonding and reduction of anxiety. Whether the decrease in gastrin levels manifested directly after birth or is the consequence of more frequent interaction and closeness during the first days of life cannot be established. Unfortunately, oxytocin levels were not measured in this study, but if they had been, they would probably have exhibited a negative association with gastrin levels in the same ways as oxytocin and cortisol levels were shown to have an inverse relationship in the skin-to-skin group of the Russian study. Perhaps gastrin levels can be used as a proxy for centrally induced oxytocinergic effects on interaction. Several studies actually indicate that low levels of gastrin are associated with high levels of social interaction (Uvnäs-Moberg & Nissen, 2005).

These results suggesting a relationship between oxytocin levels and activity in the vagal nerve fibers controlling gastrin release are consistent with other findings showing a relationship between oxytocin and heart rate variability, as an increased heart rate variability is mediated via the vagal nerves to the heart (Porges, 2009).

Milk Production Not Affected by Early Suckling or Early Skin-To-Skin Contact

The effect of different ward routines postpartum, such as skin-to-skin contact and early suckling, on the outcome of milk production and duration of breastfeeding has been investigated in several studies. Since these studies do not clearly differentiate between early suckling and early skin-to-skin contact, it is difficult to conclude whether these different routines differ as to their long-term effects (de Chateau, Holmberg, Jakobsson, & Winberg, 1977; DiGirolamo, Gummer-Strawn, & Fein, 2008; Nylander, Lindemann, Helsing, & Bendvold, 1991; Salariya et al., 1978). The results from the present studies, however, clearly show that milk production four days after birth is not promoted by early suckling. In contrast, interaction and bonding between mother and infant is promoted by early skin-to-skin contact (or even by the suckling stimulus, particularly in the absence of skin-to-skin contact). Increased interaction and bonding between mothers and infants may, of course, facilitate breastfeeding and enhance the duration of breastfeeding (Bystrova, Matthiesen, Widstrom, et al., 2007; K. Bystrova, Widstrom et al., 2007; Widstrom et al., 1990). The effect of the different

labor and maternity ward routines in the Russian study on milk production will be described more in detail in a later chapter.

Skin-to-Skin Contact in the Early Period Strengthens the Calm and Connection System

In summary, these data show that exposure to skin-to-skin contact after birth may induce long-term effects by increasing social interactive skills, decreasing the activity in the HPA axis and the sympathetic nervous system, and by increasing the activity in the parasympathetic/vagal nervous system, thereby increasing anabolic processes and growth (Uvnäs-Moberg, 1998a, 2003). This combination of effects was previously described as the calm and connection response. Obviously, there is a limited period, "a biological window," just after birth, when activity of the calm and relaxation system may be reinforced by close contact, particularly by touch and warmth. The argument in favor of stimulation of the calm and connection system by exposure to skin-to-skin contact immediately after birth may be rephrased and expressed as an inhibition of the activity in the fight or flight system.

The reason why the effect of skin-to-skin contact is so strong in the early period may be due to the unique neuro-endocrine milieu prevailing during this period. The levels of steroids are still high after pregnancy. The HPA axis is activated, as is the sympathetic nervous system and the noradrenergic systems in the brain. This neuro-endocrine pattern is consistent with learning, the establishment of conditioned reflexes, and perhaps with epigenetic imprinting. As described in more detail in a previous chapter, extra sensory stimulation during the first week of life may induce lifelong effects in rats by epigenetic imprinting. Interestingly, the effect profile is the same as in the Russian study: social interactive behavior is promoted and stress levels are reduced.

Clinical Consequences

Long-Term Relief From the Stress of Being Born or Giving Birth

According to some psychological theories, memories from birth may persist the whole life as the "trauma of birth," which may increase the risk for stress reactions. Perhaps skin-to-skin contact immediately after birth may serve not only to reduce the acute stress reaction caused by birth, "the stress of being born," but also to help resolve the unconscious memory of birth, "the trauma of birth," in the long run.

Infants are not the only ones stressed during birth. Most mothers experience birth as an extremely stressful and painful procedure, even if they may regard it as a very positive experience later on. It has been suggested that oxytocin released during labor and in the period induces a pain-relieving and amnesic effect (Heinrichs, Meinlschmidt, Wippich, Ehlert, & Hellhammer, 2004). The finding of a more persistent memory of the pain of labor in women having received an epidural analgesia supports this assumption, since epidural analgesia reduces maternal oxytocin release during labor (Waldenstrom & Schytt, 2009). This effect will be described in more detail in a subsequent chapter.

It is also possible that oxytocin released by skin-to-skin contact in the period transforms the negative experiences during birth and memories from birth into more positive ones. Skin-to-skin contact in the period may, therefore, be important in decreasing the occurrence of PTSD or other types of anxiety and stress reactions, which may occur as a consequence of a difficult and painful labor.

Kangaroo Care

When childbirth was moved from homes to hospitals, the spontaneous routine of closeness after birth was substituted by separation of mothers and infants after birth. Recently, the practice of skin-to-skin contact after birth has been re-introduced, since results from scientific studies show that it gives rise to several positive short- and long-term effects for both mother and infant.

Skin-to-Skin Contact May Also Be Used Therapeutically in the Treatment of Premature Infants

Repeated or sometimes continuous skin-to-skin contact may be used in the care of premature infants. Small, preterm babies were wrapped next to their mothers' chests in Colombia, instead of being kept in incubators, and were found to thrive and grow more quickly. The treatment was named Kangaroo Care. Several controlled clinical studies have verified the beneficial effects of kangaroo care. Kangaroo care has been associated with increased growth and development in the premature babies. The mother produces more milk, and her interaction and bonding to the child is reinforced.

In principle, the same effects as induced by skin-to-skin contact after birth are induced each time the infant is in skin-to-skin contact with a parent. Social interactive behavior is stimulated as a consequence of oxytocin release, e.g., in the amygdala. Oxytocin decreases cortisol levels and some aspects of sympathetic nervous tone, leading to lowered blood pressure in mothers and increased skin temperature in infants. These effects are induced by oxytocinergic nerves projecting within the PVN and to brainstem areas involved in the control of autonomic nervous tone. The NTS plays an important role as oxytocin released in this area increases the function of alpha-2 adrenoceptors and thereby reduces the stress reactivity. In addition, oxytocin facilitates the release of further oxytocin by an effect on incoming sensory nerves. Vagal nerve activity is also stimulated by actions in the DMX, which leads to optimized digestion and increased capacity for storing of nutrients and growth. Finally, the increased milk production is a consequence of the facilitation of prolactin release from the lactotrophs in the anterior pituitary.

Both Mothers and Fathers

One of the most important aspects of kangaroo care is that both the father and the mother may give skin-to-skin contact to their infants. Skin-to-skin contact with the father gives rise to similar positive effects in the infant as skin-to-skin contact with the mother, with the exception for the possibility of breastfeeding (Erlandsson, Dsilna, Fagerberg, & Christensson, 2007).

Co-sleeping

Before the big changes in the routines of mother care, instituted when births were moved from home to hospital, newborn babies stayed with their mothers and slept with them. Mothers intuitively positioned themselves around the infant in the bed in a way that protected them, but also allowed the mother to notice when they were hungry and needed food. In this way, the babies were kept calm (McKenna, Ball, & Gettler, 2007).

Co-sleeping, like kangaroo care, reinforces the interaction between mother and infant, and increases the duration of breastfeeding. Due to the closeness, the release of oxytocin should be stimulated continuously as long as mother and infant sleep together. It is also possible that anti-stress effects and stimulation of anabolic metabolism and growth were stimulated at the same time, just as in response to kangaroo care. The mechanisms by which these effects are induced should be analogous to those described above for kangaroo care.

Summary

- Four days after birth, mothers who were allowed both skin-to-skin contact with their newborns and breastfeeding communicated more with their babies during breastfeeding and spent more time with them as a sign of enhanced bonding than did mothers who only had skin-to-skin contact.

- In addition, they had lower gastrin levels as an expression of increased vagal nerve tone. In this way, digestive and metabolic processes were facilitated. The lower the gastrin levels the more time the mothers spent with their newborns, indicating an association between gastrin levels and bonding.

- One year after birth, mothers and infants who had skin-to-skin contact after birth interacted more and in a more intuitive way than those separated after birth.

- The infants who had skin-to-skin contact handled stress more efficiently than those who did not have skin-to-skin contact.

- Pulsing maternal breast skin temperature and high infant skin temperature during the first hours after birth predict the increase in social competence and stress buffering competence one year later.

- Skin-to-skin contact may serve to decrease the stress of being born in infants and perhaps the stress of giving birth in mothers.

- Oxytocin released during interaction between mother and infant postpartum and enhanced by skin-to-skin contact may have played an integrative role in the effects caused by skin-to-skin contact. Activation of parvocellular oxytocinergic neurons might have increased social interaction, decreased activity in the HPA axis and some aspects of the sympathetic nervous system, and increased activity in some aspects of the vagal parasympathetic system. Prolactin release may also be stimulated. The immediate effects may have turned into long-term effects by epigenetic mechanisms.

- Kangaroo care and co-sleeping act in the same way as skin-to-skin contact. The activity of the oxytocinergic effect increases by closeness, which leads to positive effects on social interaction, stress levels, and growth.

Chapter 15

Expressions of Maternal Caring Behavior in Breastfeeding Mothers

The previous chapters have described how oxytocin is released into the circulation in breastfeeding mothers to stimulate milk ejection and production. Oxytocin is released into the anterior pituitary to promote prolactin secretion.

Breastfeeding is not only about the giving of milk and warmth to newborns, it is also about care and protection of the infant, just as in other mammals. Some of the psychological and/or behavioral adaptations that occur during lactation help the mother transition to motherhood. These adaptations do not occur at a conscious level. They take place at deeper levels in the brain and reflect subtle remnants of the more programmed maternal behavior expressed during lactation in other mammalian mothers. Oxytocin released into the brain during breastfeeding plays an important regulatory role for these maternal adaptations.

The expression of maternal adaptations in human mothers is stimulated during pregnancy and labor, during skin-to-skin contact with the newborn the first hours after birth, and during breastfeeding. In this chapter, the aspects of maternal adaptations that manifest themselves during breastfeeding will be described (Figure 15.1). Those related to labor and skin-to-skin contact are described in other chapters.

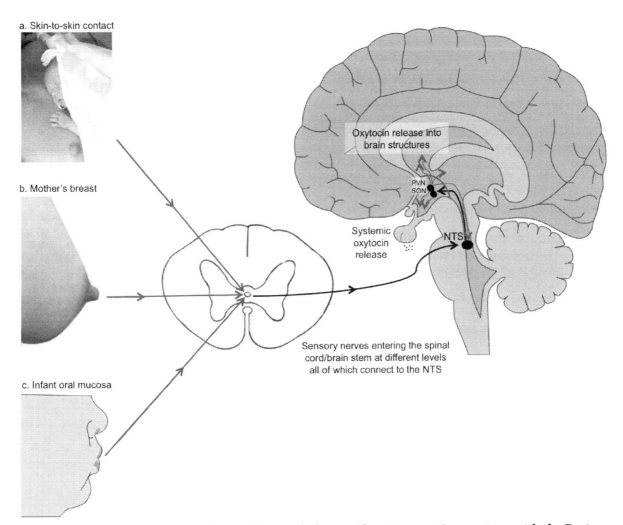

a. Skin-to-skin contact

b. Mother's breast

c. Infant oral mucosa

Oxytocin release into brain structures

PVN
SON

Systemic oxytocin release

NTS

Sensory nerves entering the spinal cord/brain stem at different levels all of which connect to the NTS

Figure 15.1. Mother and Baby, Suckling and Skin-to-Skin Contact, Connections with the Brain

Source: Uvnäs-Moberg & Prime, 2013. Reprinted with permission.

Maternal Adaptations During a Breastfeed

Approach and Social Interaction

Before breastfeeding, the mother holds her baby, looks into its eyes, and maybe talks to it and touches it. Sometimes the baby lies on her skin for a while before breastfeeding. The mother's wish to approach the baby is facilitated by the release of oxytocin and by the sight, sound, smell, and touch of the baby. Oxytocin neurons from parvocellular neurons emanating from the PVN project to the amygdala, and axon collaterals from magnocellular neurons projecting to the posterior pituitary project to the amygdala. When oxytocin is released in the amygdala, social interaction is stimulated. This approach phase of breastfeeding will be described in more detail in the chapters on the effects of skin-to-skin contact.

Decreased Anxiety and Decreased Reactivity to Stress

When mothers breastfeed and hold their infants, their level of anxiety is reduced for about one hour, as determined by questionnaires which document how the mothers' feel now (state anxiety; Heinrichs et al., 2001). When the mothers were subjected to a psychosocial stress test called The Trierer Social Stress Test, the release of cortisol was reduced (a sign of reduced stress levels) if the stress test occurred within one hour after suckling. The levels of anxiety and negative feelings, which were caused by the stress test, were not reversed and occurred to the same extent in breastfeeding and non-breastfeeding women (Altemus et al., 2001; Heinrichs et al., 2001; Heinrichs, Neumann, & Ehlert, 2002). This is important, as mothers must retain their capacity to protect themselves and their newborns.

Positive Feelings

During breastfeeding the mother may experience love and happiness. When interacting with the infant, the mother may find the infant irresistible and more beautiful than all the other children in the world. If brain function is visualized by a technique called FMRI, when a mother looks at a picture of her infant, the same areas in the frontal lobe of the cortex in the brain are activated as when lovers look at pictures of a beloved partner (romantic love). The brain's reward system, which is full of oxytocin and dopamine receptors, is activated, and areas linked to negative emotions and social judgment in the frontal cortex are deactivated (Bartels & Zeki, 2004). Just looking at the baby gives rise to activation of areas linked to reward and peripheral oxytocin levels rise. The changes in dopamine function in areas linked to reward parallel that of the rise in oxytocin levels in plasma, suggesting that a parallel release of oxytocin has occurred in the brain in order to increase the activity in the reward systems (Strathearn et al., 2009).

Long-Term Behavioral Adaptations in Breastfeeding Women

In order to characterize possible long-term changes in the psychology or behavior of breastfeeding women, a validated personality inventory called the Karolinska Scale of Personality (KSP) was used (Almay, von Knorring, & Oreland, 1987; Gustavsson, 1977). The KSP consists of 135 items referring to various aspects of anxiety, aggression, and social skills. The questions refer to how you normally feel (trait), rather than to how you feel right now (state), and, of course, reflect the subjective experience of the women tested.

Five different studies have been performed in which breastfeeding women filled in the KSP inventory. All women breastfed exclusively, i.e., the infants were not given any formula. The scores obtained in the KSP by the breastfeeding women were then compared with the scores of a normative, non-pregnant, non-breastfeeding group of women of the same age.

Clinical Studies

1. Fifty-two mothers filled in the KSP inventory four days after giving birth. They were all primipara and had undergone a normal vaginal birth. Repeated blood samples were collected in these mothers in connection with breastfeeding experiments performed at four days and four months postpartum. Blood levels of oxytocin, prolactin, and somatostatin levels were analyzed (Uvnäs-Moberg, Widström, Nissen & Björvell, 1990).

2. The KSP inventory was filled in by 161 women on three different occasions—during the third trimester of pregnancy, breastfeeding at three months after delivery, and breastfeeding at six months after delivery (Sjogren, Widstrom, Edman, & Uvnäs-Moberg, 2000).

3. Thirteen primipara and 16 multipara having undergone normal vaginal deliveries filled in the KSP inventory two days postpartum. Eight blood samples were collected in the postpartum period. Oxytocin, gastrin, somatostatin, and cholecystokinin levels were analyzed in these samples (Uvnäs-Moberg & Nissen, 2005).

4. Twenty women, who delivered vaginally, and 17 women, who delivered by Cesarean Section, filled in the KSP two days after birth. Twenty-four blood samples were collected during a breastfeeding experiment two days after birth. Plasma levels of oxytocin, prolactin, and cortisol were measured in these samples (Nissen et al., 1998).

5. Sixty-nine breastfeeding mothers filled in the

KSP inventory two days after birth and at two and six months after birth. All these women were primipara, had a vaginal delivery, and had skin-to-skin contact after birth, but some of them had been exposed to different medical interventions during labor, such as epidural analgesia and/or oxytocin infusions. Twenty-four blood samples were collected during a breastfeeding session two days after birth. Oxytocin, prolactin, and cortisol levels in plasma were measured (Jonas, Nissen, Ransjo-Arvidson, Matthiesen, et al., 2008).

Oxytocin and prolactin levels were measured in some of the studies. The results and hormone levels were related to the scores obtained in the KSP inventory in each of the participating women.

Change in Personality Profile Towards Less Anxiety and More Social Interaction

When the KSP profile of breastfeeding women was compared with the KSP profile of a "normative group" consisting of similar-aged women who were not pregnant or breastfeeding, some interesting differences appeared. The breastfeeding women described themselves as less anxious, having less somatic problems, being less aggressive, and more inclined to social interaction than the women belonging to the "normative group." In addition, they were more tolerant to monotonous tasks, i.e., they preferred a calm lifestyle. This pattern of effects, with some small variations, was demonstrated in all five studies (Uvnäs-Moberg & Nissen, 2005; Uvnäs-Moberg, Widström, Nissen, & Björvell, 1990; Jonas, Nissen, Ransjo-Arvidson, Matthiesen, et al., 2008; Nissen et al., 1998, Sjögren et al., 2000).

Since the KSP describes how somebody normally feels, we can assume that the changes in the KSP pattern occurring after a few days of breastfeeding are expressions of strong, subconscious, and powerful mental changes that make breastfeeding mothers forget how they normally feel, and instead describe the breastfeeding-related feelings as the normal state. When the mother is not breastfeeding, personality traits measured by the KSP are stable over time (Gustavsson, 1977).

Time Course of Changes

The changes in the KSP profile were not present during pregnancy, but developed gradually over the four days postpartum to be maximal at six to eight weeks postpartum. The changes persisted for at least six months postpartum if the mothers were still breastfeeding. Mothers who were breastfeeding exclusively had more pronounced changes in their KSP scores than those who did not breastfeed (Sjogren et al., 2000).

Differences Between Primipara and Multipara

Two days after birth, the changes in the KSP profile were more pronounced in multipara than in primipara, showing that the psychological adaptations developed more quickly in women with previous experiences of pregnancy and breastfeeding (Uvnäs-Moberg & Nissen, 2005).

Influence by Medical Interventions During Labor

The results of the KSP inventory filled in four days after birth were influenced by medical interventions during labor. The changes versus controls in the KSP profile were less developed in mothers who had a Cesarean section or an epidural analgesia, but were reinforced in women who had received oxytocin infusions (Jonas, Wiklund, Nissen, Ransjo-Arvidson, & Uvnäs-Moberg, K., 2007). These effects will be described in more detail in the chapter on medical interventions.

Relationships Between KSP Scores and Oxytocin Levels

Blood samples were collected and oxytocin levels were measured in three of the above-mentioned studies in which the breastfeeding women filled in the KSP formula. An immediate pulsatile rise of oxytocin levels was documented in response to breastfeeding, particularly within the first week postpartum, whereas a more coherent release was observed a few months later. The number of pulses recorded during the first ten minutes of breastfeeding varied between zero and five. A more detailed description of the oxytocin pattern is presented in chapter 10.

In the studies in which oxytocin levels were measured with RIA, correlations were found between the scores obtained in certain items of the KSP inventory and oxytocin levels/pulsatility. The increase of oxytocin caused by breastfeeding was found to correlate positively with items in the KSP reflecting social skills, and negatively with items reflecting anxiety, aggression, and fear of monotony (Uvnäs-Moberg, Widström, Nissen, et al., 1990). The scores of items reflecting social skills were positively related to the number of oxytocin peaks induced by suckling during the first ten minutes, and basal oxytocin levels were associated with calm (Nissen et al., 1998).

By contrast, in the study in which oxytocin levels were measured with EIA, no correlations between the scores of items reflecting anxiety and social skills and the rise of oxytocin levels were obtained (Jonas, Nissen, Ransjo-Arvidson, Matthiesen, et al., 2008). RIA more specifically measures the nonapeptide oxytocin than does EIA, which may record other substances or non-specific material. Therefore, correlations between oxytocin levels and KSP scores were only found in experiments in which oxytocin levels were measured with RIA. In some cases, correlations were also found with prolactin levels. These correlations were quite similar to the ones obtained with oxytocin, probably reflecting the fact that oxytocin stimulates the release of prolactin (Uvnäs-Moberg et al., 1990; Nissen et al., 1998).

Parallel Release of Oxytocin in the Blood Stream and into the Brain

The correlations in the studies above between the scores obtained in the KSP regarding social interaction, anxiety and aggression, and oxytocin levels support an important role for oxytocin in these changes. Still, the relationships must be indirect since circulating oxytocin levels released into the circulation from the posterior pituitary correlated with psychological changes induced by oxytocin released from neurons in the brain. Therefore, it must be assumed that oxytocin is released in parallel into both the circulation and the brain in response to breastfeeding. As described previously, oxytocin may even be released into the anterior pituitary from collaterals from the magnocellular oxytocinergic nerves originating in the SON and PVN, which project to the posterior pituitary. Some studies indicate that axon collaterals from the magnocellular neurons also reach the amygdala (Knobloch et al., 2012). The study in which changes in dopamine activity, as measured with FMRI, was found to correlate with circulating oxytocin levels also supports this assumption (Strathearn et al., 2009).

Oxytocin and Generosity

The anatomic arrangements of the oxytocin neurons is consistent with the strong correlations between oxytocin levels in the circulation and the decrease of anxiety and increase in social interaction induced by oxytocinergic nerves in the amygdala. It would also explain the relationship between the recorded levels of social interaction and the amount of milk ejected (Nissen et al., 1998). It is interesting to note that not only do the scores of social interactive skills relate positively to the number of oxytocin peaks observed during the ten minutes after the start of suckling, but they also relate to the amount of milk the mother gave to the baby during that breastfeed (Nissen et al., 1998). These findings may be related in a very basic sense, since both the level of social interaction and the amount of milk ejected are expressions of generosity directed to the baby.

Breastfeeding and Increased Emotional Intelligence

Another way of summarizing the changes observed in the KSP profile in breastfeeding women is to say that they are consistent with an increased emotional intelligence. As oxytocin increases the capacity for social interaction in many ways and also reduces anxiety and stress levels, oxytocin is a facilitator of emotional intelligence or E.Q.

On the other hand, there are studies showing that the memory of breastfeeding women is not as good as in non-breastfeeding women, particularly if the tests involve learning meaningless combinations of letters (Silber, Almkvist, Larsson, & Uvnäs-Moberg, 1990). It is, therefore, possible that some aspects of brain function, which are irrelevant in mothers caring for babies, are less well expressed during breastfeeding in some women. Some women have difficulty concentrating and have become less interested in theoretical and analytical work during this time period. Others feel less competitive and ambitious. These changes are temporary and vanish after weaning.

The Changes in the KSP Profile—A Result of Repeated Exposure to Oxytocin

The changes in the KSP profile most likely reflect effects of oxytocin released not only during the particular breastfeeding session when oxytocin levels were measured, but rather an accumulated effect based on oxytocin released into the brain during labor, skin-to-skin contact after birth, and during the breastfeedings preceding filling in the KSP inventory. Still, the correlations between the KSP scores and oxytocin levels suggest that immediate psychological effects may also occur in connection with a breastfeed.

Comparison Between Breastfeeding and Bottle-Feeding Mothers

The long-term changes of some personality traits in breastfeeding women, described above, may be a consequence of the repeated exposure to oxytocin taking place at each individual breastfeed. The immediate changes occurring in response to each individual breastfeeding session may have been changed into a more sustained effect pattern. There are studies in which other types of endpoints were measured demonstrating such long-term changes. Breastfeeding mothers are often compared with bottle-feeding mothers. The bottle-feeding mothers are not being exposed to as much oxytocin as the breastfeeding mothers, as they don't receive the suckling stimulus from the baby. Oxytocin release is still promoted by closeness with the baby in the bottle-feeders, but some differences between breastfeeders and bottle feeders have been demonstrated.

Breastfeeding Mothers Perceive Less Stress and Negative Feelings

Breastfeeding women perceive less stress and negative moods than bottle-feeding women and react less intensely to stress (Altemus, 1995; Mezzacappa & Katlin, 2002).

Breastfeeding Mothers Interact More Than Bottle-Feeding Mothers

Other studies show that breastfeeding increases the interaction between mothers and infants. Breastfeeding mothers have been found to interact more with their babies than do bottle-feeding mothers. They hold them more and they smile and look at their babies more while they feed them than bottle-feeding mothers do (Dunn & Kendrick, 1980; Wiesenfeld, Malatesta, Whitman, Granrose, & Uili, 1985). This difference in social interaction between breastfeeding and bottle-feeding mothers may be due to the suckling-induced oxytocin release occurring in breastfeeding mothers.

Breastfeeding Mothers Have a Higher Parasympathetic Tone and Lower Sympathetic Tone Than Bottle Feeders

Breastfeeding mothers have lower blood pressure than bottle-feeding mothers, and they have a lower skin conductance. These differences may be linked to a lack of oxytocin release in the bottle-feeding mothers, since oxytocin decreases blood pressure and increases skin conductance by decreasing sympathetic nervous tone (Mezzacappa, Kelsey, & Katkin, 2005). Also, heart rate variability (HRV) is increased during breastfeeding.

Oxytocin Levels and Maternal Interaction

The results of observations performed by other researchers show that maternal oxytocin levels actually reflect the intensity of the mother's interaction with her baby. The higher the maternal oxytocin level, the more the mother (and father) smiles, looks at, and interacts with her baby during breastfeeding (Feldman, Gordon, Schneiderman, Weisman, & Zagoory-Sharon, 2010; Feldman, Gordon, & Zagoory-Sharon, 2011). These observations were based on single blood or salivary samples collected during pregnancy and breastfeeding, and EIA was used to measure oxytocin levels in this study. RIA and EIA do not give identical results, and, therefore, these results should be regarded with some caution (Grewen & Light, 2011; Handlin et al., 2009; Jonas et al., 2009).

Interestingly, synchronization of skin temperature was observed between mothers and infants in skin-to-skin contact (Bystrova, Matthiesen, Vorontsov, et al., 2007). As increased skin temperature reflects a decrease in sympathetic nervous tone, it is tempting to suggest that the "oxytocin levels" recorded by Feldman and collaborators, with the more nonspecific recording technique EIA, may reflect a substance similar to oxytocin, which reflects vasodilation.

Still, the data cited above suggest an important role for oxytocin in the expression of maternal-infant interaction. With the RIA technique, mothers with high oxytocin levels have been shown to breastfeed longer than those that have lower levels of oxytocin (Nissen et al., 1996; Silber et al., 1991). This effect may be related to a more intense bonding to the child in mothers with high oxytocin levels. The role of oxytocin for the development of bonding and attachment will be described more in detail in the chapters on skin-to-skin contact.

Oxytocin Levels State and Trait

Oxytocin levels can be raised in response to breastfeeding, and also in response to labor and skin-to-skin contact in the period. Obviously, oxytocin-related effects may be induced in all these specific situations.

Still, each woman seems to have a certain oxytocin level. Maternal oxytocin levels measured at different time-points during pregnancy and breastfeeding have been shown in several studies to correlate within individual women (Feldman et al., 2007; Silber et al., 1991).

The reason why certain women have higher oxytocin levels and, therefore, breastfeed longer and interact more with their children is not known. Genetic and epigenetic factors, negative or positive experiences in early life, together with present close relationships and social status may all influence oxytocin levels.

As we shall discuss in later chapters, oxytocin released during breastfeeding, the massive release of oxytocin occurring during labor, and oxytocin released during skin-to-skin contact in the period are important for the maternal adaptations to develop and become established. As medical interventions during birth may influence maternal oxytocin release, aberrations in the oxytocin levels may be created during these periods. This possibility will be discussed later in this book.

Reflections of Maternal Behavior in Women

Humans are mammals. From a genetic point of view, they are strongly related to other mammals and to the big apes in particular. Human mothers should, therefore, be expected to express some type of innate maternal adaptations. In Western culture, it is accepted that human mothers share the same basic regulatory mechanisms that govern pregnancy, labor, and milk production in other mammals. It has been more difficult to gain acceptance for the idea that human mothers also have some remnants of an inborn biologically rooted mammalian maternal behavior that helps them to care for their babies. Other explanations of sociological and/or psychological nature have been completely domineering.

Still, it has always been agreed that there is the existence of some expressions of "maternal behavior" in human mothers. Everybody "knows" that human mothers may exhibit some nest-building behavior, since they often like to clean the home and have everything prepared for the baby to come. Some mothers withdraw before giving birth. Women tend to give birth during the night, when it is dark, if the birthing process is not interfered with. It is also well known that human mothers will protect their infants and may become as strong as tigers if they feel something threatens their infant.

Human mothers exhibit some changes in maternal character, e.g., decreased levels of anxiety and aggression and increased social interaction and tolerance for monotony, as revealed by the repeated studies with the KSP inventory. In addition, several studies show that the activity in the sympathetic nervous system is decreased and the activity of the parasympathetic nervous system is increased in breastfeeding women. The changes observed in breastfeeding women may reflect subtle aspects of inborn human maternal adaptations aimed at facilitation of the transition to motherhood. In certain situations, an opposite reaction pattern characterized by increased anxiety and aggression may be expressed. This reaction pattern will be discussed in the next chapter on maternal protective strategies.

Table 15.1. Summary of Correlations Between Oxytocin Levels and Milk Production/Milk Ejection, as well as Other Physiological/Behavioral/ Psychological Adaptations

Milk production	**The higher the oxytocin levels:** The more milk is ejected (RIA) The higher the prolactin levels (EIA) The longer the total period of breastfeeding (RIA)
Gastrointestinal and metabolic function	**The higher the oxytocin levels:** The lower the somatostatin levels (RIA) The higher the birth weight of the infant (RIA) **The lower the somatostatin levels:** The higher the oxytocin levels The more milk is ejected The higher the birth weight of the infant
HPA axis	**The higher the oxytocin levels:** The lower the levels of ACTH (EIA)
Psychological adaptations	**The higher the oxytocin levels:** The lower the levels of anxiety (RIA) The higher the levels of social interaction (RIA) The lower the levels of monotony avoidance (RIA) The more maternal interaction (single samples EIA) **The higher the gastrin levels:** The less maternal bonding The higher the levels of anxiety The lower the levels of social interaction

Table 15.2. Differences Between Primipara And Multipara With Regard to Breastfeeding-Related Parameters

Parameter	Primipara	Multipara
Earlier start of milk secretion		✔ (in some studies)
Quicker development of psychological adaptations, such as calm and social skills, after birth		✔
Lower blood pressure in the beginning of pregnancy		✔
Lower cortisol levels		✔
Higher oxytocin levels at day four		✔ (when measured with EIA, not RIA)

Taken together, these data imply that mechanisms involved in milk production and in the control of the HPA axis, the sympathetic nervous system, and the parasympathetic nervous system are primed in multipara by previous experiences of pregnancy and breastfeeding. The effects are likely to involve activation of oxytocinergic mechanisms within the brain.

Summary

- In addition to giving milk to their offspring, all mammals exhibit maternal behavior, and mother and young bond and attach to each other soon after birth. Oxytocin released during labor, skin-to-skin contact, and suckling is of prime importance for the development of maternal care and bonding.

- Human mothers do not exhibit a stereotyped maternal behavior, but some remnants of it can be identified. During each breastfeed, mothers become less anxious and more socially interactive. They experience love, warmth, and well being.

- In addition to short-term changes, the mothers' mentality is changed in a more sustained way during breastfeeding. In short, they become less anxious, less aggressive, more inclined for social interaction, and more tolerant of monotony. In comparison with bottle-feeders, breastfeeding mothers feel more content, they are more interactive with their infants, and they have a shift in their autonomic nervous tone towards decreased sympathetic and increased parasympathetic dominance. These changes last for the entire breastfeeding period and represent adaptations aimed at helping women transition to motherhood.

- Since oxytocin is released in response to suckling and the psychological adaptations are correlated with oxytocin levels, the maternal psychological adaptations are likely to be induced by oxytocin released from parvocellular neurons in the brain projecting to areas involved in the control of anxiety and social interaction. The finding of an association between circulating levels of oxytocin and the maternal psychological adaptations demonstrate that oxytocin is released in parallel from parvocellular neurons into the brain and from magnocellular neurons into the circulation during breastfeeding.

Chapter 16

Breastfeeding and Skin-to-Skin Contact: Maternal Protective Strategies

Most women know that breastfeeding a baby is not only about feeling happy, relaxed, and calm. Breastfeeding itself is not always easy, and practical problems in connection with breastfeeding may cause worry and concern. Mothers may become anxious and even aggressive in certain situations in order to protect their newborns. The worry and the tendency to wish to defend and protect the baby is another aspect of the maternal adaptations that occur in all mammalian species, including breastfeeding women. The maternal protective strategies are, like the maternal caring behaviors and the psychophysiological adaptations linked to breastfeeding, promoted by oxytocin.

Protective Strategies in Mammalian Mothers

Synchronization of Birth, Hiding, and Building of Nests

Both mother and offspring are extremely vulnerable in connection with birth and during lactation, and they may become easy victims of prey. Therefore, mammalian mothers use different strategies to protect their offspring.

Females of some herd-living species give birth at the same time of the year. Synchronizing female reproduction is one mechanism by which mothers, infants, and the whole group are protected. In this way, the vulnerable period around birth and lactation, when the mothers and newborns are defenseless and easily fall prey to predators, is kept as short as possible.

Inhibition of Oxytocin Release During Labor and Milk Ejection in an Unfamiliar Environment

Mammalian mothers often give birth during the night, when the mother and her offspring are difficult to detect by their enemies. In addition, they often give birth in a sheltered place, perhaps in a nest they have built. Sometimes, depending on how mature they are at birth, the offspring stays in the nest during the first period of lactation.

The release of oxytocin that occurs in connection with labor and lactation to stimulate uterine contractions and milk letdown is inhibited in unfamiliar environments or in other situations when the mother feels threatened or unsafe, and constitutes another protective mechanism

for the vulnerable mother and young. The release of oxytocin reappears when the mother has moved to a safe place or when she has become accustomed to unfamiliar surroundings. Cows being milked by milking machines don't let down their milk if moved to another stable until they feel familiar with the new environment.

Maternal Aggression

When mammalian mothers have given birth, they develop species-specific maternal behaviors involving feeding and caring behaviors. Maternal aggression is another important aspect of the more global concept of maternal behavior. During lactation, mothers become extremely wakeful, and when exposed to potentially dangerous situations, they may attack intruders who threaten their newborns. In this way, they defend their young (Mayer & Rosenblatt, 1987; Rosenblatt, Mayer, & Giordano, 1988).

The neuroendocrine regulation of maternal protective and aggressive behaviors is complex. But oxytocin plays an important coordinating role, not only for milk ejection, maternal caring behaviors, and bonding, but also for the maternal defensive and protective behaviors (Febo et al., 2005; Numan, 2006). Vasopressin, which is chemically related to oxytocin and also produced in the PVN, together with oxytocin via actions in the brain, contributes to the maternal aggression observed in lactating animals (Bosch & Neumann, 2011).

Different strains of rats express more or less "maternal defensive and aggressive behaviors," suggesting that there is a genetic component to the intensity of the expression of these behaviors (Clinton, Bedrosian, Abraham, Watson, & Akil, 2010). Recently, it has been established that epigenetic mechanisms are also involved in shaping the character of newborns. Depending on the signals from the environment, the newborns may become defensive and aggressive or social and relaxed (Caldji, Hellstrom, Zhang, Diorio, & Meaney, 2011). These mechanisms are discussed in more detail in other chapters.

Stress, Unfamiliar Environments, Danger, and Separation Change the Effect Spectrum of Repeated Oxytocin Exposure Towards Increased Anxiety and Stress

How is it possible that oxytocin release may promote anxiety, wakefulness, and aggression during lactation if oxytocin is a substance that induces calm and friendly interaction? The truth is that the effect spectrum that oxytocin induces is context dependent. The effects of oxytocin are always aimed at protecting the offspring. Therefore, exposure to oxytocin can induce aggression and stress effects under certain conditions necessary to ensure the survival of the offspring.

High Stress Levels During Birth

A high activity in the HPA and in the sympathetic nervous system is necessary during labor. Mothers need high cortisol and adrenaline levels to recruit and use energy for labor and high blood pressure to keep the blood flow up in the placenta during contractions to deliver sufficient oxygen and nourishment to the fetus. At the same time, oxytocin levels are high in order to stimulate uterine contractions. Under these conditions, oxytocin promotes high blood pressure. The ability of oxytocin to raise blood pressure is facilitated by the high estrogen levels that prevail during pregnancy and birth (Petersson, Lundeberg, et al., 1999b). The high blood pressure disappears after birth, as estrogen levels drop and oxytocin is released by suckling and tactile stimulation (Jonas, Nissen, Ransjo-Arvidson, Wiklund, Henriksson, et al., 2008; Matthiesen et al., 2001a; Nissen, Lilja, Widstrom, et al., 1995; Nissen et al., 1996; Uvnäs Moberg et al., 1990). As discussed in detail in this book, the anti-stress effects of oxytocin are facilitated when oxytocin is released in response to sensory nerves, as during skin-to-skin contact and breastfeeding.

Increased Stress Reactivity in Unfamiliar Environments

Female (and male) rats that are under the influence of oxytocin become even more afraid and cautious, and more easily stressed in new environments than animals that have not been subjected to oxytocin treatment.

Study rats given five injections of oxytocin had a sustained decrease in blood pressure, which persisted for weeks after the last injection. They were also calmer. If the oxytocin-treated rats were moved to a new environment, they became extremely nervous and started to explore the cage much more than rats that had not received oxytocin. The oxytocin-treated rats were calmer than the control rats, as long as they stayed in their home cage, but became more anxious and explorative than the control rats in an unfamiliar surrounding. As soon as the rats became accustomed to the new environment, their blood pressure resumed to the levels observed in the familiar environment and the animals became calm again and stopped exploring

(Petersson, Ahlenius, Wiberg, Alster, & Uvnäs-Moberg, 1998).

When these two groups of rats were subjected to an unexpected sound while staying in their home cage, the pulse rate and blood pressure of the oxytocin-treated rats rose more than in the control rats. Again, these results show that the oxytocin-treated rats are more anxious and react more to certain types of stressors than do the control rats. The stressors that cause this over-reaction are probably perceived as extremely threatening (Petersson & Uvnäs-Moberg, 2007).

Taken together, it seems as if repeated injections of oxytocin calms rats and lowers their blood pressure, as long as they are close to their offspring in their home cage and nothing unexpected happens. In contrast, they become over-anxious in an unfamiliar surrounding, but as they get used to it, they become calmer than usual in this setting, too. If something potentially dangerous happens suddenly, they overreact. Any lactating female is subject to an intense exposure to endogenous oxytocin and is therefore more cautious in unfamiliar surroundings and is sensitized to stressors. These basic oxytocin-linked stress reactions are most probably biological precursors of the more elaborated maternal aggressive behaviors that occur during lactation.

Separation from Pups

When a rat mother is separated from her pups, she gets anxious and even aggressive after a while. In contrast, closeness to the offspring calms the mother, lowers her cortisol levels, and buffers her stress reactions (Lonstein, 2005). The feeling of anxiety and stress may be one of nature's ways of keeping mothers close to their offspring in the nest, as this will be linked to calm, in addition to pleasure. By contrast, they will become anxious when they are in an unknown, potentially dangerous environment and when something unexpected happens which may endanger them and their offspring.

Protective Strategies in Human Mothers

Remnants of the "synchronizing, hiding, and nest-building strategies" used by other mammals during birth occur in humans, too.

The fact that women who live close together, e.g., in a family or in a dormitory, coordinate their ovulations and menstrual cycles may be a remnant from a time when early humans lived in small groups and were exposed to dangers from big predators (Weller & Weller, 1993, 1997). Synchronized ovulations may have increased the chance of women becoming pregnant at the same time and giving birth at the same time. The mothers and newborns were extremely vulnerable in connection with birth and needed protection. If women gave birth at approximately the same time of the year, the total time needed for defense and protection of the group was restricted.

Human mothers often withdraw before birth, and they still often give birth at night if nature has its way. It is well known that expecting mothers spend time cleaning the house and preparing the nest for the baby to come, a reflection of an innate nest-building behavior.

Inhibition of Oxytocin Release During Labor and Milk Ejection in an Unfamiliar Environment

An inhibition of oxytocin release during labor and breastfeeding, and consequent arrest of labor and milk ejection, may also be observed in women when they are in unfamiliar environments or feel unsafe. It is not uncommon for women who have experienced regular contractions at home to note that the contractions disappear, at least for a while, when they come to the hospital to give birth. This temporary arrest of labor may be a completely natural reaction to the unfamiliar hospital environment. Similarly, many women find that it is easier to breastfeed at home with family and friends than in a public domain with strangers, at least in the beginning of breastfeeding. In some women, oxytocin is simply not released in unknown surroundings to induce milk letdown (Newton, 1992).

From an evolutionary perspective, mothers who give birth or breastfeed are extremely vulnerable and defenseless, and, therefore, it is better to postpone labor and milk ejection until the environment is perceived as safe and familiar.

Increased Levels of Anxiety, Wakefulness, and Aggression in Mothers

In human mothers, several subtle subjective experiences have their roots in the maternal protective behaviors.

Being Close to the Baby is Calming, Separation Causes Anxiety

It is important for the mother to stay close to her newborn child, not leave it, to provide it with food and care, and to protect the newborn from unpredictable dangers. Nature has taken care of this by making mothers feel contented, calm, and relaxed, not only when breastfeeding, but also when close to their infants. When mothers leave their children to go to work or do other things, they experience a kind of separation anxiety. When leaving their baby, they feel as if they have lost something important, as if something is missing. This type of separation anxiety is one, sometimes painful, expression of being bonded or attached to the baby and, of course, it serves to keep or bring mothers and babies together.

Maternal Worry and Responsibility

A mother has to feel responsible for her baby, to be sure that it gets enough food and is well taken care of in every aspect. Feelings of worry and responsibility may resemble feelings of anxiety or guilt. These feelings are expressions of the mother's bonding or attachment to the baby. The more attached a mother is to her baby, the more anxious she may feel in certain situations.

Mothers Who Had Skin-To-Skin Contact After Birth Experience More Worry About Their Infants

The mothers who participated in the St. Petersburg study, which was described in the chapters on skin-to-skin contact, were asked about their levels of anxiety two days after birth when they were not in the presence of their infants. It turned out that the mothers who had skin-to-skin contact with their baby immediately after birth were not only more loving and caring of their babies, they were also more anxious and worried about their infants' wellbeing (Bystrova, Widstrom, Ransjo-Arvidsson, & Uvnäs-Moberg, 2014). As skin-to-skin contact gives rise to increased release of oxytocin during the period after birth and induces oxytocin-related long-term effects, the increased concern about the infant's wellbeing is likely to be due to the increased exposure of oxytocin in the period (Bystrova et al., 2009; Matthiesen et al., 2001a; Nissen, Lilja, Widstrom, et al., 1995). The worry expressed by the mother is yet another expression of a strong maternal bonding to the child.

A similar increase of maternal levels of anxiety was noted in mothers of preterm infants that were allowed more closeness (treatment based on NIDCAP) than in mothers receiving conventional care. In these mothers, more oxytocin was released as a consequence of the increased close contact between mother and infant, which, in turn, caused both an increased sense of closeness to the infant and increased anxiety and worry about the unknown (Kleberg, Hellstrom-Westas, & Widstrom, 2007).

Maternal Aggression and Wakefulness

It is well known that mothers of newborns can become extremely angry, aggressive, and forceful if they experience a threat to their babies. The saying is that they could even move a car that is driving towards their babies.

Even if the mothers don't become overtly aggressive, they may become extremely anxious and tense in situations where the mother thinks the infant is threatened. The triggers may be quite subtle and even non-specific. The stress-related effects are not only activated when the mothers actually feel that they are threatened, but also when they feel that something might happen. The mothers simply become more cautious and wakeful, and they may even look for signs in the sky.

Some women experience anxiety when something unexpected happens. Meeting strangers or being in unknown places may cause severe anxiety and a strong wish to protect or perhaps defend the baby. Phobic reactions never experienced before might appear, such as fear of heights, being in elevators, or being in market places. Some mothers avoid situations that could be potentially dangerous.

In an evolutionary perspective, this makes sense. To be in an unknown place, to climb a high mountain, and to meet people you do not know in a market place involves a certain risk for a mother with her newborn baby. Some mothers simply prefer to stay at home to avoid the unpleasant feelings linked to leaving home.

The horrible news presented by newspapers, radio, and television becomes extra threatening, and mothers of newborns may avoid reading about frightening news or seeing films with violent content.

Stronger Positive and Negative Emotions

Mothers who are bonded to their baby actually have more intense feelings, both positive and negative. As described above, mothers who are close to their infants feel extremely happy and calm. On the other hand, they feel more anxious and unhappy when they are away from their children than those that are not so bonded. Obviously, both pleasant and unpleasant feelings are stronger. Interestingly, these feelings serve to keep the contact between mother and infant. When the mother is separated from her infant, she becomes anxious and feels stressed, which makes her want to be close to the infant to dampen these unpleasant sensations. When she is close to the infant, she feels well, happy, and content, which makes her want to stay close. These are expressions of positive and negative consequences of attachment or bonding.

Opposite Reactions in Human Mothers in Familiar or Unfamiliar Surroundings

In the breastfeeding experiments referred to in chapter 10, maternal blood pressure fell in response to breastfeeding. These measurements were performed at the maternity ward, which provided a very home-like setting, or in the homes of the mothers (Jonas et al., 2009; Nissen et al., 1996). In contrast, when breastfeeding experiments were performed in an unfamiliar surrounding after a short separation between mothers and infants, blood pressure rose in response to breastfeeding (Mezzacappa, Kelsey, Myers, & Katkin, 2001). These results show that mothers who feel safe respond with oxytocin-linked anti-stress effects in response to breastfeeding, whereas a stress response is triggered in unfamiliar surroundings.

Exaggerated Stress Reactions

Women who were breastfeeding also overreacted in a very basic stress test. When they put their hands in cold water, their blood pressure rose more than the controls (Mezzacappa et al., 2001). These reactions probably represent the deep physiological aspects of a maternal defense behavior, since increased blood pressure is linked to aggression. In this way, she not only defended the baby, she also defended herself, because she most likely withdrew her hands more quickly from the cold, potentially dangerous water.

This pattern of exaggerated reactions in breastfeeding

mothers to the known and unknown or safe and unsafe, to closeness or separation, are in line with the results of the basic experiments referred to above in which animals had been exposed to repeated oxytocin administration. Rats subjected to repeated oxytocin treatment were calmer than untreated rats in a well-known environment, but more anxious in a strange environment than animals not treated with oxytocin. They overreacted to some types of intense stressors, and they avoided long-term separations from their offspring (Petersson, Ahlenius, et al., 1998; Petersson & Uvnäs-Moberg, 2007). The effects of oxytocin always favor saving life.

Increased Need of Support

Mothers are not only sensitive to the negative, they are also more open to the positive. They actually need "maternal support" themselves. Positive attitudes and a warm and supportive interaction can create wonders during this period of openness. Supportive care, not only during labor, but also during breastfeeding, increases the wellbeing and self-esteem of the mother and makes her interaction with her child more positive (Ekstrom, Widstrom, & Nissen, 2003). By seeking support, the mothers increase the chance of a positive outcome for herself and the baby.

When Anxiety and Depression Become a Problem

Maternity Blues

Almost all mothers experience a period of sadness and gloom the first days after birth. Maternity blues is a consequence of the big neurohormonal changes that occur during the transition between pregnancy, birth, and breastfeeding. The falling levels of estrogen and progesterone have been implicated in this process. The falling levels of oxytocin are important in the development of maternity blues, which in a sense is a withdrawal or abstinence reaction. It has been claimed that if mothers are allowed skin-to-skin contact after birth, the severity of maternity blues is reduced. If so, the continued release of oxytocin caused by this treatment may be responsible for these positive effects, as they counteract the fall of oxytocin occurring after birth.

Depression and Anxiety

Some mothers are more sensitive to the anxiety/aggression-related aspects of the breastfeeding adaptations. In fact, 20% of breastfeeding mothers suffer from anxiety and depressive symptoms six to eight weeks after birth. These reactions can be severe and very painful to the mothers, and may sometimes need to be treated with medication. The symptoms of anxiety and depression that develop after a few weeks of breastfeeding should not be mixed up with the slight, transient depressive systems or maternity blues that many mothers experience the first days after labor.

There may be several reasons why some women develop

anxiety and depression a few weeks after birth. It is not uncommon that these women have experienced similar episodes of depression and anxiety before. Previous negative life experiences or current stress may facilitate the development of such symptoms.

It is, however, also possible that some women are genetically predisposed to have problems with anxiety and depression during breastfeeding. It is known that some genetic variations in the structure of the serotonin and dopamine may predispose mothers to anxiety and depression. Aberrations in the oxytocin system have also been linked to anxiety and depression. Perhaps the oxytocin-mediated increased sensitivity to certain types of stressors becomes more problematic in individuals that carry certain genetic traits (Jonas et al., 2013; Kim et al., 2013).

Obviously, current environmental factors are also of great importance since the caring and calming aspects of the oxytocin-effect spectrum are preferentially activated in well-known and home-like situations. Therefore, the positive, calming aspects of oxytocin may be more easily triggered and more firmly developed in mothers who are allowed to stay at home with their newborns and receive support from their families.

In contrast, the oxytocin-related anxiety and aggression-related effects are more likely to develop in an unfamiliar environment. What happens to sensitive breastfeeding mothers who have to go back to work within a few weeks after birth? Do these mothers experience more of the negative, stress-related effects of oxytocin, such as anxiety and depression, than those who stay at home? If so, not only genetic programming, but also the mothers' previous and present experiences of stress or support will influence her reaction to oxytocin. Also, economic, cultural, and even political factors may influence the type of oxytocin-related effects that develop in breastfeeding women.

Post Traumatic Stress Disorder (PTSD)

Mothers exposed to high levels of oxytocin are not only calmer in certain situations, they are also more sensitive to certain kinds of stress. What happens if mothers are exposed to severe stress during labor when they are also exposed to high levels of oxytocin? Perhaps some of the severe long-term consequences of very painful and difficult labor or an emergency Cesarean Section, such as post traumatic stress disorder, may be an example of an oxytocin-mediated reinforcement of the stress reactions (Soderquist, Wijma, Thorbert, & Wijma, 2009; Wijma, Soderquist, & Wijma, 1997).

Perhaps the oxytocin influence during labor and in the period actually opens up for both increased calm and social interaction and also for stress reactions. The environment decides the direction. The warmer and more supportive the environment is, the less the chance of negative consequences of birth. In contrast, a cold and hostile environment may increase the chance of developing negative consequences

after birth and in the period (Ford & Ayers, 2009, 2011).

Summary

- All mammals use different protective strategies in the care of their young. They hide and build nests, and they defend their offspring from environmental dangers and intruders—maternal aggression.

- Oxytocin plays an important role in several of these aspects of maternal aggression since repeated exposure to oxytocin increases the sensitivity and reaction to separation from the infant, and to novel environments. Further, it increases the stress reaction to certain kinds of life-threatening stress.

- Human mothers express similar adaptations. Labor, skin-to-skin contact, and breastfeeding are associated with oxytocin release and, therefore, an increased propensity for not only caring, but also protective behaviors. As the mother becomes bonded to the infant, separation from the infant gives rise to anxiety, which is relieved upon reunion.

- The mothers feel calm when they are at home or in a familiar or "safe" environment. If they are in an environment that they consider unsafe and if they feel that something threatens their baby, an opposite reaction pattern develops. They may become cautious, suspicious, and sometimes overtly aggressive. All these adaptations, which are reinforced by oxytocin, are aimed at protecting the infant.

- Skin-to-skin contact immediately after birth, i.e., during the sensitive period, stimulates both mothers' and infants' future interaction and dampens their stress reactivity. It is possible that stress in connection with birth may cause an opposite reaction pattern, i.e., inhibition of social interaction, increased anxiety, and increased stress reactivity.

- Genetic vulnerability and previous experiences of anxiety and stress increase the chance of developing anxiety and depression during breastfeeding.

Chapter 17

Anti-Stress Effects During Lactation: Role of Suckling and Oxytocin

Not only milk production and milk ejection are driven by the suckling stimulus, maternal physiology and behavior/psychology are also subjected to many changes during the lactation period in order to facilitate adaptation to motherhood. In the previous chapter, some maternal protective strategies were described that may create aggression or defense reactions in the mother, e.g., certain types of stress which are or may be perceived as threatening to the newborn. The mother may also overreact to some types of physical stress.

In contrast, maternal reactions to some types of stress are reduced and her basal stress levels are reduced. The reason for this is that the mother should focus her attention on the newborn and direct her energy towards milk production. Oxytocin released in response to suckling participates in the control of some of these adaptations. For example, oxytocin released from nerves projecting from the PVN to areas involved in the control of autonomic nervous function and of the HPA axis in the brainstem area and in the hypothalamus are involved in these anti-stress effects. The following two chapters will be devoted to the role of suckling-related oxytocin release in the regulation of stress levels.

Anti-Stress Effects in Lactating Animals

Increasing the levels of calm and reducing stress levels and stress reactions during lactation may serve many functions. It may divert maternal interest from irrelevant stimuli in the environment, thereby helping the mother focus her attention on the offspring. It may serve an even more basic function. By being calm and avoiding unnecessary stress reactions or physical movement, energy is saved. In this way, more calories may be used for milk production and the caloric demands of the offspring are ensured. Reduction of unnecessary energy expenditure is also achieved by a decrease of some aspects of the activity of the HPA axis and the sympathetic nervous system, and thereby unnecessary heat production or catabolic processes. The expressions of these adaptations vary between species as they are linked to the reproductive style of the different species and to how and under what circumstances they live.

Calm

Some lactating animals have to stay still for varying periods of time when they are giving milk to their offspring. The suckling stimulus activates mechanisms related to calm in the mother, which "helps" the mother stay in her nest. In some species, milk ejection is related to decreased consciousness. Rat mothers exhibit a slow wave EEG during suckling, and no milk can be ejected unless the mother is "partly unconscious" (Lincoln et al., 1980; Voloschin & Tramezzani, 1979). This is not the case in pigs or rabbits, probably because they have to be more watchful during milk letdown than rat mothers, who hide in a dark place while nursing (Neve, Paisley, & Summerlee, 1982; Poulain, Rodriguez, & Ellendorff, 1981).

Reduced Physical Activity

Some lactating animals reduce their physical activity and stay in the nest for long periods of times during lactation. By reducing physical activity during the lactation period, they focus on their offspring and save large amounts of calories that can be used for milk production and growth of the pups. When weaning, these animals leave their offspring and return to normal activities. For example, hamsters kept in a cage spend large amounts of their time running on a wheel. Lactating hamsters spend most of their time with their pups and avoid running on the wheel. As soon as they wean their offspring, they resume running on the wheel. The decreased motor activity during lactation is linked to decreased activity in dopaminergic neurons in the striatum.

Reduced Reactivity to Certain Types of Stress

In addition, the reactivity to certain types of stressors is reduced in lactating animals. Rat mothers exposed to unexpected noise or light react less to these stimuli than non-lactating rats. The importance of some stressors, which are not linked to the protection of the offspring are down regulated (Neumann, 2001, 2002). The calming and reduced reactivity to the stress-reducing effect of suckling has been described in previous chapters.

Reduced Activity in the Sympathetic Nervous System and the HPA Axis

Rats have lower blood pressure during lactation than during pregnancy or other periods of life. The lowering of blood pressure is driven by the suckling stimulus and is mediated by a decreased tone in the aspects of the sympathetic nervous system that controls blood pressure. Still, blood flow to the mammary glands is increased, illustrating the complex change in the function of the cardiovascular system during lactation.

Cortisol Levels

In several mammalian species, such as rats and cows, cortisol levels are increased in response to suckling (Gorewit, Svennersten, Butler, & Uvnäs-Moberg, 1992). Cortisol is important for recruitment of energy for milk production and contributes to the stimulation of milk production.

In contrast, regular stroking of the abdominal area decreases both pulse rate and cortisol levels in cows, and in some species, suckling also decreases cortisol levels. Lowering of cortisol levels is linked to saving energy.

This complicated energy equation has been solved in sometimes opposing ways in different mammalian species, depending on how they live, how many pups they need to feed, and so forth. In some species, cortisol levels are higher than during other periods of life and in some they are lower. In both cases they represent adaptations to provide energy to the offspring in the best way.

Role of Suckling and Oxytocin in the Inhibition of the Sympathetic Nervous System and the HPA Axis During Lactation

The structure and function of the sympathetic nervous system and the HPA axis, and the inhibitory effects exerted by oxytocin on these systems, as well as how oxytocin is released in response to suckling, was described in great detail in previous chapters. A short summary of these mechanisms will be given below to allow understanding of the mechanisms behind the oxytocin-mediated anti-stress effects caused by suckling.

The Sympathetic Nervous System and the HPA Axis

The sympathetic nervous system and the HPA axis represent two individual aspects of the stress system. The neurogenic sympathetic nervous system induces very quick responses, whereas the endocrine HPA axis reacts more slowly. The mechanisms involved have been described in great detail in previous chapters and only a short summary will be given here.

The sympathetic nerves innervate and activate the function of the cardiovascular system, the lungs, and the gastrointestinal and genitourinary organs. Noradrenaline is the main transmitter substance in the sympathetic nervous system. The adrenal medulla, which produces adrenaline, is part of the sympathetic system.

Cortisol is secreted from the adrenal cortex and is of major importance for all reactions linked to activity and stress. It is released by adrenocorticotrophic hormone (ACTH) from the anterior pituitary and the secretion of ACTH is regulated by corticotrophin-releasing hormone (CRF), which is produced in parvocellular neurons in the paraventricular nucleus of the hypothalamus (PVN). The release of CRF is under inhibitory control from neurons

in the hippocampus. The HPA axis is under inhibitory control by cortisol released from the adrenal cortex, as it inhibits the secretion of CRF and ACTH via feedback (inhibitory loops).

The activity of the sympathetic nervous system and the HPA axis is influenced from many brain regions. The noradrenergic fibers that originate in the Locus Coeruleus (LC) and which are activated in response to stress, play an important regulatory role in both systems. In addition, noxious or painful sensory stimuli may activate noradrenergic fibers in the nucleus tractus solitarius (NTS), which stimulate the activity of the HPA axis and the sympathetic nervous system.

Reciprocal Activation of Brainstem and Hypothalamic Stress Systems

The noradrenergic neurons from the LC and NTS exert a strong influence on the secretion of CRF from the hypothalamus and thereby the activity of the HPA axis. At the same time, CRF-containing nerve fibers, projecting from PVN to areas in the brainstem, exert a stimulatory effect on areas involved in the control of the function of brainstem areas involved in stress regulation, e.g., the LC, the rostroventrolateral medulla (RVLM), an important center for regulation of blood pressure, and the NTS. In this way, the function of the hypothalamic and the brainstem stress systems are interrelated.

Administration of Oxytocin Inhibits the Effect of the Sympathetic Nervous System and the HPA Axis

Oxytocin and Blood Pressure

Administration of oxytocin may increase or decrease blood pressure, depending on experimental conditions, by acting on different sites involved in the control of blood pressure. When oxytocin is administered into the brain, blood pressure decreases after a certain delay. After repeated administration of oxytocin, a long-term decrease of blood pressure is induced (Petersson et al., 1996b; Petersson, Hulting, Anderson, et al., 1999).

The oxytocin-mediated decrease of blood pressure is induced as a consequence of decreased activity in the sympathetic nerves, which regulate the function in the cardiovascular system. Oxytocinergic neurons originating in the paraventricular nucleus (PVN) project to many regions involved in cardiovascular control, such as the nucleus tractus solitarius (NTS), nucleus ambiguus, Locus Coeruleus (LC) the dorsal motor nucleus of the vagus nerve (DMX), the raphe nuclei, the rostroventrolateral medulla (RVLM), and the intermediolateral cell column in the thoracolumbar segments of the spinal cord and, therefore, these areas may have been involved in the decrease of blood pressure induced by oxytocin (Petersson et al., 1996b; Petersson, Lundeberg, et al., 1999b).

Oxytocin and the HPA Axis

Administration of oxytocin results in a decrease of cortisol levels (Petersson, Hulting, & Uvnäs-Moberg, 1999). Oxytocin may decrease cortisol secretion by several parallel mechanisms. Oxytocin released within the PVN decreases CRF secretion. Oxytocin released from nerves in the anterior pituitary decreases the secretion of ACTH. Oxytocin in the circulation decreases cortisol secretion directly from the adrenals. As will be described more in the chapters on skin-to-skin contact, oxytocin also influences cortisol secretion by actions in areas in the brainstem involved in the control of sympathetic nervous tone.

Long-Term Effect on Blood Pressure and HPA Axis

Repeated exposure to oxytocin is associated with sustained anti-stress effects, e.g., a decrease of blood pressure and cortisol levels. The long-term decrease of blood pressure caused by repeated exposure to oxytocin seems to be mediated by activation of a specific kind of receptors, alpha-2 adrenoceptors, which exert inhibitory actions on noradrenergic transmission in the brain. This effect of oxytocin has been demonstrated by neurophysiological, immunohistochemical, pharmacological, and physiological techniques (Petersson, Eklund, & Uvnäs-Moberg, 2005; Petersson, Lundeberg, et al., 1999a; Petersson, Uvnäs-Moberg, Erhardt, & Engberg, 1998).

The sustained decrease of cortisol levels may involve an increased function of alpha-2 receptors discussed above and also a change in the function of other mechanisms involved in the regulation of the HPA axis in the brain. For example, the function of the GR and MR receptors in the hippocampus is changed after repeated exposure of oxytocin (Petersson, Hulting, Andersson, et al., 1999; Petersson & Uvnäs-Moberg, 2003).

Decreased Activity in the Noradrenergic Neurons of the LC

Administration of oxytocin has been demonstrated to induce an anxiolytic effect (Uvnäs-Moberg et al., 1994). The anxiolytic effect is exerted in the amygdala and the reaction to stress is reduced. As a consequence of the reduced stress reactivity, the activity of the noradrenergic nerves in the LC is decreased, and thereby the activity in the sympathetic nervous system and the HPA axis, as the activity of both these systems are stimulated by noradrenaline.

Suckling Stimulates Oxytocin Release via Activation of Somatosensory Nerves

Oxytocin is released from magnocellular neurons in the SON and PVN into the circulation in response to suckling to induce the milk ejection reflex. It is also released from oxytocinergic nerves originating from parvocellular neurons in the PVN, which project to many different areas in the brain. Some oxytocinergic nerves project to the hypothalamus and areas in the brainstem involved

in the control of the HPA axis and the sympathetic nervous system. These oxytocinergic nerves are of utmost importance for the oxytocin-mediated anti-stress effects caused by suckling.

Neurogenic Pathways Involved in Oxytocin Release by Suckling

During suckling, both somatosensory nerves, originating in the nipple and entering the central nervous system via the spinal cord, and sensory nerves, that bypass the spinal cord and project directly to the NTS—"the vagal nerve afferents"—are activated (Eriksson, Lindh, et al., 1996).

On their way to the hypothalamus, the neurogenic impulses induced by suckling relay in the NTS. In this area, afferent nervous pathways that connect with the SON and PVN of the hypothalamus are activated. As the magnocellular oxytocin-containing neurons are activated, oxytocin is released into the circulation, and as the parvocellular oxytocin-containing neurons are activated, oxytocin is released into the brain.

Suckling Induces Oxytocin Release from Parvocellular Neurons Projecting to the Hypothalamus and Brainstem

Some of the anti-stress effects induced by suckling, e.g., the lowering of blood pressure in nursing rats, are due to a release of oxytocin from parvocellular neurons emanating in the PVN, projecting to brainstem areas involved in the control of the activity of the sympathetic nervous system, such as nucleus tractus (NTS), nucleus ambiguus, Locus Coeruleus (LC), the dorsal motor nucleus of the vagus nerve (DMX), the rostroventrolateral medulla (RVLM), and the intermediolateral cell column in the thoracolumbar segments of the spinal cord (Buijs, 1983; Buijs et al., 1985; Sofroniew, 1983; Stern & Zhang, 2003; Zerihun & Harris, 1983; Zimmerman et al., 1984).

Oxytocin released from oxytocinergic fibers emanating from parvocellular neurons in the PVN in response to suckling may also be involved in the control of the HPA axis. Oxytocin-containing fibers reach areas in the hypothalamus and the anterior pituitary involved in the control of the HPA axis (Buijs et al., 1985; Sofroniew, 1983).

Decrease of Stress Levels and Stress Buffering

As the noradrenergic tone in the LC is lowered by suckling, the reactivity to certain types of stress responses will also be decreased. In this way, oxytocin released in response to suckling not only induces a direct anti-stress effect on the HPA axis and the sympathetic nervous system, it also dampens the effects of stress in the LC and may therefore also exert a stress-buffering effect.

Long-Term Effects

When the LC, the NTS, and adjacent areas involved in the control of autonomic tone are repeatedly exposed to oxytocin during suckling, the function of the alpha-2 receptors gradually increases. As a consequence, the activity in the central noradrenergic system and the sympathetic nervous system is reduced in a long-term way and the function of other transmitter systems may also be increased (Diaz-Cabiale et al., 2000; Petersson, Eklund, et al., 2005; Petersson, Hulting, Andersson, et al., 1999; Petersson, Uvnäs-Moberg, et al., 1998).

Summary

- Suckling induces calm in lactating animals.

- Suckling may reduce physical activity in lactating animals.

- Suckling reduces reactivity to stressors that do not activate protection of the offspring.

- Suckling reduces basal energy expenditure.

- All these adaptations help the mother focus on her offspring and use energy for milk production.

- The effects are induced via suckling-induced oxytocin release in the brain.

- Oxytocinergic fibers projecting to brainstem areas involved in the control of stress reactions and sympathetic nervous tone, and oxytocinergic fibers within the hypothalamus, play a major role in these anti-stress reactions.

Chapter 18

Anti-Stress Effects in Breastfeeding Mothers

As described in the last chapter, lactating animals become calmer, reduce their physical activity, and react less intensely to certain kinds of stressors. In addition, lactation is linked to decreased blood pressure and sometimes reduced activity of the HPA axis. As described in a previous chapter, breastfeeding mothers are less anxious and calmer than non-breastfeeding mothers both in a short-term and a more long-term perspective.

In this chapter, we will focus on the effect on blood pressure and the HPA axis in response to suckling in breastfeeding mothers. These effects are induced by a suckling-induced release of oxytocin into the hypothalamus and, above all, into the brainstem areas involved in the control of autonomic nervous tone.

Clinical Studies

In order to characterize suckling-related anti-stress effects in breastfeeding women, Nissen et al. and Jonas et al. have studied the effect of breastfeeding on blood pressure and cortisol levels in a short- and long-term perspective.

1. Seventeen mothers with emergency Cesarean section and 20 mothers with normal vaginal delivery participated in the study. The children were put directly to the breast after a period of separation and helped to initiate breastfeeding by the midwife. Twenty-four blood samples were collected before, during, and after breastfeeding. Cortisol levels were measured in nine of the samples. (As mentioned previously, oxytocin and prolactin levels were analyzed in all of the samples.) Blood pressure was measured before breastfeeding and 60 minutes after breastfeeding (Nissen et al., 1996).

2. Seventy-two primiparous women were included in the study. Some had received medical interventions, such as epidural analgesia and administration of oxytocin, during labor, which will be described in detail in a later chapter. The infants were put in skin-to-skin contact on the mothers' chest before breastfeeding, and they initiated breastfeeding themselves. Twenty-four blood samples were collected in 63 mothers. Oxytocin and prolactin levels were determined. In addition, cortisol levels were measured in eight samples and ACTH levels in nine samples. Oxytocin levels were measured by ELISA. The duration of skin-to-skin contact before suckling and the duration of suckling were measured. Blood pressure was measured four times before and after breastfeeding in 66 of the

women. In a subgroup of these mothers (33), blood pressure was measured repeatedly before and after breastfeeding during a six-month period (Handlin et al., 2009; Jonas, Nissen, Ransjo-Arvidson, Wiklund, et al., 2008).

Main Results

- Blood pressure is decreased in response to suckling at each breastfeeding episode (Nissen et al., 1996; Jonas, Nissen, Ransjo-Arvidson, Wiklund, et al., 2008).
- Cortisol levels are decreased in response to suckling at each breastfeeding episode (Nissen et al., 1996; Handlin et al., 2009).
- ACTH levels decrease in response to suckling during each breastfeeding episode (Handlin et al., 2009).
- The decrease of ACTH levels is larger, the longer the period of breastfeeding (Handlin et al., 2009).
- ACTH levels are inversely related to oxytocin levels (Handlin et al., 2009).
- Blood pressure and cortisol levels, but not ACTH levels, decrease in response to skin-to-skin contact before breastfeeding (Handlin et al., 2009; Jonas, Nissen, Ransjo-Arvidson, Wiklund, et al., 2008).
- The decrease of blood pressure and cortisol levels in response to skin-to-skin contact is associated with each other (Handlin et al., 2009).
- Basal levels of blood pressure decrease after six weeks of suckling and remain decreased during the entire period of breastfeeding (Jonas, Nissen, Ransjo-Arvidson, Wiklund, et al., 2008).

Influence of Suckling on Blood Pressure, Cortisol, and ACTH Levels

Blood Pressure

In both of the above studies, blood pressure fell in response to suckling. The results from the study, in which blood pressure was monitored more frequently, demonstrate that blood pressure fell within minutes of starting breastfeeding and continued to fall during the 30- to 60-minute observation period. A significant fall in both systolic and diastolic blood pressure, amounting to around 10 mm Hg, was noted (Jonas, Nissen, Ransjo-Arvidson, Wiklund, et al., 2008; Nissen et al., 1996).

Cortisol and ACTH Levels

The results from both studies in which cortisol levels were measured repeatedly during a 60-minute breastfeeding period showed that each time a mother breastfeeds her cortisol levels decrease. In both studies, the fall of blood pressure was preceded by a brief increase in cortisol levels (Handlin et al., 2009; Nissen et al., 1996). ACTH levels were shown to parallel cortisol levels in the sense that they also fell after an initial rise, which preceded that of cortisol (Handlin et al., 2009).

Suckling-Related Anti-stress Effects

Both studies demonstrate that blood pressure and cortisol levels fall in response to a breastfeeding session, reflecting a decreased activity of those aspects of the sympathetic nervous system that are involved in the control of blood pressure, as well as a lower activity in the HPA axis. These results are in line with data published by other authors showing that blood pressure and cortisol levels fall in response to breastfeeding (Amico, Johnston, & Vagnucci, 1994; Heinrichs et al., 2001; Light et al., 2000).

Skin-to-Skin Contact Decreases Blood Pressure and Cortisol Secretion

Skin-to-skin contact before actual suckling contributed to the fall in blood pressure and the decrease in cortisol levels during breastfeeding (Jonas, Nissen, Ransjo-Arvidson, Wiklund, et al., 2008). The mechanism underlying suckling and skin-to-skin-induced anti-stress effects are partly the same and partly different. These mechanisms and the differences between them will be highlighted below.

Suckling Stimulates Oxytocin Release in the Anterior Pituitary

The Decrease of ACTH Levels Related to the Duration of Suckling

Interestingly, the decrease of ACTH levels was related to the duration of suckling. The longer the period of suckling the lower the ACTH levels were. A similar but positive association between the levels prolactin and duration of suckling has also been established and was described in a previous chapter. These data suggest that suckling activates pathways in the anterior pituitary, which both decreases the secretion of ACTH and increases prolactin secretion (Nissen et al., 1996; Handlin et al., 2009).

Inverse Relationship Between Oxytocin and ACTH

The ACTH levels were inversely correlated to the oxytocin levels, i.e., the higher the oxytocin levels were in response to suckling the lower the ACTH levels. As oxytocin inhibits the secretion of both CRH in the hypothalamus and ACTH from the anterior pituitary, this inverse relationship may reflect the inhibitory action of oxytocin on the HPA axis at the hypothalamic and/or pituitary level (Handlin et

al., 2009).

Positive Relationship Between Oxytocin and Prolactin

As described in a previous chapter, oxytocin and prolactin levels in response to suckling are positively correlated (Jonas et al., 2009). As oxytocin exerts stimulatory actions on the lactotrophs in the pituitary whereby prolactin is released, the correlation reflects a stimulatory effect of oxytocin on prolactin release (Samson et al., 1986).

Oxytocin the Key

The nervous pathways by which oxytocin inhibits the secretion of ACTH and stimulates the secretion of prolactin may be identical. Recent findings demonstrate that some oxytocin neurons, which project to the posterior pituitary and release oxytocin into the circulation, send axon collaterals to the anterior pituitary (Pittman et al., 1981; Knobloch et al., 2012). This anatomical arrangement would explain why changes in circulating oxytocin levels parallel oxytocin-induced effects in the anterior pituitary, since oxytocin would induce a parallel decrease in ACTH and an increase in prolactin levels by nervous actions in the anterior pituitary. Another possibility would be that oxytocin fibers from the PVN, which project to the anterior pituitary, decrease the levels of ACTH and stimulate prolactin secretion and that oxytocin is released into the circulation from the posterior pituitary at the same time. In either case, the release of oxytocin into the circulation represents a parallel phenomenon to the release of oxytocin occurring in the anterior pituitary, which is responsible for the influence on the release of ACTH and prolactin.

Oxytocin Inhibits the Secretion of CRH in the Hypothalamus

As oxytocin also inhibits the secretion of CRH in the hypothalamus, the inverse relationship between oxytocin and ACTH levels may also reflect the inhibitory action of oxytocin on the HPA axis at the hypothalamic level.

Suckling and Skin-to-Skin Contact Stimulate Oxytocin Release in the Anterior Pituitary and in the Brainstem

Breastfeeding consists not only of suckling, but also of different types of tactile interaction.

The fall in cortisol levels, as well as the fall of blood pressure during breastfeeding, was related to duration of skin-to-skin contact before breastfeeding (Handlin et al., 2009).

No relationship was established between the duration of skin-to-skin contact before suckling and the levels of ACTH and oxytocin (Handlin et al., 2009).

Skin-to-Skin Contact Induces Oxytocin Effects at the Brainstem Level

The decrease in cortisol levels in response to skin-to-skin

contact was closely linked to the decrease in blood pressure, indicating a correlation between decrease in sympathetic nervous tone involved in the regulation of blood pressure and the decreased activity in the HPA axis (Agren, Lundeberg, et al., 1997).

As described in great detail in the previous chapter, the activity of the HPA axis, the LC, and other areas involved in sympathetic nervous tone are linked in several ways. The noradrenergic systems, originating in the LC and the NTS, not only promote the activity in the sympathetic nervous system, they also potentiate the activity of the CRF neurons, which regulate the activity in the HPA axis. The effect is reciprocal and, a sub-population of CRF neurons emanating in the PVN project to and stimulate the activity in the LC, NTS, and other areas involved in stress reactions. Thus, the function of the stress systems in the hypothalamus and the brainstem is highly integrated.

Sympathetic nerve activity may influence the HPA axis in yet another way. The sympathetic nerves innervating the adrenal cortex potentiate the function of the ACTH receptors in the adrenal cortex. In this way, the ACTH receptors on the adrenal cortex become more sensitive to the effects of ACTH and less ACTH is needed to release cortisol.

Release of Oxytocin in Response to Skin-to-Skin Contact

Touch or skin-to-skin contact results in a release of oxytocin, not always from the magnocellular neurons, but particularly from the oxytocin-producing neurons projecting from the PVN to the areas in the brainstem involved in stress regulation—the LC, the RVLM, and the NTS.

As described in detail in previous chapters, sensory stimulation, such as touch and skin-to-skin contact, results in a direct inhibitory effect of sympathetic nervous tone by actions in the brainstem nuclei involved in the regulation of this function, an effect which is then potentiated by oxytocin released from the oxytocinergic fibers projecting from the PVN to these regulatory areas in the brainstem. In addition, the release of oxytocin is promoted as the activity of the sensory nerves in the NTS is promoted. Thirdly, oxytocin released into the brainstem by increasing the function of alpha-2 adrenoceptors induces a profound inhibition of the activity in the noradrenergic fibers, which emanate in the NTS, LC, and other areas in the brainstem area and are involved in the control of the HPA axis and the sympathetic nervous system.

By these different mechanisms, oxytocin will decrease the activity of the HPA axis and the sympathetic nervous system. One consequence of the decreased function of the sympathetic nervous system is that cortisol secretion from the adrenal cortex decreases. As the activity in the sympathetic nervous system decreases, the ACTH receptors become less sensitive and less cortisol is released in response to ACTH (Stachowiak et al., 1995). Activation

of this mechanism may explain why cortisol levels, but not ACTH levels, were influenced by skin-to-skin contact during breastfeeding.

By this web-like effect pattern, sensory stimulation emanating in the skin results in an oxytocin-mediated profound reduction of stress levels without necessarily involving the oxytocin neurons that secrete oxytocin into the circulation and, at the same time, via axon collaterals that influence the release of hormones in the anterior pituitary.

Decreased Sympathetic Nervous Tone also Involves Facilitation of the Milk Ejection Reflex

As was described in the chapter on neurogenic control of milk ejection, the suckling stimulus not only induces milk ejection by releasing oxytocin, it also facilitates the role of oxytocin by local neurogenic mechanisms (activation of axon reflexes) and by decreasing sympathetic nervous tone. In fact, the suckling-related decrease of the activity in the sympathetic nerves innervating the milk ducts and blood vessels of the mammary glands reflects just one aspect of a more generalized decrease in sympathetic nervous tone aimed at facilitating lactation.

Contribution of Sensory Fibers from the Skin

As was pointed out in the chapter in which the neurogenic control of milk ejection was described, stimulation of sensory nerves contributes to the decreased sympathetic tone facilitating the milk-ejection reflex. The same is true for the anti-stress effects of suckling, i.e., decreased blood pressure, lowered activity in the HPA axis, and other types of sensory stimuli contribute to the effects. Touch and warm temperature stimulates afferent nerves originating in the skin overlying the mammary glands and the chest to trigger oxytocin release. Therefore, touch-induced effects contribute to the anti-stress effects observed during lactation.

Paradoxical Increase in Blood Pressure During Breastfeeding

Not all studies demonstrate a decrease of blood pressure in response to breastfeeding. In one study, blood pressure actually increased in response to breastfeeding. This study was performed in a laboratory setting, which was unfamiliar to the breastfeeding women and might have been considered unsafe. As a result, release of oxytocin is linked to activation of defense reactions, which involve an increase in blood pressure (Mezzacappa et al., 2001). The studies performed by Nissen, Jonas, and Handlin were all performed in a very home-like setting in the maternity ward and, therefore, the oxytocin-related anti-stress pattern was promoted in response to suckling (Handlin et al., 2009; Jonas, Nissen, Ransjo-Arvidson, Wiklund, et al., 2008; Nissen et al., 1996). This reversed type of reaction is discussed in more detail in the chapter on maternal protective strategies. When mothers feel threatened or simply are in an unfamiliar environment, oxytocin release and effects in response to breastfeeding are changed and may be linked to activation of defense mechanisms. An increase in blood pressure is part of such a defense reaction.

Long-Term Anti-stress Effects

After some weeks of breastfeeding, basal blood pressure had decreased by around 10-15 mm Hg and stayed low during the entire period of breastfeeding. Still, blood pressure continued to fall in connection with each breastfeeding session (Jonas, Nissen, Ransjo-Arvidson, Wiklund, et al., 2008).

Basal blood pressure continues to decrease as breastfeeding goes on. Some studies also demonstrate that it becomes difficult for breastfeeding mothers to recruit cortisol in response to physical activity, a sign of a long-term inhibition of the function in the HPA axis (Altemus et al., 2001).

Other Expressions of a Long-Term Decreased Sympathetic Nervous Tone in Breastfeeding Women

As described above, the decrease in blood pressure, both during a breastfeed and during the entire breastfeeding period, is due to a decreased sympathetic nervous tone in response to oxytocin released by skin-to-skin and by suckling.

There are other expressions of a changed balance in the autonomic nervous system, suggesting that breastfeeding women have a higher parasympathetic tone and a lower sympathetic tone. These effects were described in a previous chapter and will only be summarized here.

Breastfeeding Versus Bottle Feeding

One way to establish such effects on autonomic nervous function is to compare breastfeeding women with bottle-feeding women. Breastfeeding women are repeatedly exposed to a release of oxytocin in response to suckling and touch, whereas bottle-feeding mothers are only exposed to touch and skin-to-skin contact. Therefore, breastfeeding can be expected to be associated with a more pronounced pattern of oxytocin-mediated anti-stress effects. Breastfeeding is related to an increased parasympathetic modulation of heart function. It is also associated with a lower heart rate than bottle feeding, which may be due to an increased parasympathetic tone and a decreased sympathetic tone. Further evidence of a decreased sympathetic nervous input on cardiovascular function in breastfeeding women is that they have a longer pre-ejection period when compared to bottle feeders (Mezzacappa et al., 2001). Breastfeeding women also have increased electrodermal reactivity and greater skin conductance than bottle-feeding women, a further sign of reduced sympathetic tone (Mezzacappa et al., 2005). The levels of catecholamines in the circulation are lower in breastfeeding women, probably as a consequence of reduced sympatho-adrenal activity (Altemus et al., 2001). All these effects are linked to the frequent release of oxytocin in breastfeeding women as discussed previously.

Lifelong Effects of Breastfeeding?

No doubt most physiological adaptations linked to breastfeeding disappear after some time. Still, it is possible that some of the effects remain, albeit in a weakened form for a very long time.

It has been shown that pregnant women have lower blood pressure in the beginning of their second pregnancy compared to their first (Strevens, Kristensen, Langhoff-Roos, & Wide-Swensson, 2002; Strevens, Wide-Swensson, & Ingemarsson, 2001). This may be due to the fact that their alpha-2 adrenoceptors or other mechanisms involved in autonomic nervous tone have been sensitized during the first pregnancy and breastfeeding, and that they are then more easily reactivated when estrogen and oxytocin levels rise during the second pregnancy. Also, long-term inhibition of cortisol secretion and perhaps of other functions may have been induced, but not yet demonstrated.

A long-term enhancement of alpha-2 adrenoceptor sensitivity, including a facilitated insulin secretion, may be linked to enhanced weight gain, since more of the ingested calories are used for storing and anabolic purposes, unless catabolic mechanisms are activated at the same time. Some women notice that it is not only difficult to get rid of the extra weight gained during pregnancy and breastfeeding, they may also put on weight more easily after childbirth. Perhaps the tendency to put on weight is another consequence of sensitized alpha-2 receptors. The effect of breastfeeding on metabolism will be discussed in more detail in the subsequent chapters.

Long-Term Health-Promoting Effects

Another sign of long-lasting anti-stress effects of breastfeeding are the findings that women who have given birth to and breastfed children have a reduced chance of developing several types of stress-related diseases, e.g., cardiovascular disease, many years later. The risk for hypertension, stroke, heart infarction, and diabetes type 2 is reduced in a "dose dependent" manner in women who have breastfed. The more children a woman has given birth to and the longer she has breastfed, the stronger the preventive effect. Perhaps an increased activity in some of the alpha-2 receptor populations or long-term changes of the activity in other transmitter systems in the brain protects them by buffering their reactions to stressful experiences long after the end of breastfeeding (Lee, Kim, Jee, & Yang, 2005; Stuebe, Rich-Edwards, Willett, Manson, & Michels, 2005; Stuebe et al., 2011).

Summary

- Breastfeeding is associated with potent anti-stress effects.

- Each breastfeeding session is followed by a decrease in blood pressure, ACTH, and cortisol levels.

- Breastfeeding consists of both suckling and touch or skin-to-skin contact.

- The duration of suckling is associated with the decrease in ACTH levels.

- Circulating oxytocin is elevated by suckling, and oxytocin levels correlate with a lowered level of ACTH. These results suggest that oxytocin is released into the anterior pituitary during suckling to decrease ACTH secretion (and to increase prolactin secretion). Oxytocin is released in parallel into the circulation.

- The duration of skin-to-skin contact is associated with lower blood pressure and cortisol levels and the size of these effects correlate strongly. These effects mainly involve activation of oxytocin neurons projecting from the PVN to the regulatory centers in the brainstem, such as the LC and the NTS.

- Basal blood pressure decreases over the entire breastfeeding period.

- The long-term effects of breastfeeding are induced by oxytocin-mediated changes in the function of other signaling and receptor systems, e.g., alpha-2 adrenoceptors.

- The anti-stress effects induced by breastfeeding may serve to help mothers concentrate on breastfeeding the infant and saving energy.

- The anti-stress effects may last for a long time after breastfeeding ends, and may protect against stress for a very long time. Such effects may explain why women who have breastfed have a lower risk of developing certain types of cardiovascular disease, such as stroke, hypertension and heart infarction, and diabetes type 2.

Chapter 19

Effects on Digestion and Metabolism During Lactation: Role of Oxytocin and Neurogenic Mechanisms

Need for Efficient Handling of Nutrients

Pregnancy and lactation are energy-demanding processes. Therefore, the mother needs extra calories in order to allow the unborn and born offspring to grow. The mother's appetite may increase during gestation and lactation, and she may eat more to cover the need for extra calories. But if sufficient supplies of food are not available, there are several other ways the mother can use her own energy in a more efficient way. This may be achieved by reducing unnecessary energy expenditure, e.g., by reducing stress levels and the use of calories as fuel in the muscles as was discussed in the previous chapter. Another way is by optimizing digestion, absorption, and metabolism of food. In the following chapters, these physiological adaptations will be described and how they are linked to the suckling stimulus and oxytocin release during lactation will be explained (Uvnäs-Moberg, 1989, 1996; Uvnäs-Moberg, Widstrom, Marchini, & Winberg, 1987).

The Endocrine System of the Gastrointestinal Tract

The endocrine system of the gastrointestinal tract is the largest hormone-producing gland in the body. The gastrointestinal hormones, such as gastrin, cholecystokinin (CCK), and secretin, facilitate and optimize digestion of food by actions in the gastrointestinal tract. They also reinforce the release of insulin from the pancreas, thereby stimulating the storage of nutrients (the incretin effect). In contrast, the pancreatic hormone glucagon stimulates recruitment of energy. The hormone somatostatin, which is present in both the gastrointestinal tract and the pancreas, inhibits gastrointestinal and pancreatic function, and thereby growth, since the availability of nutrients needed for growth is diminished.

Some of the gastrointestinal hormones, e.g., CCK, influence functions in the brain by activation of afferent, sensory fibers in the vagal nerve. In this way, food intake releases CCK in the small intestine, which, in turn, activates vagal afferents. As a consequence of the afferent vagal nerve activity, satiety, and postprandial sedation is induced. In addition, oxytocin is released and some oxytocin-related functions are induced in the brain.

The release of gastrin, CCK, and insulin are partly under positive control by the vagal nerve (part of the parasympathetic nervous system), whereas somatostatin is mainly under inhibitory control by the vagal nerves. The vagally mediated inhibition of somatostatin release is mediated by cholinergic mechanisms. In contrast, the release of somatostatin is increased by sympathetic nerve activity, which is associated with decreased digestive and metabolic function (Uvnäs-Moberg, 1989, 1994).

All gastrointestinal hormones and insulin are released during a meal by local effects of food in the gastrointestinal tract and by the presence of nutrients, e.g., glucose, in the circulation. Vagal nerve activity also contributes to the control of the release of these hormones (Uvnäs-Moberg, 1994).

Suckling-Related Release of Gastrointestinal and Pancreatic Hormones

The endocrine system of the gastrointestinal tract is not only activated during feeding, but also by suckling in lactating animals. In this way, the function of the gastrointestinal tract is adapted to the increased food intake necessary during lactation in order to compensate for the energy expenditure of milk production.

Studies performed in dogs, sows, and rats demonstrate that suckling is related to a release of gastrointestinal and pancreatic hormones. The levels of gastrin, cholecystokinin, insulin, and glucagon rise and somatostatin levels fall or rise in response to suckling in dogs, pigs, and rats (Eriksson et al., 1994; Eriksson, Linden, Stock, & Uvnäs-Moberg, 1987; Eriksson, Linden, & Uvnäs-Moberg, 1987; Eriksson & Uvnäs-Moberg, 1990; Linden, Carlquist, Hansen, & Uvnäs-Moberg, 1989; Linden, Eriksson, Carlquist, & Uvnäs-Moberg, 1987; Uvnäs-Moberg et al., 1985).

The Number of Suckling Piglets and Massage of the Udder Contributes to the Decrease of Somatostatin Levels

In lactating sows, the decrease in somatostatin levels was, like the increase in prolactin levels, related to the number of suckling piglets and to the duration of udder massage given by the piglets before and after milk letdown. In this way, the function of the gastrointestinal tract was adapted to the amount of food needed to feed the young (Algers, Madej, Rojanasthien, & Uvnäs-Moberg, 1991; Algers & Uvnäs-Moberg, 2007).

Mechanisms Involved in the Suckling-Induced Release of Gastrointestinal and Pancreatic Hormones

The mechanisms and pathways involved in the suckling-related release of gastrointestinal hormones were investigated in a series of animal experimental studies performed by Eriksson, Björkstrand, Linden, Stock and Smed.

Role of the Vagal Nerves

The suckling-related release of gastrin, insulin, and cholecystokinin and the decrease in somatostatin levels were demonstrated to be mediated via the vagal nerves, since the effects were abolished in animals in which the vagal nerves had been cut. Decreased activity in the sympathetic nerves also contributed to the decrease of somatostatin levels (Eriksson et al., 1994; Linden, Eriksson, Hansen, & Uvnäs-Moberg, 1990). The suckling-induced rise of glucagon levels involved both increased vagal nerve activity and a direct effect in the pancreas by an increase of circulating oxytocin levels (Bjorkstrand, Eriksson, et al., 1996; Stock et al., 1990).

Role of Oxytocinergic Pathways in the Brain

The rise of insulin, gastrin, and cholecystokinin levels and the decrease of somatostatin levels induced by suckling involve activation of oxytocinergic pathways in the brain. This has been demonstrated in several types of experiments.

Lesions of Afferent Pathways in the Brain

Studies have been performed in which the pathways in the brain that link the suckling stimulus to milk ejection, and thereby to activation of the oxytocin-producing nuclei in the hypothalamus, are disconnected. Under these circumstances, no CCK or gastrin was released in response to suckling (Linden, Eriksson, et al., 1990).

Administration of Oxytocin into the Brain

The role of oxytocin in the regulation of the release of gastrointestinal hormones in the CNS is further supported by experimental findings, which show that administration of oxytocin into the brain influences the release of gastrointestinal hormones in rats. Insulin levels increase in response to administration of oxytocin into the brain, and gastrin, CCK, and somatostatin levels are reduced (Bjorkstrand, Ahlenius, et al., 1996; Bjorkstrand, Eriksson, et al., 1996). After repeated administration, a decrease of basal, but increased feed-induced levels of gastrointestinal hormones are observed (Petersson, Hulting, Andersson, et al., 1999).

Oxytocinergic Innervation of the DMX and NTS

Efferent vagal nerve activity is controlled from the DMX. The data reported above suggest that the effects of oxytocin are exerted in the DMX, the site for efferent vagal nerve activity. Parvocellular oxytocinergic fibers, emanating in the paraventricular nucleus, project to the DMX and NTS, where the gastrointestinal function is regulated and is also richly provided with oxytocin receptors (Buijs, 1983; Buijs et al., 1985; Buijs & Swaab, 1979; Rogers & Hermann, 1987; Sofroniew, 1983; Zimmerman et al., 1984).

A parallel release of oxytocin from magnocellular and parvocellular neurons has also been demonstrated (Zerihun & Harris, 1983), supporting the assumption that suckling is associated with a release of oxytocin both into the circulation and from parvocellular neurons innervating brainstem areas.

Some effects, in particular those induced by repeated administration of oxytocin, may also be exerted in the NTS, the vagal sensory nucleus, which is strongly interconnected with the DMX.

Effects of Oxytocin Antagonists

In further support of a role for oxytocin in the suckling-mediated effects on the release of gastrointestinal hormones, administration of an oxytocin antagonist increased the suckling-induced release of somatostatin (Eriksson et al., 1994; Uvnäs-Moberg & Eriksson, 1996). This finding implicates that an inhibitory effect on somatostatin release was blocked by the oxytocin antagonist.

In addition, the elevation of blood glucose and glucagon levels induced in response to suckling was counteracted by an oxytocin antagonist. These effects are likely to have been exerted via oxytocin receptors on the glucagon cells in the pancreas (Eriksson et al., 1994).

Role of Serotonin

When the release of endogenous oxytocin was induced indirectly by administration of a serotonin agonist (5 HT 1a), a rise of insulin levels and a decrease of CCK and somatostatin levels were observed. The link between the central release of oxytocin and a decrease of somatostatin levels was supported by the finding that the effect of the 5 HT 1a-agonist on somatostatin release disappeared if the animals were pretreated with oxytocin antagonists (Bjorkstrand, Ahlenius, et al., 1996).

Suckling Influences the Release of Gastrointestinal Hormones in Two Steps

The suckling-mediated effects are mediated via activation of somatosensory nerves that reach the brainstem via the spinal cord and possibly by the vagal nerve afferents that originate in the mammary gland and project directly to the NTS (Eriksson, Lindh, et al., 1996). The release of gastrointestinal hormones may be influenced via short brainstem reflex loops, i.e., via neurons that connect the NTS with the DMX, the motor centers of the vagal nerves.

In addition, suckling activates pathways that, e.g., contain B-inhibin as a transmitter substance, which connect the NTS with the oxytocin-producing neurons in the SON and PVN. As a result of such activation, parvocellular oxytocinergic pathways that project to areas involved in the control of the gastrointestinal tract, e.g., the DMX and NTS, are activated. This hypothalamic reflex may act together with and reinforce the effects induced by the shorter brainstem reflexes described above on the release of gastrointestinal hormones.

The Effect on Gastrointestinal Hormones in Response to Suckling Part of a Broad Pattern of Adaptive Changes

Taken together, these data show that when oxytocin is released from the magnocellular neurons into the circulation in response to suckling, it is also released from parvocellular neurons projecting to the DMX and NTS. These effects, however, only reflect one aspect of a broad pattern of adaptive changes occurring in response to a suckling-induced activation of oxytocinergic neurons projecting into different parts of the brain.

As mentioned in the previous chapters, the release of prolactin is facilitated and the release of ACTH and CRH are decreased by oxytocin released from oxytocinergic neurons in the anterior pituitary and the PVN. Blood pressure and cortisol levels are decreased by oxytocin released from oxytocinergic neurons projecting from the PVN to the LC, RVLM, and NTS. Oxytocin is also released from nerves projecting to the amygdala, the hippocampus, the raphe nuclei, the PAG, and the NAC to influence social behavior, decrease the levels of anxiety, increase wellbeing, and decrease the levels of pain.

Functional Changes Induced by Suckling in the Gastrointestinal Tract

Lactation is an energy-demanding process. Several physiological mechanisms, which act to optimize digestion and metabolism in order to save energy, are activated during this period.

Increased Digestive Capacity

An increased size and an increased functional capacity of the gastrointestinal tract have been demonstrated in several species during lactation, which ascertains an optimal digestion of ingested food. As the gastrointestinal hormones, such as gastrin and cholecystokinin, stimulate the growth of the gastrointestinal mucosa, the suckling-related release of these hormones is responsible for the hypertrophy of the gastrointestinal tract and, consequently, for its optimized functional capacity (Fell, Smith, & Campbell, 1963; Lichtenberger & Trier, 1979).

Energy Saving

Role of Insulin

Insulin, being in several aspects an essential hormone, exerts many important effects. It stimulates transport of nutrients into the cells and facilitates storage of ingested nutrients. As insulin is released by suckling, it promotes an efficient handling of nutrients during lactation.

The Incretin Effect

Since some of the gastrointestinal hormones reinforce the release of insulin—the incretin effect—gastrointestinal hormones released by suckling further stimulate nutrient assimilation and anabolic metabolism during lactation (Uvnäs-Moberg, 1989).

Mobilization and Transfer of Energy for Milk Production

It is not only important to save and use energy efficiently during lactation in order to produce milk, it is equally important to be able to recruit energy from the maternal stores and transfer it to the mammary glands for milk production.

Role of Glucagon in Mobilization and Transfer of Nutrients

The pancreatic hormone, glucagon, which plays a key role in mobilization of energy, has been demonstrated to be released by suckling in animal experiments (Algers et al., 1991; Eriksson et al., 1994; Eriksson, Linden, & Uvnäs-Moberg, 1987). There is a difference between the suckling-related release of insulin and glucagon. Suckling-related insulin release is mainly mediated via the vagal nerve, whereas the elevation of glucagon levels seems to be exerted both vagally and by oxytocin that reaches the pancreas via the circulation (Eriksson et al., 1994).

Oxytocin contributes to the suckling-related glucagon release in two ways: 1. by an effect in the vagal centers in the NTS and DMX in the medulla oblongata via oxytocin released from nerve endings projecting from the paraventricular nucleus to this area, and 2. by a local effect in the pancreas after having been released into the circulation from the posterior pituitary.

When glucagon is released, energy, e.g., glucose, is recruited from its stores, allowing it to be transported to the mammary gland to be used for milk production. The elevation of blood glucose levels observed in lactating animals is reversed by oxytocin antagonists (Eriksson et al., 1994), demonstrating the important role of oxytocin in the control of glucagon secretion and mobilization of energy.

Not only glucose levels are increased in lactating animals. The levels of non-esterified fatty acids (NEFA) also rise in the circulation of lactating sows. This could be an effect of oxytocin, as administration of oxytocin has been demonstrated to increase the levels of NEFA (Suva, Caisova, & Stajner, 1980). In lactating sows, oxytocin levels correlated with the levels of NEFA. Further, the important role of oxytocin in the transfer of nutrients from the sow to the litter was indicated by associations between oxytocin levels and weight loss in the sow and increase of weight of the litter (Algers et al., 1991; Algers & Uvnäs-Moberg, 2007; Valros et al., 2004).

Differences in the Balance Between Storing and Recruitment of Energy (Energy Partitioning)

In sows, genetic variations exist as to the balance between storing and recruitment of energy. Some sows produce more milk and lose a lot of weight in the beginning of lactation in order to feed more piglets, whereas others tend to produce less milk and keep their own energy stores to a greater extent (Algers & Uvnäs-Moberg, 2007).

The balance between stimulation of storing and recruitment of energy also changes during lactation, as more energy is needed as the piglets grow and require more milk. As will be described in the next chapter, suckling-induced oxytocin levels increase during the breastfeeding period in women. As glucagon, to a larger extent than insulin, is controlled by circulating oxytocin levels, the higher oxytocin levels later on during lactation will influence the ratio between glucagon and insulin, insulin release will change in favor of glucagon. This means the recruitment of energy becomes more prominent in comparison to the storing mechanisms during the lactation period. This makes sense as more energy is needed for the offspring as they grow.

Direct Effects of Oxytocin on Metabolism

Oxytocin may also influence metabolism directly via effects in the circulation. Oxytocin can increase the production of glucose from the liver, thereby elevating glucose levels. It may also exert insulin-like effects by increasing the storage of fat (Bjorkstrand, Eriksson, & Uvnäs-Moberg, 1992).

Transfer of Nutrients to the Mammary Glands

Role of Insulin

Insulin contributes to the transfer of energy to the mammary gland by preferentially increasing the storage of energy in this area. Insulin has also been demonstrated to stimulate milk production more directly by increasing the function of prolactin receptors on the milk-producing lactocytes, and thereby milk production (Bolander, Nicholas, Van Wyk, & Topper, 1981; Hartmann, Sherriff, & Mitoulas, 1998; Uvnäs-Moberg et al., 1987).

Somatostatin—A Break in Metabolism and Growth

Somatostatin produced in the hypothalamus inhibits the release of growth hormone from the anterior pituitary. In this way, somatostatin levels inhibit growth. Somatostatin can, however, inhibit growth in another way, i.e., by inhibiting the function of the gastrointestinal tract and the pancreas.

Somatostatin inhibits the release of all gastrointestinal and pancreatic hormones. Since somatostatin is released in response to stress, stress is related to low levels of gastrointestinal and pancreatic hormones, and, therefore, to a decreased function of the gastrointestinal tract, as well as a decreased metabolic function. Consequently, anabolic processes and growth are retarded. By contrast, all these functions increase when somatostatin levels are low (Uvnäs-Moberg, 1989, 1994).

Somatostatin Levels Reflect a Balance Between Vagal and Sympathetic Nerve Activity

Somatostatin levels in the circulation mainly represent somatostatin originating in the gastrointestinal tract. Somatostatin levels decrease in response to activation of the vagal nerve and increase in response to an enhanced activity of the sympathetic nerves.

Oxytocin released from nerves projecting from the PVN in the hypothalamus to the DMX decreases the secretion of somatostatin via a vagal mechanism. In contrast, CRF released from the PVN, which stimulates the activity in the HPA and the sympathetic nervous system, is released from nerves by decreasing the activity in the vagal nerve and increasing the activity in the sympathetic fibers that innervate the gastrointestinal tract. Obviously, the balance between CRF secretion and oxytocin secretion in the areas regulating autonomous nervous tone, e.g., the DMX, is important for the release of somatostatin, and, therefore, for the function of the gastrointestinal and pancreatic endocrine systems (Smedh & Uvnäs-Moberg, 1994; Uvnäs-Moberg, 1994).

CRF is released in response to stress, e.g., induced by painful or noxious somatosensory stimulation, whereas oxytocin is released by less intense somatosensory stimulation, e.g., suckling or touch. Therefore, the oxytocin-related effects increase during suckling. The levels of somatostatin will be decreased, and as a consequence, the function of the gastrointestinal tract, including the pancreas, will be stimulated, and digestive and metabolic processes optimized.

Somatostatin in Milk Production

Somatostatin levels are decreased in a piglet in a "dose dependent" way in response to suckling and massage of the udder in sows at the same time as prolactin levels increase. In this way, prolactin secretion and the metabolic processes that facilitate milk production change in a synchronized way according to the number of suckling piglets and the duration of suckling (Algers et al., 1991).

endocrine system of the gastrointestinal tract and the pancreas are adapted to the nutritional needs caused during lactation.

Summary

- Suckling stimulates the release of the gastrointestinal hormones gastrin and CCK.

- Suckling stimulates the release of insulin and glucagon.

- Suckling inhibits the release of somatostatin.

- The suckling-induced effects on the release of all hormones are mediated via the vagal nerves.

- Suckling also stimulates glucagon release via circulating oxytocin levels.

- Oxytocinergic pathways projecting from the PVN to the DMX and NTS are involved in the suckling-induced effects on gastrointestinal and pancreatic hormones.

- Gastrin released in response to suckling stimulates the growth and thereby the function of the gastrointestinal tract.

- Insulin, together with the gastrointestinal hormones, facilitates storing of nutrients.

- Glucagon facilitates recruitment of nutrients from maternal stores.

- Insulin and glucagon together facilitate transfer of nutrients to the mammary gland and thereby stimulate milk production.

- Somatostatin inhibits the function in the gastrointestinal tract and the pancreas. Lowered somatostatin levels induced by suckling therefore stimulates gastrointestinal and pancreatic function. In this way, milk production is facilitated and stimulated, as the function of the

Chapter 20

Effects on Digestion and Metabolism in Breastfeeding Mothers

In order to nourish the fetus in the womb and to give milk to the child during breastfeeding, perhaps for several years, the mother has to transfer large amounts of calories to the fetus or infant. During pregnancy, the mother transfers about 150,000 calories to the fetus. During breastfeeding, a mother who exclusively breastfeeds transfers about 1,000 calories per day to her baby via the milk.

The mother has to cope with this extra energy demand. In our Western world, the need for extra calories during pregnancy and breastfeeding is easily compensated. Food is available, often in abundance, and pregnant and breastfeeding women may eat as much as they want and need in order to compensate for the calories they transfer to the fetus or the baby. This has, however, not always been the case. In order to help women create and feed children when the supply of food is short, women, like other mammals, are provided with a multitude of physiological adaptations, which were described in the previous chapters and which help them use energy more efficiently.

Clinical Studies

Some clinical studies were performed to investigate the role of breastfeeding on the endocrine system of the gut in women and possible associations between the levels of gastrointestinal hormones and breastfeeding variables. Also, the relationship between the levels of the different gastrointestinal hormones and breastfeeding variables were assessed.

1. Six blood samples were collected in connection with breastfeeding in six women during established lactation. The mothers' experiences of the milk-ejection reflex were noted. The third blood sample was collected one minute after the occurrence of the milk-ejection reflex. Gastrin, insulin, and prolactin levels were measured with RIA (Widstrom et al., 1984).

2. This study was performed on 15 multiparous women in connection with a breastfeed. Gastrin and somatostatin levels were measured in 11 blood samples collected during the breastfeeding session. The amount of milk received by the infants during the breastfeed was recorded (Widstrom, Winberg, et al., 1988).

3. Fifty-two primiparous women participated in the study. Eighteen blood samples were collected in connection with a breastfeed on day four after birth. Thirty-six women who were still breastfeeding were subjected to a second experiment three- to four-months postpartum. The women's smoking habits were recorded. Somatostatin levels were measured by RIA. (Oxytocin and prolactin levels were also measured as described in a previous chapter.) Milk yield in connection with the breastfeeding session and the duration of breastfeeding was recorded. In addition, the weight of the infant at birth as well as placental weight was noted (Widstrom, Matthiesen, Winberg, & Uvnäs-Moberg, 1989; Widstrom, Werner, Matthiesen, Svensson, & Uvnäs-Moberg, 1991).

4. Repeated blood samples were collected during pregnancy and breastfeeding. Oxytocin, somatostatin, gastrin, and insulin levels were measured and linked to the outcome of breastfeeding (Silber et al., 1991).

Main Results

- Gastrin and insulin levels exhibited a peak-shaped rise within a few minutes after onset of breastfeeding (Widstrom et al., 1984; Widstrom, Winberg, et al., 1988).

- Somatostatin levels sometimes rose and sometimes fell in response to suckling. Somatostatin fell in response to suckling four-days after birth, particularly in those mothers having low somatostatin levels, and tended to rise at four-months postpartum. Median somatostatin levels fell during the 60-minute observation period four-days postpartum (Widstrom et al., 1991).

- Somatostatin levels more often rose in response to breastfeeding in smoking women, and they also breastfed for a shorter time (Widstrom et al., 1991).

- The more the maternal somatostatin levels fell in the response to breastfeeding, the more milk was given to the infants during that particular breastfeeding session (Widstrom, Winberg, et al., 1988).

- Maternal somatostatin levels obtained four days after birth were strongly and inversely correlated with the birth weight of the infants and also with placental weights (Widstrom et al., 1989).

- Somatostatin levels obtained at four days after birth and four-months postpartum correlated strongly with each other, indicating that each mother has a certain somatostatin level (Widstrom et al., 1991).

- Somatostatin levels obtained four days after birth and four-months postpartum were inversely related to oxytocin levels (Uvnäs-Moberg, Sjogren, Westlin, Andersson, & Stock, 1989).

- Somatostatin levels were inversely and negatively related to oxytocin levels during pregnancy and breastfeeding (Silber et al., 1991).

Maternal Digestive Capacity Increases During Breastfeeding

The results from the clinical studies demonstrate that suckling does indeed influence the levels of gastrointestinal hormones in human mothers in a similar way to that observed in the animal studies.

Optimized Digestive Function; The Mother "Eats" When The Baby Eats

The release of gastrin observed implies that the vagal nerves are activated in response to suckling in breastfeeding women and that the function of the gastrointestinal tract is stimulated each time a mother breastfeeds, as in other mammals (Widstrom, Winberg, et al., 1988). The more gastrin, CCK, and other gut hormones that are released in response to breastfeeding, the more the growth of the gastrointestinal mucosa will be stimulated. In this way, the size and function of the gastrointestinal tract is adapted to the increased demands for digestive capacity during lactation in breastfeeding women.

More Efficient Handling of Energy During Breastfeeding

Increased Storing of Energy

The release of insulin caused by breastfeeding suggests that the maternal capacity for storing nutrients is reinforced as insulin promotes storing of nutrients (Widstrom et al., 1984). As mentioned above, the increased release of gastrointestinal hormones reinforce the secretion of insulin further (the incretin effect), thereby contributing to stimulation of the anabolic metabolism induced by insulin.

Stimulation of Milk Secretion

As insulin preferentially stimulates storing of nutrients in the mammary glands and facilitates prolactin-induced milk secretion, the breastfeeding women's capacity to produce milk is enhanced by the release of insulin linked to suckling.

Increased Recruitment of Energy

Glucagon levels were not measured in the present studies,

but are likely to be elevated during suckling as in other mammalian species (Algers et al., 1991; Bjorkstrand, Eriksson, et al., 1996; Stock et al., 1990). An elevation of glucagon and glucose levels has been recorded in other studies in lactating women (Altemus et al., 1995). It is likely that not only glucose, but also fatty acids, are recruited from fat tissues during breastfeeding, although this has not been demonstrated.

Breastfeeding Counteracts Weight Gain Obtained During Pregnancy

Long-term breastfeeding is often linked to weight loss, in particular to loss of the extra weight accumulated during pregnancy. In fact, breastfeeding may be important to normalize the metabolic effects and consequences caused by breastfeeding (Stuebe et al., 2010; Uvnäs-Moberg, 1996). A suckling-induced release of gastrointestinal and, in particular, pancreatic hormones may contribute to recruitment of energy from maternal stores.

The Ratio Between Energy Recruitment and Storing of Energy Increases Over Time

Interestingly, the release of oxytocin into the circulation in response to suckling is more pronounced after three to four months of breastfeeding compared to the first days after birth (Uvnäs-Moberg, Widstrom, Nissen, et al., 1990). As circulating oxytocin levels are important for the release of glucagon, the catabolic effect of suckling may become stronger over time in breastfeeding women as more glucagon is released during a breastfeed. In the beginning of breastfeeding, stimulation of prolactin release and milk production is relatively more important. During this period, when milk production increases, the release of insulin and gastrointestinal hormones, and consequent stimulation of maternal digestive and anabolic-storing capacities, may be of relatively greater importance than recruitment and transfer of energy from maternal stores.

As discussed in the previous chapter, different strains of sows vary as to their capacity to store energy versus to recruit and transfer nutrients into the mammary glands for milk production. Similar inborn differences in the balance between maternal storing of nutrients versus recruitment and transfer of nutrients for milk production may also exist in breastfeeding women. Such differences in the partitioning of energy may explain why some women lose weight during breastfeeding, whereas others do not lose weight until they stop breastfeeding.

Breastfeeding Reduces Somatostatin Levels, The Break of Metabolism and Growth

Somatostatin Levels and Milk Yield

The size of the fall in maternal somatostatin levels in the response to suckling was associated with the amount of milk ejected during the breastfeed; the more the somatostatin levels fell, the more milk was given to the infants during that particular breastfeeding session (Widstrom, Winberg, et al., 1988).

The decrease in somatostatin levels is not likely to be associated with the milk ejection process per se, but rather reflects a parallel process in the gastrointestinal tract aimed at optimizing digestive and metabolic functions for milk production. As somatostatin inhibits the function of the gastrointestinal tract by inhibiting the release of gastrointestinal hormones, insulin, and glucagon, low somatostatin levels facilitate milk production indirectly by increasing digestive capacity and optimizing metabolic activity (both energy storage and transfer).

Decreased Somatostatin Levels and Increased Oxytocin Levels Associated With Milk Yield

The number of oxytocin peaks in the circulation recorded during a breastfeed is related to the amount of milk ejected (Nissen et al., 1996). Obviously, both a rise in oxytocin levels and a decrease in somatostatin levels are related to a high milk yield in connection with a breastfeed the first days after birth.

These findings point to an association between the release of oxytocin in the circulation from the magnocellular neurons in the SON and PVN in the hypothalamus and the decrease of somatostatin levels. As described in the previous chapter, oxytocinergic neurons project from the PVN to the vagal motor nucleus (DMX), from which gastrointestinal function is controlled. In addition, administration of oxytocin into the brain gives rise to lowering of somatostatin levels and administration of oxytocin antagonists gives rise to higher levels of somatostatin (Björkstrand et al., 1996, Eriksson et al., 1994). These effects are mediated via the autonomic nervous system; stimulation of the vagal nerve decreases somatostatin levels and activation of the sympathetic nerves increase somatostatin levels (Uvnäs-Moberg & Eriksson, 1996).

Therefore, the results indicate that oxytocin is not only released from the magnocellular neurons of the SON and PVN into the circulation to induce milk ejection during breastfeeding, but is, at the same time, released from oxytocinergic nerves originating in the PVN that terminate in the DMX to influence somatostatin secretion. They also reflect different functions. The rise of oxytocin levels is involved in milk ejection and the decrease in somatostatin levels adapts mechanisms involved in growth and metabolism to the needs of milk production.

Higher Somatostatin Levels in Smoking Women

Somatostatin levels were linked to the outcome of breastfeeding in another way. As presented above, smoking women had higher somatostatin levels and more often responded with a rise in somatostatin levels following a breastfeed than non-smokers. They also breastfed for a shorter time than non-smokers (Widstrom et al., 1991).

Since somatostatin levels are decreased by vagal, cholinergic activity and increased by activity in the sympathetic nervous system, the results suggest that women who smoke are more "stressed" and have a higher sympathetic tone than non-smokers.

As summarized above, somatostatin levels are decreased by oxytocin via an increased vagal nerve activity and a decreased sympathetic nerve activity. Increased stress levels, e.g., induced by smoking, will create an opposite effect pattern. An increased release of CRF into the centers in the brain regulating vagal and sympathetic nerve activity will increase somatostatin levels (Smed & Uvnäs Moberg, 1994). Both a decreased oxytocin release and an increased release of CRF from the PVN in the hypothalamus may lie behind the increase in somatostatin levels in smoking women.

The lower the somatostatin levels, the more energy efficient the mother becomes, which enables them to store, mobilize, and transfer more energy for milk production. Consequently, the higher somatostatin levels in smoking women make them less energy efficient, which might have an adverse effect on milk production. This may explain the shortened period of breastfeeding observed in smoking mothers (Widström et al., 1991).

Somatostatin Levels a Trait

Somatostatin levels measured in response to breastfeeding were found to be significantly lower four-days postpartum than after four months. Yet, somatostatin levels obtained at both investigations correlated strongly with each other, indicating that each mother has a certain somatostatin level (Widstrom et al., 1991).

Somatostatin Levels and Birth Weight of Infants

Average maternal somatostatin levels obtained four days after birth were strongly and inversely correlated with the birth weight of the infants and with placental weights (Widstrom et al., 1989). These data indicate that the lower the maternal somatostatin levels were at four days after birth, the more energy had been transferred to and stored in the fetus during pregnancy. This is consistent with the role of somatostatin to act as a brake to digestion, metabolism, and growth.

As the somatostatin levels obtained during the early phases of breastfeeding correlated with the birth weight of the infants, the results indicate that a metabolism consistent with a high potential for growth must have already prevailed in these women during pregnancy.

Indeed, women who have low levels of somatostatin during pregnancy also have low levels of somatostatin during breastfeeding (Silber et al., 1991). These data further indicate the presence of low and high somatostatin mothers. The mothers with low somatostatin levels give birth to bigger babies, and eject more milk during breastfeeding.

Inverse Association Between Oxytocin and Somatostatin Levels

An inverse correlation was established between average oxytocin and somatostatin levels in the breastfeeding women (Uvnäs-Moberg, 1989). A similar relationship was found in a study performed by Silber et al. (1991). Oxytocin levels were found to be inversely related to somatostatin levels, i.e., the higher the maternal oxytocin levels, the lower their somatostatin levels during pregnancy and breastfeeding.

As described in the paragraphs above, somatostatin levels decreased in response to suckling in the breastfeeding mothers, and this fall coincided with a rise of oxytocin levels. The findings of inverse correlations between average oxytocin and somatostatin levels obtained during the entire breastfeeding period and also during pregnancy suggest that oxytocin plays a more general role in the control of somatostatin levels during these periods.

The functional link between oxytocin and somatostatin is further supported by the findings that the birth weight of the child was not only negatively associated with somatostatin levels, but was positively associated with oxytocin levels.

The findings also support the assumption of a functional relationship between mechanisms involved in the control of the two hormones. As discussed above, the effect of oxytocin on somatostatin levels during a breastfeed is not mediated via the circulation, but via oxytocinergic projections from the PVN to the DMX, which are activated in parallel with the magnocellular oxytocinergic neurons projecting to the posterior pituitary, which release oxytocin into the circulation. These data suggest that not only suckling-related somatostatin levels, but also basal somatostatin levels during pregnancy and breastfeeding are regulated by oxytocinergic nervous projections from the PVN to the NTS.

Inverse Relationship Between Oxytocin and Somatostatin During Other Circumstances

The link between oxytocin and somatostatin levels seems to be of general importance. An inverse relationship between oxytocin and somatostatin levels was also demonstrated during the menstrual cycle and during treatment with low doses of estrogen (HRT), suggesting that somatostatin levels are, in part, controlled by oxytocinergic functions in the brain under these circumstances (Silber et al., 1991; Uvnäs-Moberg et al., 1989; Uvnäs-Moberg, Widstrom, Werner, et al., 1990).

Estrogen Promotes Oxytocin Release

Some of the oxytocinergic fibers that innervate areas involved in the control of autonomic nervous functions are provided with estrogen receptors (Stern & Zhang, 2003). Therefore, estrogen may decrease somatostatin release by

stimulating the activity of oxytocinergic parvocellular neurons. This mechanism may be of particular importance during pregnancy and also during treatment with estrogen.

Symptoms of Increased Vagal Nerve Tone and Decreased Sympathetic Nervous Tone

Milk Ejection and Dizziness

Some mothers may experience hunger, thirst, dizziness, and sometimes weakness when they are breastfeeding, particularly in connection with the milk ejection reflex. These subjective phenomena may be related to the fact that suckling not only stimulates milk production and ejection, it is associated with an activation of the vagal nerves, the major neurogenic regulator of the endocrine system of the gastrointestinal tract, and with a decrease of sympathetic nervous tone. An influence on gastrointestinal motility, blood sugar, and blood pressure may lie behind the symptoms and may explain the inner sensations.

Morning Sickness

The levels of gastrointestinal hormones are influenced in early pregnancy. In studies, oxytocin and insulin levels were higher and somatostatin levels were lower during pregnancy (Silber et al., 1991). The levels of CCK were raised during pregnancy (Frick, Bremme, Sjogren, Linden, & Uvnäs-Moberg, 1990).

Some of the symptoms of morning sickness experienced by women during the first months of pregnancy may be related to a change in the function of the autonomic nervous system. During early pregnancy, the levels of estrogen rise and oxytocin levels increase in the circulation. As the oxytocinergic fibers projecting to the brainstem are provided with oxytocin receptors, the function of some aspects of the autonomic nervous system is changed. Elevated insulin levels and a tendency to hypoglycemia are important factors behind the symptoms of early pregnancy, together with a changed motility of the gastrointestinal tract and lower blood pressure.

Energy saving is reinforced, which is reflected by a tendency to increased weight gain during this period. This often occurs in spite of sickness and a reduced food intake (Frick et al., 1990; Silber et al., 1991).

Summary

- Breastfeeding in women is associated with a release of several gastrointestinal hormones, such as gastrin and insulin, and a decrease of somatostatin levels, suggesting that gastrointestinal function and metabolism is adapted to the energy needs of milk production.

- The lower the maternal somatostatin levels were in response to suckling, the more milk was ejected during a breastfeeding episode.

- The lower the maternal somatostatin levels were during pregnancy, the higher the birth weight of the infant.

- Somatostatin levels measured at different occasions during pregnancy and breastfeeding correlated with each other suggesting that each mother has a certain somatostatin level.

- Oxytocin levels were negatively associated with somatostatin levels, i.e., the higher the oxytocin levels the lower the somatostatin levels were during pregnancy, in connection with milk ejection, and also during an entire breastfeeding session.

- These data suggest that oxytocin lowers somatostatin levels. Estrogen during pregnancy and suckling during breastfeeding increase oxytocin release into both the circulation and the brain. Oxytocinergic nerves projecting to the DMX decrease somatostatin levels.

Chapter 21

Effect of Suckling in the Offspring on Digestion, Metabolism, and Growth

As presented in the previous chapter, suckling/breastfeeding in lactating mothers is associated with a release of oxytocin and gastrointestinal and pancreatic hormones. The suckling stimulus activates the vagal nerve via actions in the brainstem, and this effect is mediated by oxytocin released from parvocellular neurons in the brain that project to the dorsal vagal motor nucleus (DMX) in the brainstem. In this way, maternal digestion and metabolism are optimized to meet the energy demands of milk production and feeding of the newborn.

The effect induced by the suckling stimulus is reciprocal, and a similar effect on oxytocin release and the function of the gastrointestinal tract is induced in the offspring/infant. Suckling not only provides the offspring/infant with food, it optimizes the function of the gastrointestinal tract and adapts the metabolism to promote storing of energy and growth (Figure 21.1).

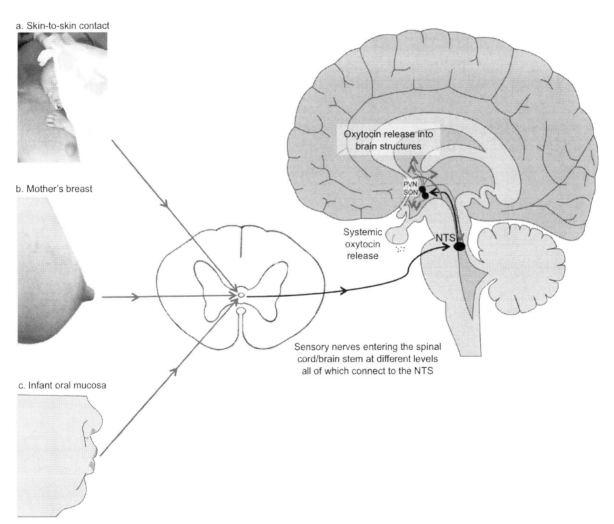

Figure 21.1. Mother and Baby, Suckling and Skin-to-Skin Contact, Connections with the Brain

Source: Uvnäs-Moberg & Prime, 2013. Used with permission.

Suckling-Induced Effects on Oxytocin Levels

Feeding has been demonstrated to induce a release of oxytocin into the circulation in several species, such as sows, dogs, and dairy cows. This effect is due to the presence of food in the gastrointestinal tract and to the stimulation of sensory nerves in the oral mucosa, which project to the NTS centers in the brainstem (Rojkittikhun, Uvnäs-Moberg, & Einarsson, 1993; Svennersten et al., 1990; Uvnäs-Moberg et al., 1985).

Oxytocin is released as a result of suckling in the offspring, as evidenced by rising oxytocin levels, e.g., in suckling calves. In experiments in which the effect of suckling and bucket feeding in calves were compared, more oxytocin was released in response to the suckling stimulus. These data implicate that the suckling stimulus, not just the ingested nutrients, was important for release of oxytocin (Lupoli et al., 2001). Suckling is not related to a rise in circulating oxytocin levels in all species. This does not exclude that oxytocin is released from parvocellular neurons originating in the PVN, as activation of such neurons is not necessarily linked to activation of magnocellular neurons from the SON and PVN, which would result in elevated levels of circulating oxytocin.

Suckling-Induced Effects on Gastrointestinal Hormones

In the experiments referred to above in which calves obtained milk either by suckling the cows or by drinking milk from a bucket, the levels of gastrin, insulin, and cholecystokinin (CCK) were measured in plasma. The levels of all hormones rose in response to feeding, irrespective of suckling or bucket feeding, but CCK levels were significantly higher in calves that were suckling. In addition, cortisol levels were significantly lower after suckling than after bucket feeding (Lupoli et al., 2001). These results show that suckling reinforced the increase of CCK levels and the decrease of cortisol levels induced by food ingestion, as a consequence of the more intense tactile stimulation within the oral mucosa caused by suckling, when compared to bucket feeding.

Link Between Suckling-Related Release of Oxytocin and Gastrointestinal Hormones

A strong correlation was observed between the amounts of oxytocin and insulin released in response to suckling, suggesting that oxytocinergic activity might have influenced insulin secretion (Lupoli et al., 2001). As oxytocin administered into the brain releases insulin, a release of oxytocin from parvocellular neurons projecting to the DMX in the brain induced in parallel to a release of oxytocin from magnocellular neurons into the circulation might have triggered the secretion of insulin in the calves. A similar oxytocin-mediated mechanism may have been involved in

the rise of CCK levels, as CCK levels are also influenced by oxytocinergic mechanisms in the brainstem (Bjorkstrand, Eriksson, et al., 1996; Buijs et al., 1985; Linden et al., 1989; Sofroniew, 1983).

The lower cortisol levels seen in the suckling calves, when compared to those that were bucket feeding, indicates that oxytocin induced in response to suckling within the PVN or from nerves in the anterior pituitary may have inhibited the HPA axis by decreasing the release of CRF in the hypothalamus or of ACTH from the anterior pituitary.

Stimulation of Growth

There is data showing that suckling calves grow more quickly than bucket-fed calves. The growth-promoting effect of suckling in the calves may be due to the more intense exposure to oxytocin, gastrointestinal hormones, and insulin in response to the suckling stimulus, and a consequent stimulation of anabolic metabolism and growth (Krohn, 1999; Uvnäs-Moberg, 1989).

Integrative Role of Oxytocin in Stimulation of Growth

Just like in the mother, oxytocin released by the suckling stimulus in the offspring may play an integrative, facilitating role on growth processes by stimulation of vagal nerve activity caused by suckling. The release of hormones, such as gastrin, CCK, and insulin, is increased and levels of somatostatin, which acts as a brake on metabolism and growth, are lowered. In this way, processes that promote growth, such as an optimized digestion and metabolism, will be stimulated.

If newborn rats are given repeated injections of oxytocin, they grow more quickly than those that were treated with saline. They also have lower blood pressure and cortisol levels, higher pain thresholds, and more expression of alpha-2 adrenoceptors as adults, suggesting that oxytocin-induced growth and anti-stress effects become permanent (Diaz-Cabiale et al., 2004; Holst et al., 2002; Olausson et al., 2003; Uvnäs-Moberg et al., 1998). Repeated intense stimulation of oxytocin in response to suckling might be considered to be an analogous treatment to giving repeated oxytocin injections and may explain the growth-promoting effects of suckling.

Chain of Events in the Suckling-Related Stimulation of Gastrointestinal Hormones in Mother and Offspring

The Mother

In the mother, suckling activates receptors on the nipple, which activate sensory nerves that project to the NTS in the brainstem.

Vago-vagal or Brainstem Reflexes

As described in the previous chapter, sensory nerves originating in the mammary gland area, particularly the special vagal afferents (ingoing fibers), which project directly to the vagal sensory nucleus (NTS), may induce a "reflex" activation of vagal efferent (outgoing) nerve activity via an action in the vagal motor area (DMX). This "vago-vagal reflex" is exerted at the brainstem level and may influence the secretion of gastrointestinal function (Eriksson et al., 1994; Eriksson, Lindh, et al., 1996; Uvnäs-Moberg, 1994; Uvnäs-Moberg & Eriksson, 1996).

Hypothalamic Oxytocinergic Reflexes

The NTS and oxytocin-producing nuclei, the SON and the PVN, are connected by nervous pathways, which are activated by suckling. Oxytocin is not only released into the circulation in response to suckling in mothers, but also from oxytocinergic nerves originating in the PVN, which project to many important regulatory areas in the brain, e.g., to the areas involved in control of the autonomic nervous system. Oxytocin released from nerves in the DMX and NTS influence the function of the vagal motor neurons, and thereby influence gastrointestinal function (Buijs et al., 1985; Rogers & Hermann, 1987; Sofroniew, 1983; Zimmerman et al., 1984).

Oxytocin released from nerves projecting to the NTS and DMX increase vagal nerve activity, and at the same time, reinforce the effect of the vago-vagal reflex exerted at the brainstem level (Olson, Hoffman, Sved, Stricker, & Verbalis, 1992).

As described in great detail in previous chapters, oxytocin influences the release of gastrointestinal hormones by actions in the DMX in the brainstem. In fact, the effect of suckling on maternal gastrointestinal hormones was abolished when the function of the oxytocinergic system was blocked (Linden, Eriksson, et al., 1990).

The Offspring

The mechanisms by which oxytocin and gastrointestinal hormones are released by suckling in the offspring and the possible role of oxytocin in this context has not been investigated as extensively as in the mothers. Still, the fact that suckling stimulates the release of oxytocin and gastrointestinal and pancreatic hormones in the offspring suggests that similar mechanisms are activated in mothers and offspring.

In the offspring, suckling activates receptors in the oral mucosa, which via activation of sensory nerves project to the NTS (Lupoli et al., 2001; Uvnäs-Moberg, 1989; Uvnäs-Moberg et al., 2001, Uvnäs-Moberg et al., 1987).

Nervous pathways connect the NTS with the DMX where vagal afferent nerves projecting to the gastrointestinal tract are activated. In addition, nervous pathways, which connect the NTS with parvocellular neurons in the PVN (and sometimes magnocellular neurons in the PVN and SON), stimulate the release of oxytocin from oxytocinergic fibers projecting to the DMX and the NTS, where oxytocin may stimulate the activity of vagal efferent neurons, thereby facilitating the direct effect exerted by suckling in the DMX on gastrointestinal function.

Not Always a Parallel Release of Oxytocin from Magno- and Parvocellular Neurons

Suckling in ewes induced a rise of maternal oxytocin levels into the circulation and the brain (Kendrick et al., 1986). Oxytocin released into the circulation induces milk letdown. Oxytocin released into the brain induces maternal behavioral and physiological adaptations.

Suckling in calves also induces a rise of oxytocin into the circulation, but a suckling-induced rise of oxytocin is not seen in all species. In fact, the circulating oxytocin may not play as important a role during suckling in the offspring as in the mother, in which oxytocin induces milk ejection. This difference regarding the function of oxytocin in mothers and offspring may explain why a rise of circulating oxytocin levels is not always seen in response to suckling in the offspring. Still, oxytocin may be released from parvocellular oxytocinergic neurons in order to induce oxytocin-linked effects in the brain in the offspring.

Effects of Suckling in Human Newborns

The effect of suckling on the release of gastrointestinal hormones has been studied in a series of experiments performed in human newborn infants. The levels of gastrointestinal hormones can be measured in blood samples. As some gastrointestinal hormones are not only released into the circulation, but also into the lumen of the gastrointestinal tract, it is also possible to record the release of gastrointestinal hormones by recording hormone levels in gastric aspirates (Uvnäs-Wallensten, Efendic, & Luft, 1977).

Clinical Studies

In breastfeeding infants, both the suckling stimulus and ingested food stimulate the release of gastrointestinal and pancreatic hormones. In order to study the effects of suckling on the release of gastrointestinal hormones and avoid the stimulatory effects of ingested food, studies were also performed on infants sucking a pacifier.

1. Gastric aspirates were collected from 25 newborns immediately after birth. The volume and the pH of the contents were analyzed. In addition, gastrin and somatostatin levels were analyzed in the aspirates (Widstrom, Christensson, et al., 1988).

2. Eight preterm infants were tube-fed twice with maternal milk—once without and once with sucking on a pacifier 15 minutes before, during, and after tube feeding. Gastric aspirates were withdrawn. Volume and pH, as well as gastrin and somatostatin levels of the aspirates were measured (Widstrom, Marchini, et al., 1988).

3. Blood samples were collected from an umbilical catheter from premature and full-term newborns in response to sucking on a pacifier. Insulin, gastrin, and somatostatin levels were measured with radioimmunoassay (Marchini, Lagercrantz, Feuerberg, Winberg, & Uvnäs-Moberg, 1987).

4. Blood samples were collected in 58 newborn infants. Each child contributed one blood sample collected before, just after, or at ten, 30, and 60 minutes after breastfeeding. Determination of plasma levels of CCK was performed by high performance liquid chromatograpy (HPLC) and radioimmunoassay (Uvnäs-Moberg, Marchini, & Winberg, 1993).

Main Results

• The volume of the gastric contents obtained by gastric suction in the newborns averaged 4 ml and varied between 0 and 11 ml; pH of the gastric aspirates averaged 7.0 and varied between 2.8 and 9.6. There was a relationship between the volume and the pH of the gastric aspirates, the lower the volume of the gastric aspirate, the lower the pH (Widstrom, Christensson, et al., 1988).

• Both gastrin and somatostatin levels could be detected in gastric aspirates by radioimmunoassay and their chemical identity was established by HPLC and gel filtration chromatography (Widstrom, Christensson, et al., 1988).

• The concentration of somatostatin in the gastric aspirates was influenced by the pH of the gastric contents. More somatostatin was found when pH of the gastric aspirates was low (Widstrom, Christensson et al., 1988).

• The somatostatin levels were lower and gastrin levels higher in the group of infants allowed to suck a pacifier when compared to infants that were bolus fed without sucking a pacifier (Widstrom, Marchini, et al., 1988).

• Insulin levels were shown to rise within minutes in connection with sucking a pacifier. In contrast, no effect on gastrin or somatostatin levels was observed in this particular experiment (Marchini et al., 1987).

• Cholecystokinin levels rose in breastfed infants. Interestingly, the release of CCK was found to be biphasic, an initial almost immediate peak was followed by a later, more protracted release (Uvnäs-Moberg, Marchini, et al, 1993).

Drinking Cycles in Utero

The finding of low pH in some of the aspirates demonstrates that fetuses produced gastric acid. The finding of an association between pH and the volume of the gastric aspirates, i.e., the higher the pH of aspirates the larger the volume, and the lower the pH of the aspirates the smaller the volume, suggests that the fetus has established cycles of drinking behavior in utero. When the stomach is almost empty, pH of the stomach is low because it contains gastric acid, but when the fetus drinks amniotic fluid, the acid contents of the stomach become gradually diluted and pH rises. When the volume of the gastric content reaches 10 ml, the gastric contents are emptied (Widstrom, Christensson, et al., 1988).

Secretion of Gastric Acid and Hormones in Utero

The finding of higher somatostatin levels in gastric aspirates with low pH is consistent with the fact that somatostatin produced in the stomach is released by low pH (Uvnäs-Wallensten, Efendic, Johansson, Sjodin, & Cranwell, 1980). The results clearly demonstrate that the drinking spells of the fetus are associated with both gastric exocrine (HCL) and endocrine (gastrin and somatostatin) secretions similar to those triggered by feeding (Widstrom, Christensson, et al., 1988).

Sucking a Pacifier Activates the Vagal Nerves

Shortened Feeding Time

The experiments where feeding time was reduced when the infants received a pacifier, suggest that the stomach relaxed more efficiently to receive the ingested milk when the bolus feeding was linked to sucking a pacifier. This "gastric relaxation" is mediated via specific nerve fibers in the vagal nerve (Widstrom, Marchini, et al., 1988).

Lower Levels of Somatostatin and Increased Function of the Gastrointestinal Tract

The decrease of somatostatin levels caused by sucking a pacifier is due to a suckling-induced activation of vagal nerves that inhibit somatostatin release (Uvnäs-Wallensten, Efendic, Roovete, & Johansson, 1980). As described above, somatostatin release from the stomach is influenced by both vagal nerve activity and intragastric pH. When the vagal nerves are activated during suckling, the release of somatostatin in response to low pH is diminished, and thereby the pH-dependent inhibitory effect of somatostatin is weakened.

As somatostatin inhibits the release of gastrin, gastrin levels rise as the "somatostatin break" is inhibited by vagal nerve stimulation (Uvnäs-Wallensten et al., 1977).

Suckling Increases the Release of Insulin and CCK

Suckling was associated with an immediate rise of both insulin and CCK into the circulation. CCK levels exhibited a second more protracted peak. The rise of insulin levels and the initial rise of CCK are likely to have been mediated by a suckling-induced activation of efferent vagal nerves. The latter, more protracted release of CCK is likely to have been mediated by the presence of food in the stomach (Uvnäs-Moberg, Marchini, et al., 1993).

Suckling Stimulates Vagal Nerve Activity

As described in detail in the chapter 7, suckling in breastfeeding women is associated with activation of the vagal nerve. The present data show that the effect of suckling is mutual and that reciprocal effects are induced in the sucking infant. When the nipple is in contact with the oral mucosa, receptors that respond to touch and pressure are activated, and afferent sensory nerves are activated. These sensory nerves connect to the NTS (the vagal sensory nucleus) and then to the DMX to activate vagal nerve activity. The enhanced vagal nerve activity, in turn, influences the release of gastrointestinal hormones and insulin (Uvnäs-Moberg et al., 1987).

Role of Oxytocin

Circulating oxytocin levels do not rise in response to suckling in human infants (Marchini, Lagercrantz, Winberg, & Uvnäs-Moberg, 1988). Whether oxytocin released from parvocellular neurons projecting to the NTS and DMX in response to the suckling stimulus contributes to the activation of the vagal nerve has not been demonstrated in humans, but is very likely given the similarities in the control of vagal functions in different mammalian species. Parvocellular oxytocin neurons may well be activated without a concurrent release of oxytocin into the circulation following activation of magnocellular neurons (Uvnäs-Moberg et al., 1987).

Suckling Promotes Growth of the Gastrointestinal Mucosa

The in utero drinking behavior of the unborn may contribute to the maturation of the gastrointestinal tract by allowing gastrin, CCK, and other hormones and growth factors, which are released into the gastrointestinal lumen, to be transported along the gastrointestinal canal and, therefore, to come in contact with the gastrointestinal mucosa and stimulate growth. Such a growth-promoting effect of gastrointestinal contents has been demonstrated both in animal models and in human fetuses (Uvnäs-Moberg, 1989).

Sucking Promotes Anabolic Metabolism and Increases Weight Gain

Infants that are allowed to suck a pacifier during bolus feeding have been demonstrated to increase in weight more efficiently than infants that are only tube fed, even if they do not ingest more milk, suggesting that they handle their energy in a more efficient way (Bernbaum, Pereira, Watkins, & Peckham, 1983).

The effects observed on the levels of gastrointestinal and pancreatic hormones in response to suckling may have contributed to efficient use of energy and weight-promoting effect. The decrease of somatostatin levels is consistent with enhanced vagal nerve activity and increased digestive and metabolic function, as somatostatin inhibits the secretion of gastrointestinal and pancreatic hormones. When somatostatin levels are lowered, the levels of the other hormones rise (Widstrom, Marchini, et al., 1988).

The finding of a vagally mediated release of insulin in response to suckling may play an important part in the energy-saving effect induced by suckling, as insulin stimulates anabolic metabolism and exerts growth-promoting effects (Marchini et al., 1987). Other gastrointestinal hormones, such as gastrin and cholecystokinin which are released by suckling and breastfeeding, may contribute, as the gastrointestinal hormones promote the release of insulin and, in this way, reinforce the effects of insulin (Uvnäs-Moberg, 1989; Uvnäs-Moberg, Marchini, et al., 1993; Uvnäs-Moberg et al., 1987).

Suckling Gives Rise to Calm

Breastfeeding is not only satisfying, but also calming. Some of these effects are secondary to the food ingested, but the sucking stimulus by itself plays a part and is why pacifiers induce calm in human babies. These effects may involve central effects and a release of oxytocin from parvocellular neurons into areas in the brain, but may also involve activation of the vagal nerves.

As will be described in detail in a subsequent chapter describing the effects of food intake on oxytocin-related mechanisms, CCK, which is released in response to ingestion of food, has been demonstrated to exert calming effects in the brain via activation of afferent vagal nerves (Uvnäs-Moberg, 1994). Also, the vagal impulses generated by the presence of CCK in the small intestine activate oxytocin release, and thereby induce an oxytocin-related effect spectrum.

Basal levels of CCK are particularly high soon after birth. The high levels of CCK obtained after birth may be related to the fact that newborns stay quiet and calm in spite of receiving very little food the first days of life (Uvnäs-Moberg, Marchini, et al., 1993).

Breastfeeding Versus Bottle Feeding

It is obvious from the results described above that the procedure of suckling is active and exerts important physiological and behavioral effects. This, of course, raises some questions as to the short and long-term consequences of bottle feeding. It is difficult to compare breastfeeding and bottle feeding from the perspective of the infant, since the composition of formula differs from that of breastmilk. Still, some studies show that bottle feeding with expressed mother's milk may influence the infants differently than breastfeeding.

Recently, it has been shown that the risk of developing obesity in adulthood is increased in bottle-fed infants, irrespective of if they receive formula or expressed maternal milk (Spatz, 2014). Given the strong effect of suckling on vagal nerve activity, and thereby the function of the gastrointestinal tract, it is tempting to suggest that the suckling stimulus is important not only for growth and metabolism, but also for regulation of food intake. As CCK is an important satiety hormone, which will be described in the next chapter, the release of CCK repeatedly induced by the suckling stimulus may, in the long term, result in a balanced intake of food.

Mutual Regulation of the Gastrointestinal Tract During Breastfeeding

Taken together, the results from this and the previous chapter show that mother and baby influence each other's gastrointestinal function in a reciprocal way. The mutual regulation adapts the physiology of the digestive and metabolic systems of both the mother and infant, and the needs of calories for milk production and growth of the infant. Suckling in mothers is associated with nutrient storage and recruitment and transfer of nutrients from maternal stores to the mammary glands, whereas suckling in infants is related to storing of nutrients and growth.

Summary

- The fetus has cycles of drinking and gastric emptying, which are accompanied by secretion of gastric acid and gastrointestinal hormones.

- Suckling increases the release of gastrin and decreases the release of somatostatin into the gastric lumen. The lower the pH in the gastric lumen, the more somatostatin is released.

- Suckling shortens the feeding time.

- The suckling-related release of gastrointestinal hormones released into the lumen of the gastrointestinal tract promotes growth of the gastrointestinal tract via the gastrointestinal lumen.

- Suckling induces a release of gastrointestinal

hormones and insulin into the circulation, which may promote digestive and anabolic metabolic functions resulting in growth.

- The sucking-induced release of oxytocin and stimulation of vagal nerve activity are induced by touch and pressure on the oral mucosa induced by sucking of the nipple.

- Suckling-induced release of CCK may be involved in postprandial sedation.

- Suckling activates the release of oxytocin and activates vagal nerve activity in both the mother and the infant. The suckling-induced release of oxytocin participates in the stimulation of vagal nerve activity. The suckling-induced release of gastrointestinal hormones promotes efficient handling of nutrients to promote metabolism and growth in both.

Chapter 22

Breastfeeding: Increased Food Intake and Effect of Food on Oxytocin-Mediated Effects

Food is Necessary for Growth and Reproduction

To provide offspring with adequate amounts of milk is important for the survival of all mammalian species. Milk production is energy consuming for the mother. Chapters 19 and 20 included a description of how mothers optimize the use of energy by optimizing their digestive capacity and their ability to store and transfer nutrients to the mammary glands. They also save energy by reducing their stress levels. These effects are obtained by increased activity in the vagal efferent nerves and decreased activity in the HPA (hypothalamic-pituitary-adrenal) axis and the sympathetic nervous system in response to the suckling stimulus. Oxytocin plays an integrative role in the suckling-mediated modulation of the activity in the autonomic nervous system.

A more direct mechanism to cover the energy expenditures of milk production is to increase the intake of food. Most mammalian mothers eat more during the energy-demanding period of lactation unless they have large stores of fat, e.g., seals or whales, which can be mobilized and used for milk production. The increased food intake during lactation is linked to oxytocin released by the suckling stimulus. This process will be described in this chapter.

In addition, ingested food influences milk production and maternal interaction with the infant. The presence of food in the gastrointestinal tract stimulates oxytocin release by activation of vagal sensory or afferent neurons. In this way, the presence or absence of food in the gastrointestinal tract will adapt milk production and interaction with the offspring to access calories. This facilitatory effect by food in the gastrointestinal tract on the release and effects of oxytocin will also be described in this chapter.

Role of Oxytocin in Food Intake

Oxytocin-Mediated Increase in Food Intake During Lactation

Oxytocin may influence food intake in several ways, and these effects are differently expressed in lactating and non-lactating animals. Lactating rats eat more than non-lactating animals. The increased food intake is induced by the suckling stimulus and involves pathways in the brain that mediate the milk ejection reflex. Lesions in the lateral midbrain, which abolish suckling-activated oxytocin release and milk ejection, are followed by a 50% reduction in food intake and a loss of weight in lactating rats (Hansen & Ferreira, 1986).

In support of a role for oxytocin in the increased food intake observed during lactation, administration of oxytocin into the brain of non-lactating female rats has been demonstrated to give rise to increased food intake. This effect, however, was not observed in all rat strains (Bjorkstrand & Uvnäs-Moberg, 1996).

The rats that increased their food intake in response to administration of oxytocin also increased in weight. The increase in weight was most likely due to a combination of an increased intake of calories and an increased anabolic-storing metabolism. Administration of oxytocin increased weight gain in some strains of rats without increasing food intake (Uvnäs-Moberg, Alster, & Petersson, 1996). As previously mentioned, administration of oxytocin may induce a rise of insulin levels and a decrease in the levels of CCK and somatostatin, an endocrine pattern which is consistent with increased weight gain, even in the absence of enhanced food intake (Bjorkstrand, Ahlenius, et al., 1996; Bjorkstrand, Eriksson, et al., 1996; Uvnäs-Moberg, 1989). The metabolic effects of oxytocin were discussed in more detail in chapters 19 and 20.

Role of Female Sex Steroids

The reason why some rat strains responded to administration of oxytocin with increased food intake and weight gain and not others is probably related to the physiological potential for these events to occur. The responsive rats had a low spontaneous growth rate, which might have been innate or stress induced. In addition, the effects were only observed in females. Therefore, the presence of female sex steroids might have been important for the weight gain to occur. Female rats in which the ovaries and, consequently, the production of estrogen and progesterone had been taken away decreased in weight in response to oxytocin compared to rats with intact ovaries (Petersson, Eklund, & Uvnäs-Moberg, 2005).

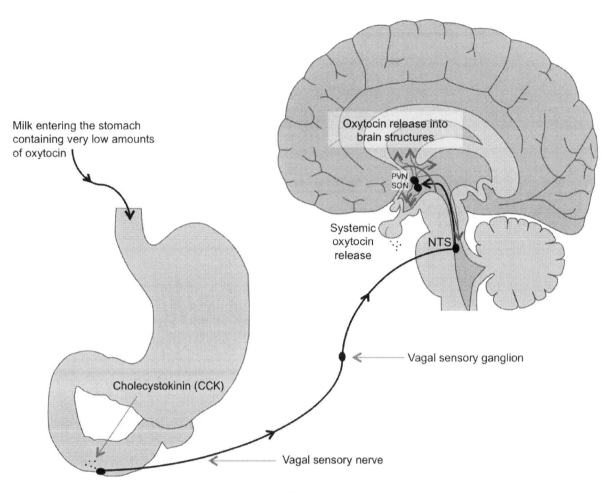

Figure 22.1. Stomach – Brain Connection

Source: Uvnäs-Moberg & Prime, 2013. Reprinted with permission.

The Role of Oxytocin as a Satiety Hormone

The role of oxytocin as a hyperphagic hormone contrasts with current opinions that oxytocin is a satiety hormone. Oxytocin has been demonstrated to decrease food intake for some hours after administration into the brain in male rats (Olson et al., 1991). This effect is induced via a reflex loop involving CCK released from the gastrointestinal tract in response to food intake and consequent activation of vagal nerve afferents (ingoing fibers). The sensory nucleus of the vagal nerves, the nucleus tractus solitarius (NTS), is an important relay station in this reflex. Neurons projecting from the NTS to the vagal motor nuclei (DMX) activate efferent vagal neurons (outgoing fibers) that inhibit gastric emptying. In addition, the nerve impulses from the NTS reach the hypothalamus and oxytocin is released from magnocellular and parvocellular neurons of the SON and PVN (Buller & Day, 1996; Luckman, Hamamura,

Antonijevic, Dye, & Leng, 1993; Renaud, Tang, McCann, Stricker, & Verbalis, 1987; Rinaman et al., 1995). Oxytocin decreases food intake by several mechanisms. Oxytocin released from parvocellular neurons decreases appetite by releasing CRF, which reduces food intake by actions in hypothalamic areas involved in the control of food intake. Via parvocellular oxytocin fibers relaying back to the brainstem, oxytocin potentiates the CCK-induced inhibition of gastric emptying. Oxytocin also facilitates the leptin-induced decrease of gastric emptying by actions in the brainstem (Blevins, Eakin, Murphy, Schwartz, & Baskin, 2003; Olson et al., 1991; Olson et al., 1992; Verbalis, Blackburn, Hoffman, & Stricker, 1995). The mechanisms involved in the release of oxytocin in response to food intake will be described in more detail below, along with other functions of the feeding-induced release of oxytocin.

Oxytocin May Induce Both Short-Term Satiety and

Long-Term Hyperphagia During Lactation

Oxytocin is involved in opposing effects on food intake during lactation, a short-term inhibition after food intake initiated by the presence of food in the stomach and a long-term stimulation over the entire lactation period, which is driven by the suckling stimulus. These effects are likely to be mediated by different pathways. The release of CCK in response to feeding is decreased in lactating rats, suggesting that the function of the postprandial vagally mediated inhibition of food intake by CCK is less prominent during the lactation period (Linden, Uvnäs-Moberg, et al., 1990).

Role of Food-Induced Oxytocin Release on Milk Ejection and Milk Production, Maternal Behavior, and Attachment

As mentioned in the previous paragraph, food intake is related to a release of oxytocin, which is involved in postprandial satiety and reduction of food intake. At the same time, the release of oxytocin occurring in response to a meal influences other physiological and behavioral effects, e.g., postprandial sedation, and during lactation, it facilitates milk ejection and production. Just as the effect of oxytocin on food intake is related to the amount of calories ingested, the other oxytocin-induced effects are also linked to the amount of food ingested, since the vagal sensory (afferent or ingoing) fibers transmit important information regarding the nutritional status in the gastrointestinal tract to the oxytocin system in the brain (Figure 22.1).

Mechanisms Involved in the Release of Oxytocin in Response to Food Ingestion

Oxytocin is released into the circulation in response to food intake in many mammalian species, such as cows, sows, and dogs, and in response to suckling in calves (Lupoli et al., 2001; Svennersten et al., 1990; Uvnäs-Moberg et al., 1985). The release of oxytocin in response to food intake may be mediated by two different mechanisms.

Release of Oxytocin in Response to Touch of the Oral Mucosa

In some species, a rapid peak-shaped release of oxytocin is induced in response to activation of sensory fibers in the oral cavity, which project to the NTS, and from there to the oxytocin-producing neurons in the hypothalamus. This mechanism from a functional point of view is similar to the one induced by sucking in infants and was described in more detail in chapter 21.

CCK Released from the Gastrointestinal Tract, Activates the Vagal Nerves and Induces Oxytocin Release

When food is ingested, gastrointestinal hormones are released to stimulate digestive and metabolic processes. The hormone CCK is released by the presence of food in the gastrointestinal tract (in particular by protein and fat) and stimulates pancreatic function, contracts the gall bladder, and blocks gastric emptying. In addition, CCK activates sensory fibers in the vagal nerves, which, as described above, results in satiety and postprandial sedation (Uvnäs-Moberg, 1989, 1994). Oxytocin is released from magnocellular neurons into the circulation and from parvocellular oxytocinergic neurons in the brain in response to administration of CCK to induce a multitude of effects (Linden, Uvnäs-Moberg, Forsberg, Bednar, & Sodersten, 1989; Olson et al., 1992; Renaud et al., 1987; Verbalis, McCann, McHale, & Stricker, 1986; Verbalis, Stricker, Robinson, & Hoffman, 1991). Other gastrointestinal hormones, such as secretin, may contribute to the vagally mediated release of oxytocin following food intake (Velmurugan, Brunton, Leng, & Russell, 2010).

Oxytocin Released from the Gastrointestinal Tract

It is important to mention that large amounts of oxytocin are produced within the gastrointestinal tract; therefore, food intake may also be associated with a release of oxytocin from the gastrointestinal tract (Ohlsson et al., 2006). Oxytocin emanating from the gastrointestinal tract may contribute to the elevation of oxytocin levels after food intake.

Experiments Illustrating the Link Between Food Intake and Release of Oxytocin and Prolactin

Role of Food and Release of CCK

Food Intake During Milking Increases Oxytocin Levels and Milk Yield in Cows

The fact that food in the gastrointestinal tract stimulates the release of oxytocin, inducing milk ejection and possibly stimulating milk production, has practical implications. For example, if cows are fed just before or during being milked by a milking machine, more oxytocin is released and milk yield increases (Johansson, Uvnäs-Moberg, Knight, & Svennersten-Sjaunja, 1999; Svennersten, Gorewit, Sjaunja, & Uvnäs-Moberg, 1995; Uvnäs-Moberg et al., 2001).

Food Deprivation Decreases the Release of Oxytocin and Prolactin

If the mother does not receive food, it is simply not possible to produce milk. In cases of lack of food or large fat stores, which can be mobilized and transferred to the mammary gland, milk production ceases sooner or later.

If lactating cows or sows are not provided with food, both basal and suckling-induced levels of oxytocin and prolactin decrease, and they stop producing milk. Milk production is resumed as soon as food is ingested again (Rojkittikhun et al., 1993; Samuelsson, Uvnäs-Moberg, Gorewit, & Svennersten-Sjaunja, 1996).

This effect is not simply due to the lack of nutrients in the circulation, but to a decreased activation of the afferent or ingoing sensory fibers in the vagal nerves, as a consequence of the lack of food in the gastrointestinal tract according to the mechanism described below.

Role of the Vagal Nerves

In support of an important role for the vagal nerves in the control of oxytocin release, electrical stimulation of afferent (ingoing) vagal nerves in lactating animals gives rise not only to oxytocin release into the circulation, but also to milk ejection (Moos & Richard, 1975a, 1975b; Stock & Uvnäs-Moberg, 1988).

Effects of Cutting the Vagal Nerves

The role of the vagal nerves on the effects induced by food intake on oxytocin and prolactin levels, as well as on milk ejection and milk production, was investigated in experiments performed on lactating rats in which the vagal nerves from the gastrointestinal tract had been cut (Eriksson et al., 1994).

After this operation, the rats gradually stopped releasing oxytocin and prolactin in response to suckling, and within a few days, they stopped ejecting and producing milk. They cared less for their pups, but continued to overeat as normal lactating rats do. The reason for the inhibition of oxytocin and prolactin release and inhibition of milk ejection and milk production was not the lack of food, but rather the lack of information to the brain from the gut, which normally takes place when food has been ingested. This information is transferred via afferent or sensory fibers in the vagal nerves in response to CCK released by food intake. If the vagal nerves connecting the gut and the brain are cut, no such information will be transmitted to the brain, even if sufficient amounts of food has been ingested.

In the absence of information about the presence of food in the stomach normally mediated by the vagal nerve, the release of oxytocin from the magnocellular neurons was reduced. This effect appeared gradually over a week and resulted in an inhibition of milk ejection.

Prolactin levels, which were also reduced after cutting the vagal nerves, are normally stimulated by the suckling stimulus and mediated by a decrease of dopamine in the anterior pituitary. However, oxytocin released into the anterior pituitary from magno- or parvocellular oxytocin neurons also contributes to the stimulation of prolactin release. In the absence of oxytocin, other stimuli fail to release prolactin (Mogg & Samson, 1990; Samson et al., 1986). Therefore, the decrease in prolactin levels seen following the cutting of the vagal nerves most likely is secondary to the decreased release of oxytocin into the anterior pituitary. Taken together, not only milk ejection, but also milk production is decreased as a result of the lack of sensory information from the gastrointestinal tract normally occurring in response to ingestion of food. These results further support the integrative role of oxytocin in the control of milk ejection and production.

Continued Stimulation of Food Intake and Maternal Weight Gain

In spite of the inhibition of oxytocin and prolactin release, the suckling stimulus continued to drive the rat mothers' appetite. The lactating rats subjected to vagotomy continued to overeat, and they even increased slightly in weight when compared to lactating rats with an intact vagal nerve (Eriksson et al., 1994). In metabolic terms, the rats stopped giving out energy, they kept it for themselves in the absence of information about ingested calories from the gastrointestinal tract. Instead of being altruistic, they became more egotistic (Uvnäs-Moberg & Eriksson, 1996).

Different Types of Oxytocin Mechanisms Regulate Processes Related to Energy Expenditure and Energy Saving

The classical uterine type of oxytocin receptor is present in the brain. Oxytocin-induced effects, not only on uterine contraction and milk ejection, but also on maternal behavior and bonding, are blocked by an oxytocin antagonist, which blocks the activity of the uterine-oxytocin receptors (Gimpl & Fahrenholz, 2001). These types of oxytocin-linked effects result in loss of energy.

When oxytocin exerts anti-stress effects and stimulates anabolic metabolism, it binds to and activates another type of receptor, which can't be blocked by the antagonists directed against the classical oxytocin receptor. Higher doses of oxytocin are needed in order to induce these effects in comparison to the doses needed to induce the effects on milk ejection and social interactive behaviors. These effects are not fully blocked by the oxytocin antagonist directed to the uterine type of oxytocin receptors (Petersson et al., 1996a). This other type of oxytocin receptor seems to correspond to or be closely linked to the alpha-2 adrenergic receptor that inhibits the activity of the (nor)adrenergic system in the brain to induce anti-stress effects (Diaz-Cabiale et al., 2000; Petersson et al., 1999a; Petersson, Uvnäs-Moberg, et al., 1998; Uvnäs-Moberg, 1998a, 1998b). Stimulation of the alpha-2 adrenergic receptors, e.g., results in lowering of blood pressure and cortisol levels and in a more pronounced release of insulin in response to feeding and storing of energy (Petersson, Hulting, Andersson, et al., 1999).

Taken together, activation of the alpha-2 adrenoceptor-mediated functions results in energy saving. Indeed the alpha-2 adrenoceptor system within the brain has been labeled the energy-conserving system.

Food in the Gastrointestinal Tract Selectively Activates Oxytocin-Mediated Effects Related to Giving Energy

Severing the vagal nerves blocked the effects of oxytocin that were related to friendly interaction and giving out energy (milk ejection, maternal behavior), but not the effects related to saving of energy (anabolic processes, storing of nutrients, and increased food intake), as the rats continued to overeat and increased in weight. It, therefore, seems as if the afferent vagal nerve activity caused by food intake and via a release of CCK preferentially facilitates the oxytocinergic mechanisms related to interaction and giving, i.e., the oxytocin effects that are induced by administration of lower amounts of oxytocin, which are blocked by the oxytocin antagonist that blocks the uterine type of receptor. It makes sense from a biological perspective to stop giving out energy when no food is received, and to increase appetite and store energy.

Administration of CCK Induces Maternal Behavior

Oxytocin released in response to food intake or administration of CCK not only stimulates milk ejection and production, it is also released from parvocellular oxytocin neurons to induce physiological and behavioral adaptations.

Administration of CCK has been demonstrated to stimulate maternal behavior in rats, normally attributed to central effects of oxytocin (Numan & Sheehan, 1997), supporting the existence of a link between food-induced release of CCK and oxytocin-related behaviors. Whereas the effect induced by CCK on milk ejection is exerted by oxytocin released from the magnocellular neurons into the circulation, the effects on maternal behavior must be mediated by oxytocin released from parvocellular neurons in the brain (Linden, Uvnäs-Moberg, Eneroth, & Sodersten, 1989; Miranda-Paiva, Nasello, Yim, & Felicio, 2002; Weber, Manfredo, & Rinaman, 2009).

CCK Participates in the Development of Attachment in Lambs

In lambs suckling, particularly the first suckling episode, it is extremely important for development of recognition and attachment to the ewe. If the lamb is not allowed to suck during the first 24-48 hours after birth, the lamb fails to recognize its mother (Nowak, Murphy, et al., 1997). CCK released from the intestine in response to suckling and the presence of colostrum in the gastrointestinal tract has been demonstrated to be important for the development of the lamb's attachment to the ewe, since administration of CCK antagonists were shown to block the effect on attachment

(Linden, Carlquist, et al., 1989; Nowak, Murphy, et al., 1997). These effects of CCK must have been induced by oxytocin released from parvocellular neurons in the brain. Oxytocin has been shown to be of prime importance in the process of attachment between mother and young, presumably an analogous mechanism is operating in the bonding between the offspring and its mother (Keverne & Kendrick, 1994).

Release of CCK in Response to Sensory Stimulation

Somatosensory-Vagal Reflexes

One effect of non-noxious somatosensory stimulation is to increase the release of the gastrointestinal hormones gastrin and CCK. These effects are blocked by vagotomy and must, therefore, be mediated via neurons originating in the DMX. Obviously, there are nervous connections between somatosensory neurons originating in the skin and the vagal nerves controlling gastrointestinal function. The NTS is a relay station before the nerve impulses are transmitted to the DMX (Uvnäs-Moberg, Lundeberg, et al., 1992).

Close contact between pups and their mothers results in a release of CCK. As much CCK was released in the dog pups when they had been separated and were reunited with their mothers as when the pups were sucking (Uvnäs-Moberg, 1989).

As discussed in detail above, the gastrointestinal hormone cholecystokinin plays an important role in activation of the vagal nerve afferents from the gastrointestinal tract. CCK released in response to food intake not only influences digestive and metabolic functions (stimulation of pancreatic enzyme secretion, emptying of gallbladder, inhibition of gastric motility and emptying), it also induces central effects, such as satiety, sedation, and calm. It may also stimulate oxytocin release, milk ejection and milk production, maternal behavior, and the development of attachment between newborns and their mothers (Uvnäs-Moberg et al., 1987).

Naturally, CCK released by sensory stimulation, such as closeness, also results in activation of vagal afferents. The presence or absence of food in the gastrointestinal tract may reinforce or inhibit the nerve impulses projecting more centrally within the brain. Newborn rat pups given antagonists to CCK, failed to become sedated and calm after suckling (Weber, Manfredo, & Rinaman, 2009; Weller & Blass, 1998). When the CCK-related signals from the gastrointestinal tract were blocked by the antagonist, suckling and closeness failed to induce the sedating and calming effects.

What about Human Mothers?

Human mothers need between 500 and 1,000 extra calories per day in order to provide their infants with adequate amounts of milk. Normally, breastfeeding mothers have a good appetite to compensate for the energy expenditure caused by milk production. The mother's nutritional status during lactation is also important for human mothers, but they can continue breastfeeding for a long time, even when the food supply is short. Energy-saving mechanisms activated by suckling can cover for the loss of food for some time. However, in the absence of food, milk production will eventually deteriorate. Since so much energy is invested in each infant, every effort is made to continue milk production for as long as possible.

Food Intake and Positive Mood and Trust

Whether the amount of food intake during breastfeeding influences mothers has not been demonstrated, but it is very likely that such effects exist, albeit in a modified form.

Oxytocin is released in response to food intake or administration of cholecystokinin in humans, suggesting that oxytocin-mediated effects are induced or augmented by feeding (Borg et al., 2010; Ohlsson et al., 2002). Milk ejection and the production of prolactin might also be facilitated, as oxytocin stimulates prolactin release. Eating may induce oxytocin release in the brain, which may improve mood and increase social interaction. That food intake does improve mood and makes individuals more prone to social interaction is well known. It is also known that food intake increases trust between individuals.

Relationship Between Milk Ejection and Social Interaction

The number of oxytocin peaks observed during the first ten minutes in response to suckling in breastfeeding women is related to the amount of milk ejected. The number of oxytocin peaks is also related to level of social interactive capacities, as determined by the Karolinska Scale of Personality (Nissen et al., 1998). The more generous a mother is in terms of ejecting milk to her baby, the more social and interactive she is. These data suggest that oxytocin released into the circulation to cause milk ejection and into the amygdala to increase social skills occurs in parallel. Nerves projecting from the SON and PVN to the posterior pituitary send axon reflexes not only to the anterior pituitary to synchronize the release of oxytocin and prolactin, but also to the amygdala to synchronize oxytocin release and maternal psychological adaptations, such as increased social skills, with milk ejection. CCK released from the intestine may, via the vagal nerve, facilitate this "generosity circuit."

Inhibition by Stress

It is well known that suckling-related oxytocin release and milk ejection is easily inhibited by stress (Newton, 1992;

Nissen et al., 1996). Since the same mechanisms regulate social interactive behaviors, it is likely that the psychological components of motherhood can also be inhibited by stress. To eat too little food is certainly a stressor during lactation, and, therefore, both milk production and the psychological adaptations should be influenced to some extent.

Not Only Stress, But Also Eating Disorders

An important question to explore is whether the maternal psychological adaptations, i.e., the decreased levels of anxiety and the increased tendency for social interactive and caring behavior, are reduced as a consequence of an inhibition of oxytocin release if a breastfeeding mother eats too little. Such changes may occur long before milk production has ceased. These questions are relevant not only in countries where starvation is prevalent, but also in Western societies, since many women choose to eat too little to become slim, particularly after pregnancy. Low levels of oxytocin have been demonstrated in women with anorexia nervosa, but it is difficult to decide what is the hen and what is the egg, because both a low appetite and too little food in the stomach may be linked to low oxytocin levels (Demitrack et al., 1990).

Summary

- Suckling stimulates food intake and anabolic storing of metabolism. Both of these effects are facilitated by oxytocin released in the brain by the suckling stimulus.

- In addition to stimulating food intake in a long-term perspective, oxytocin released in response to feeding may reduce food intake in the short term by slowing down emptying of the stomach and by reducing appetite. These effects are induced by parvocellular oxytocin fibers terminating in the brainstem (DMX) and in areas in the brain involved in the control of food intake.

- Food intake stimulates oxytocin release in two different ways—when the food touches the oral mucosa and when CCK is released from the intestine by food. Both these effects are mediated by afferent vagal nerve fibers. If suckling is combined with food intake, more oxytocin is released and more milk is ejected.

- When food is present in the gastrointestinal tract, CCK is released. This activates afferent vagal nerve fibers, which induces release of oxytocin from the SON and PVN from magnocellular neurons into the circulation and from parvocellular neurons into the brain.

- If the vagal nerves are cut in lactating rats, oxytocin and prolactin release, as well as milk ejection and production, is blocked within a few days. The information normally exerted by food in the gastrointestinal tract is not transmitted into the brain. This lack of information is misinterpreted by the brain as starvation, and the oxytocin-related mechanisms involved in milk ejection and milk production are not stimulated. This probably also inhibits the oxytocin-related interactive behaviors.

- The component of the oxytocin system related to saving of energy, possibly the alpha-2 adrenoceptor system labeled the energy-saving system, is not affected by cutting the vagal nerves. Obviously, only the oxytocin effects related to the output of energy receive stimulation as to the intake of calories via afferent vagal nerves.

- Oxytocin is released following food intake in human mothers. The relationship between food intake, milk production, and maternal behavioral adaptations are not well studied in human mothers, but oxytocin levels in response to suckling reflect both the amount of milk ejected, as well as the level of social interactive behavior.

- It is very likely that low food intake, whether caused by starvation or anorexic food habits, influence oxytocin release and induce a consequent effect on milk production and interactive behavior.

Chapter 23

Skin-to-Skin Contact Facilitates Breastfeeding

Infants are not only suckling during breastfeeding, they are also in skin-to-skin contact with their mothers. A period of skin-to-skin contact may precede suckling, and after the infants have sucked, they may lie on their mothers' chests for some time. This means that some of the effects observed during breastfeeding may be induced or facilitated by skin-to-skin contact. In fact, the effects of breastfeeding and skin-to-skin contact are to a certain extent indistinguishable. Both suckling and skin-to-skin contact induce oxytocinergic mechanisms, which exert a major integrative function on the effect patterns caused by the respective stimuli.

Skin-to-Skin Contact Facilitates Suckling During Breastfeeding

Skin-to-Skin Contact Facilitates Milk Ejection in the Mother

Activation of Axon Reflexes

During the period of skin-to-skin contact preceding suckling, the blood vessels on the mother's breast and chest start to dilate, which results in increased skin temperature. At the same time, the muscles surrounding the opening of the milk ducts on the nipple start to dilate. These effects are exerted by local neurogenic reflexes. When these reflexes are activated, peptides, which relax smooth muscles, are released locally in the nipple and skin overlying the mammary gland.

Decreased Activity in Sympathetic Nerve Fibers

In addition, skin-to-skin contact decreases the tone in the sympathetic nervous system. The decreased sympathetic nervous tone caused by skin-to-skin contact is associated with facilitation of milk ejection and increased skin temperature, as the stress-induced contraction of the muscles surrounding the milk ducts and blood vessels is counteracted. The decrease in sympathetic nervous tone is induced by activation of sensory nerves from the mammary gland area and from the skin of the chest, which results in a decreased activity in brainstem centers involved in the control of sympathetic nervous tone.

Effects of Oxytocin Released in the Brainstem

The sensory stimulation induced by skin-to-skin contact also stimulates oxytocin release via nervous pathways that connect the nucleus tractus solitarius (NTS) and the oxytocin producing supraoptic and paraventricular nuclei (SON and PVN). For example, oxytocin is released from nerves projecting to areas in the brainstem where autonomic tone is regulated. Oxytocin released from these nerves reinforces the decrease in sympathetic tone caused by the short brainstem reflexes mentioned above.

Decreased Levels of Anxiety by Oxytocin Released in the Amygdala

Oxytocin is also released in the amygdala, causing the mother's level of anxiety to decrease. When the levels of anxiety decrease, sympathetic nervous tone decreases, since there is a link between the amygdala and the noradrenergic centers in the brainstem involved in the control of sympathetic nervous tone. Consequently, the relaxation of the muscles around blood vessels and the milk ducts is reinforced, which leads to further increase in skin temperature and opening of the milk ducts.

Multiple Effects at Multiple Sites of Action

When the sensory nerves are stimulated by skin-to-skin contact, effects are induced at multiple sites at different levels in the nervous system and the brain, which facilitate breastfeeding. A summary of the effects is given below.

- The circulation in the skin increases and the milk ducts start to open in response to a local release of peptides from nerves (via axon reflexes).

- The nerve impulses decrease sympathetic nervous tone by actions in the basal areas in the brainstem involved in the control of autonomic nervous tone, e.g., the NTS, thereby contributing to the increased skin temperature and opening of the milk ducts. Sensory nerves emanating in the mammary gland area and from the chest contribute to this effect.

- The nerve impulses induced by skin-to-skin contact reach the oxytocin-producing neurons in the PVN and SON in the hypothalamus. Breastfeeding is facilitated in several ways by activation of oxytocinergic nerves from the PVN.

- The sympathetic nervous tone is further decreased by oxytocin released into the NTS and adjacent areas.

- The level of anxiety is decreased by actions of oxytocin in the amygdala. This will, in turn, lead to a further decrease of sympathetic nervous tone.

- Maternal interaction is stimulated by actions in the amygdala and other areas involved in the control of social interaction.

- Milk production is facilitated as oxytocinergic fibers projecting to the anterior pituitary influence the prolactin producing cells.

Suckling Stimulates Milk Ejection and Milk Production

Milk Ejection

During suckling oxytocin is released into the circulation by the more intense suckling stimulus. The suckling-related oxytocin profile is characterized by pulses, which occur in 90-second intervals when studied two days after birth (Uvnäs-Moberg et al., 1990; Nissen et al., 1996, Jonas et al., 2009). When oxytocin peaks reach the mammary glands, the myoepithelial cells surrounding the alveoli in the mammary glands contract and milk is expressed in 90-second intervals (Uvnäs-Moberg & Prime, 2013).

Skin-to-skin contact alone gives rise to oxytocin pulses that are of longer duration and occur at irregular intervals (Nissen et al., 1995). When the infants are massaging the mothers' breasts immediately after birth, oxytocin peaks may be induced. The more intense the massage, the more oxytocin pulses are induced (Matthiesen et al., 2001a). However, this stimulation is not strong enough to cause short oxytocin peaks and milk ejection by itself, but it facilitates the suckling-induced milk ejection.

Prolactin Release

Suckling induces a release of prolactin and thereby milk secretion. The size of prolactin release is dependent on the duration of suckling. Oxytocin released from nerves in the anterior pituitary promotes prolactin release. The correlation observed between suckling-related oxytocin and prolactin release may reflect this connection (Jonas et al., 2009).

In contrast, the neurogenic stimulation caused by skin-to-skin contact does not induce an immediate prolactin release nor therefore prolactin-related stimulation of milk production. Still the release of oxytocin caused by skin-to-skin contact will facilitate prolactin release in response to suckling and thereby milk production.

The Effects of Skin-to-Skin Contact and Suckling Overlap

Suckling can induce all the effects of skin-to-skin contact and skin-to-skin contact can induce all the effects induced by suckling, with the exception of the more intense suckling stimulus needed to induce the pulsatile oxytocin pattern characterized by 90-second intervals, which gives rise to contraction of the alveoli and milk ejection. Prolactin is not released by skin-to-skin contact, but by suckling.

Skin-to-Skin Contact Facilitates Suckling in the Infant

Skin-to-skin contact also prepares the infant for breastfeeding. Sensory nerves originating in the skin are activated in the infant during skin-to-skin contact. The increased maternal skin temperature together with the tactile stimulation caused by skin-to-skin contact stimulates the infant's breast-seeking behavior (Widström et al., 1987). Pheromones released from the breasts in response to dilation of the maternal blood vessels in the skin may attract the infant's attention to the breasts and stimulate their wish to suckle.

Skin-to-skin contact may induce these effects via activation of oxytocinergic mechanisms in the brain. The skin-to-skin-induced calming effect and reduction of stress levels may also help the infant start to breastfeed.

Both Mother and Infant Profit from Skin-to-Skin Contact Before Breastfeeding

Taken together, these data show that skin-to-skin contact before breastfeeding is essential because it prepares both the mother and the infant for breastfeeding. The mothers become more interactive and physically warm, and milk ejection is facilitated by both central and local mechanisms. The infants become calmer and more relaxed, and their inborn breast-seeking behavior is activated.

Further Adaptations Caused by Skin-to-Skin Contact

In addition to facilitation of milk ejection and milk production, skin-to-skin contact before breastfeeding may adapt mothers and infants for breastfeeding in a more general way. It stimulates the interaction between mother and infant, decreases stress levels, and promotes digestive and metabolic processes related to growth.

Social Interaction, Anxiety, and Pain

Both suckling and skin-to-skin contact increase the mother's wish for and competence to interact with her child and reduce her levels of anxiety. These effects are probably caused by a release of oxytocin in the amygdala and other areas in the brain that are involved in the regulation of social behavior and anxiety.

The perception of pain is decreased both during suckling and skin-to-skin contact (Abdulkader, Freer, Fleetwood-Walker, & McIntosh, 2007). Oxytocinergic fibers originating in the PVN that project to areas involved in the control of the pain threshold, such as the PAG and the dorsal column of the spinal cord, may be involved in these effects.

Anti-stress Effects

Blood Pressure

Blood pressure falls in response to both suckling and skin-to-skin contact in breastfeeding mothers (Jonas et al., 2008). The intensity of the effect, which is related to an inhibition of the activity in the aspects of the sympathetic nervous system that control cardiovascular function, may vary between the two types of sensory stimuli. Oxytocin released from nerves projecting from the PVN to the NTS play an important role in the mediation of these effects.

Link Between Facilitated Milk Ejection and Lowered Blood Pressure

As discussed above, one mechanism that facilitates milk ejection is a lowered sympathetic nervous tone. The fall in blood pressure is also due to a lowered sympathetic nervous tone. The two effects are related and demonstrate that the decreased sympathetic tone, which results in opening of milk ducts and relaxation of blood vessels in the skin overlying the mammary glands, is just one aspect of a more generalized shift in autonomic nervous tone, from sympathetic dominance to parasympathetic dominance.

Cortisol Levels

Cortisol levels decrease in response to both skin-to-skin contact and suckling (Handlin et al., 2009). This effect involves an oxytocin-mediated inhibition of the activity in the HPA axis in several ways. Oxytocin inhibits CRF secretion in the PVN and secretion of ACTH in the anterior pituitary. It inhibits secretion of cortisol in the adrenal cortex. Together, all these sites of action allow oxytocin to have a very strong inhibitory action on the release of cortisol.

Anti-stress Effects Partly by Different Mechanisms

The anti-stress effects caused by skin-to-skin contact differ from those caused by suckling in the sense that the skin-to-skin-related mechanisms involve to a larger extent "lower or more brainstem-oriented" mechanisms, whereas the suckling-related mechanisms also involve the HPA axis.

Growth-Promoting Effects

Skin-to-skin contact and suckling increase activity in the endocrine system of the gastrointestinal tract, which, in turn, optimizes maternal digestion and stimulates anabolic metabolism. Levels of gastrointestinal hormones are lowered in response to the less intense stimulation caused by skin-to-skin contact and increased by the more intense suckling stimulus in both mothers and infants (Uvnäs-Moberg, 1989). By reducing the levels of gastrointestinal hormones, skin-to-skin contact increases the potential for the increase caused by suckling, and as a consequence, the effect on digestion and anabolism. These effects are mediated by oxytocin released from neurons originating in the PVN, which project to the vagal nuclei, the DMX and NTS.

Infants

Skin-to-skin contact gives rise to the same effects in the infants as in the mothers. Social interaction is increased, and anxiety and the perception of pain are reduced. Their stress levels decrease, as evidenced by lower cortisol levels and increased skin temperatures caused by vasodilation in the skin vessels, as a result of an inhibited sympathetic nervous tone. Basal levels of gastrointestinal hormones are decreased in infants in the same way as in the mothers. The same effects are induced when the infants are suckling, but the effects may be more strongly expressed. In addition, suckling stimulates the release of gastrointestinal hormones that stimulate digestive, metabolic, and anabolic processes.

Summary

- Suckling induces short peak-shaped pulses of oxytocin levels into the maternal circulation. Skin-to-skin contact induces more protracted rises of oxytocin levels in the maternal circulation.

- Suckling, but not skin-to-skin contact, is associated with milk ejection and prolactin release.

- Skin-to-skin contact before breastfeeding facilitates the milk ejection reflex and maternal-caring behavior.

- Skin-to-skin contact stimulates the infant's breast-seeking behavior and facilitates sucking.

- Both suckling and skin-to skin contact result in lowered cortisol levels and lowered blood pressure. The effects on cortisol levels in response to skin-to-skin contact are to a larger extent exerted at lower brainstem levels. Similar effects are induced in both mother and infant.

- Both skin-to-skin contact and suckling influence the activity of the endocrine system of the gastrointestinal tract, but the effect of suckling is stronger and mimics effects caused by food intake. Similar effects are induced in both mother and infant.

Table 23.1. Similarities and Differences Between Effects Induced by Suckling and Skin-to-Skin Contact

	Skin-to-Skin Contact	Suckling
Oxytocin pattern	A few protracted pulses at irregular intervals	Frequent 90-second interval pulses
Milk ejection	Not linked to milk ejection*	Linked to milk ejection
Milk production	Not linked to prolactin release and milk production*	Stimulates prolactin release and milk production
Mother-infant interaction and bonding/attaching	Stimulates mother-infant interaction and increases bonding/attachment	Stimulates mother-infant interaction and increases bonding/attachment
Levels of anxiety	Reduces levels of anxiety	Reduces levels of anxiety
Pain	Reduces pain in mother and baby	Reduces pain in mother and baby
Anti-stress effects	Induces anti-stress effects—lowers blood pressure and cortisol levels, increases cutaneous blood flow	Induces anti-stress effects—lowers blood pressure and cortisol levels, increases cutaneous blood flow
Digestive and anabolic processes	Stimulates digestive and anabolic processes; lowers basal levels of GI hormones.	Stimulates digestive and anabolic processes; raises levels of GI hormones

*Skin-to-skin contact may indirectly facilitate milk ejection and production via activation of local sensory reflexes in the mammary gland and by an oxytocin-mediated inhibition of anxiety and of sympathetic nervous tone. It may also stimulate milk production in the long term, as prolactin levels are stimulated by oxytocin.

Chapter 24

Factors That Influence the Success of Breastfeeding

Breastfeeding Patterns Change

Breastfeeding patterns have been subjected to dramatic changes over time. The breastfeeding pattern observed in hunter-gatherer societies living in our time is supposed to reflect that of the first humans who evolved several hundred thousand years ago. In these societies, a very intense breastfeeding is practiced, i.e., mothers breastfeed several times every hour for short periods of time, and they breastfeed frequently during the night. In these societies in which breastfeeding may continue for three to four years after the child is born, breastfeeding problems are rarely seen (Hartmann, 2007). Such intense breastfeeding plays an important role in birth control in these cultures, as the high prolactin levels induced by intense and frequent suckling patterns inhibit ovulation and thereby the ability to conceive (Labbok, 2007).

"Disappearance of Breastfeeding"

In the beginning of the 20th century, birth was moved from homes to hospitals in the Western world, and breastfeeding became the subject of "medical programming." Mothers and babies were separated after birth. Strict rules allowing breastfeeding every fourth hour were introduced instead of feeding on demand. As a result of these unnatural practices, breastfeeding became difficult. As milk formula became available as an easy and alternative way to feed newborns, some cultures have almost completely exchanged breastfeeding for bottle feeding. In other cultures, milk pumping is practiced and mothers' own milk is given by bottle.

Revival of Breastfeeding

Breastfeeding is becoming increasingly popular in some countries. Due to the scientific data that show that mothers' milk is better than milk formula, breastfeeding has been promoted and has, in some countries like Sweden, almost become the rule again.

Breastfeeding may not only be important because it supplies the newborn with the perfect nutrition and antibodies to some diseases, it also stimulates the development of bonding and social interactive behaviors in both mothers and infants. This is because oxytocin is released into the brain during suckling to induce a broad pattern of oxytocin-mediated effects. In addition, breastfeeding gives rise to long-term health-promoting effects in the mother.

To achieve an increase in the rate of breastfeeding, it became important to optimize practices in the labor and maternity wards and to give mothers optimal support. The concept of baby-friendly hospitals was created and the recommendations include breastfeeding initiation within one hour after birth, giving only breastmilk, rooming-in, and breastfeeding on demand. Today, almost 90% of Swedish women breastfeed when they leave the maternity ward, and 60% still breastfeed exclusively after six months.

The success of breastfeeding not only depends on practices around birth. Basic facts, such as the ability to obtain enough food and whether a woman has to work soon after birth, influence the rate of breastfeeding. Cultural norms and attitudes toward breastfeeding are important. For example, upper-class European women have not always breastfed themselves, but have left this task to wet nurses.

Effects of Labor and Maternity Ward Routines on Milk Production

In contrast to mothers living in hunter-gatherer societies, breastfeeding is not always easy for the mothers in our Western culture. Even if society supports breastfeeding as being the best way to feed babies and mothers want to breastfeed, milk production and milk ejection often become a problem for individual mothers. It is, therefore, important to identify scientifically based practices or other factors that increase the chance of successful breastfeeding.

It is obvious that both prolactin and oxytocin released in response to suckling play important roles in milk production and milk ejection in breastfeeding women. It therefore follows that in order to promote breastfeeding, the conditions for suckling-related prolactin and oxytocin release should be maximized. It has been established that frequent breastfeeding, particularly during the early phase of breastfeeding when milk production is established, is linked to more milk production and longer total periods of breastfeeding (Salariya et al., 1978). Baby-friendly practices improve the chances of breastfeeding at least for six weeks (DiGirolamo et al., 2008). The positive role for initiation and duration of breastfeeding caused by early skin-to-skin contact has, however, been questioned (Carfoot, Williamson, & Dickson, 2003).

The success of breastfeeding can be measured in several objective ways. Milk production can be measured by weighing the baby before and after a breast meal. The difference in weight corresponds to the amount of milk ingested by the baby and is often taken as a measure of maternal milk production. By measuring an infant's weight gain over time, it may be inferred if the infant's milk intake is adequate or not. The duration of partial or exclusive breastfeeding is often used to describe the success of breastfeeding.

Clinical Study, The Russian Study

The influence of some labor and maternity ward routines on the outcome of breastfeeding was investigated in an extensive controlled, randomized study performed by Bystrova and collaborators in St. Petersburg, Russia (Bystrova, Matthiesen, et al., 2007; Bystrova, Widstrom et al., 2007). In this study, 176 mothers and their infants participated. The mothers were randomized to have skin-to-skin contact with their infants (group 1), to hold their dressed infants (group 2), or to be separated from their infants, who were placed in a cot in a nursery in the labor ward (groups 3 and 4) from 25 to 120 minutes after birth. After that time period, the mother-infant dyads in groups 1, 2, and 4 were assigned to a four-day period of rooming-in at the maternity ward, whereas the infants of mothers in group 3 were placed in a nursery in the maternity ward. The mother-infant dyads in group 4 were only separated between 25 and 120 minutes after birth, whereas the mothers in group 3 were separated from their infants both during the stay in the labor ward and in the maternity ward.

During the four-day stay in the maternity ward, the infants were either dressed in clothes or were swaddled according to the Russian tradition, irrespective of being with their mothers or staying in the nursery. The number and duration of breastfeeds, the amount of milk ingested by the infant in connection with a breastfeed on day four, and the duration of nearly exclusive breastfeeding was recorded. The occurrence of early suckling was noted (Bystrova, Matthiesen, Widstrom, et al., 2007; Bystrova, Widstrom, Matthiesen, 2007).

Main Results

- Labor ward routines do not influence milk production four days after birth (Bystrova, Matthiesen, Widstrom, et al., 2007).

- Early suckling was associated with more milk production four days after birth within groups allowed skin-to-skin contact and early suckling, but not between groups not allowed skin-to-skin contact and early suckling (Bystrova, Widstrom, Matthiesen, et al., 2007).

- Rooming-in at the maternity ward was associated with more milk production four days after birth than nursery care (Bystrova, Widstrom,

Matthiesen, et al., 2007).

- Milk production on day four predicted the duration of breastfeeding (Bystrova, Widstrom, Matthiesen, et al., 2007).

Labor Ward Routines Do Not Influence Milk Production

The labor ward practices used in this study had no influence on milk production four days later. The mothers on the average produced 249, 263, 162, and 254 ml of milk in groups 1, 2, 3, and 4, respectively (Bystrova, Matthiesen, Widstrom, et al., 2007). It is important to notice that a short-term separation between mother and infant (from 25-120 minutes after birth) in the labor ward did not influence milk volume four days later. A short-term separation after birth did, as described previously, influence the future interaction between mother and infant, and also the infant's ability to regulate stress levels (Bystrova et al., 2009). This difference suggests that milk production and behavioral effects are regulated by different mechanisms.

Early Suckling Does Not Influence Milk Production

In the study groups in which mothers and infants were kept in skin-to-skin contact after birth (group 1) or in which the mothers held their children dressed in clothes (group 2), the infants had the possibility to suckle immediately the after birth. Not all infants did. Suckling within the first two hours postpartum was associated with increased milk ingestion/production four days after birth in groups 1 and 2, as the infants who suckled early ingested more milk. In addition, they recovered more quickly from the neonatal weight loss when compared to the non-sucklers (Bystrova, Matthiesen, Widstrom, et al., 2007).

It may seem as if early suckling stimulates milk production. However, the average amount of milk ingested by the infants who had been separated for 25-120 minutes after birth and were not able to suckle immediately after birth (group 4) was the same as the amount of milk ingested by the infants in groups 1 and 2, who were close to their mothers and allowed to suckle. These data make the effects of early suckling on milk production more difficult to interpret and suggest that early suckling does not increase milk production. Rather, it suggests that the difference in milk ingestion observed within the groups reflects differences between the infants within the group. In fact, the non-sucklers in groups 1 and 2 were not as well developed and mature as the sucklers, weighing significantly less at birth (Bystrova, Matthiesen, Widstrom, et al., 2007). Some of the non-sucklers may also have had difficulties with suckling immediately after birth, as a consequence of having endured the "trauma" of recent labor and birth. Such non-suckling infants may have continued to suckle, albeit not as well, during the four-day stay in the maternity ward, which might have led to less prolactin secretion and less stimulation of milk production observed four days later.

The non-sucklers should be represented in all four groups due to the randomized design of the study. The non-sucklers were not identified in groups 3 and 4, since these infants were not presented with the possibility of early suckling.

The suggestion that early suckling does not stimulate milk production is supported by the results from a randomized study in which early suckling was not associated with more milk production four days after birth (Widstrom et al., 1990). Other studies do, however, suggest that early suckling influences milk production in a positive way, but it is often difficult to discern the differences between the effects of early suckling, early skin-to-skin contact, and rooming-in due to the design of these studies (Nylander et al., 1991; Salariya et al., 1978). The bonding or increased interaction between mother and child induced by early skin-to-skin contact/suckling rather than increased milk production, may lie behind the prolonged breastfeeding observed in these studies (Widstrom et al., 1990).

More Milk Produced After Rooming-In Than After Nursery Care in the Maternity Ward

The only hospital practice that enhanced mothers' production of milk was rooming-in. All breastfeeding variables were significantly lower in the nursery group (group 3), i.e., the group of mothers and infants that were separated from each other both in the labor ward and in the maternity ward, than in the skin-to-skin groups (Bystrova, Matthiesen, Widstrom, et al., 2007). There was no difference in the amount of milk produced between the groups assigned to rooming-in after birth (groups 1, 2, and 4), nor did the number of breastfeeds or duration of breastfeeding during day four differ between these groups.

The difference in milk production/ingestion of milk between the nursery and the skin-to-skin groups, may be due to the negative consequences of the stay in the nursery and the positive effects caused by the practice of rooming-in. Several factors may have contributed to the lower production of milk in the mothers whose infants stayed in the nursery.

Restriction of Breastfeeding

The mothers whose infants stayed in the nursery were only allowed to breastfeed seven times per 24 hours, whereas the mothers rooming-in breastfed on demand and significantly more often and for longer periods of time. The lower frequency and duration of breastfeeding observed in the mothers whose infants stayed in the nursery, may have contributed to the lower milk production in this group. Other studies have found that breastfeeding frequency and duration, particularly during the first week after birth, influence milk production positively (Houston et al., 1983; Salariya et al., 1978). This is consistent with the fact that the release of prolactin, which stimulates milk production, is dependent on the duration of suckling (Jonas et al., 2009).

Administration of Formula

Another reason for the lower milk production in the mothers belonging to the nursery group could be that these infants were often given significantly more formula or glucose water by the staff than were babies in the rooming-in groups. (Some of the rooming-in infants also received formula, and these mothers produced less milk.) These data are in line with previous studies that found that any supplementary food the infant receives in the maternity ward may cause a reduction in milk volume (Widstrom et al., 1990). In addition, the more supplementary food the infant was given during day one to day five, the shorter the duration of exclusive breastfeeding (Houston et al., 1983; Nylander et al., 1991). By restricting the use of supplementary food in the maternity ward, the frequency of early breastfeeding failure diminished (de Chateau et al., 1977). Taken together, these data suggest that giving supplementary food may impact the amount of milk produced in the maternity ward and possibly the duration of exclusive breastfeeding.

One possible explanation for the reduced milk production in mothers of babies who received formula could be that these babies were less hungry and, therefore, did not suckle as well as those who did not receive formula. In this way, less prolactin was released and maternal milk production was not stimulated as efficiently as in the infants who did not receive any supplement(s) (Jonas et al., 2009).

Closeness and Release of Oxytocin During Rooming-In

The practice of rooming-in may be associated with an enhanced milk production since frequent suckling and continuous closeness between mother and infant might have increased maternal oxytocin levels. As described earlier, both suckling and skin-to-skin contact are associated with increased oxytocin levels. More prolactin is released in response to frequent breastfeeding, and the effect of the inhibitory factor FIL is reduced in response to frequent milk ejections. Oxytocin released in the anterior pituitary during suckling promotes prolactin secretion. All these factors together may explain why milk production may be increased by the practice of rooming-in and, consequently, contribute to the success of long-term breastfeeding.

Predictors of Duration of Breastfeeding

None of the interventions in the Russian study had any positive long-term effects on the duration of nearly exclusive breastfeeding. Nor did skin-to-skin contact after birth, early suckling, or the practice of rooming-in predict the duration of the entire breastfeeding period in this study. Taken together, these data did show that modifications of the routines around birth did not influence the process of milk production. It is to be expected that minor stressors or short-term separations between mother and infant after birth should not influence milk production. From an evolutionary perspective, a stable milk production has been vital for survival of the infant and, in a more long-term perspective, for the human species.

Milk Production Four Days After Birth

Still, the amount of milk produced by the mother and ingested by the infant four days after birth correlated with the total breastfeeding duration (Bystrova, Widstrom, et al., 2007). This relationship may be due to the fact that some mothers simply produce more milk than others, irrespective of early routines and practices. The reason for this might be that the newborn suckles very well or that the mother is a good milk producer. The more milk a mother produces, the easier it will be for her to continue to breastfeed for a long time.

High Oxytocin Levels

Some of the mothers who breastfed for a long time might have had high oxytocin levels, either as a trait or a state. Several studies show that high oxytocin levels are linked to long periods of breastfeeding (Nissen et al., 1996; Silber et al., 1991). The high oxytocin levels would facilitate prolactin secretion and milk production, and stimulate milk ejection and maternal bonding to the infant.

Support

Unless the society and culture where a women lives support breastfeeding as a natural and important way of feeding, breastfeeding will not be practiced. A positive and supportive attitude from family members, the presence of the partner or a friend during labor and birth, and a friendly and supportive attitude of the staff are all important factors for a positive outcome of breastfeeding (Cernadas, Noceda, Barrera, Martinez, & Garsd, 2003; Ekstrom et al., 2003; Sikorski, Renfrew, Pindoria, & Wade, 2003).

Trust and Self-Confidence

A very important factor for successful breastfeeding is that the mother trusts her own ability to breastfeed and feels absolutely confident that she can do it.

Re-lactation

Suckling may even induce milk secretion in women who have not given birth to the child that is going to be breastfed. The phenomenon of "re-lactation" is often used in some African countries when a mother for some reason can't breastfeed. Instead, a female relative takes on the role of breastfeeding. Frequent suckling and a good supply of water and food to the mother is important to stimulate milk production, which most often occurs within one week of suckling (Amimo Amola, personal communication, 2011). Interestingly, the infants are allowed small amounts of food until the re-lactating woman's milk production is established. This fact implicates that other factors besides suckling are important for the mother's milk production. Instead, a positive view on the ability to breastfeed and absence of negative thoughts and worry seem to be extremely important for breastfeeding mothers. It is not known how mental activity influences the ability to breastfeed in Western cultures. Perhaps negative thoughts, worry, and lack of confidence influence the mother's ability to breastfeed to a greater extent than previously thought.

Summary

- Labor ward routines, including early suckling, have a minor impact on milk production during the stay in the maternity ward.

- In contrast, the practice of rooming-in is associated with more milk production four days after birth than separating mothers and infants by keeping the infants in a nursery. Multiple factors may lie behind this difference. The fact that infants kept in a nursery are often given milk formula by the staff is associated with a negative impact on milk production.

- On the other hand, rooming-in is related to more frequent breastfeeding sessions, as well as to continuous closeness between mother and infant, which stimulate milk production.

- Long-term breastfeeding is positively linked to the amount of milk produced four days after birth and to high maternal oxytocin levels, possibly related to maternal bonding.

- Support from family, staff, and society are of utmost importance for successful breastfeeding. Perhaps the most important factor of all is the mother's positive view on breastfeeding and her own unquestioned belief in her capacity to breastfeed.

Chapter 25

Interventions During Labor: Cesarean Section

It has become increasingly popular to introduce technical and medical interventions of different kinds during birth. Vaginal birth can be avoided by performing Cesarean sections. Pain during delivery may be relieved by administration of analgesic drugs, such as meperidine or sufentanil, or by blockade of nervous transmission by local anesthetics, e.g., marcaine in spinal blocks, epidural analgesia, or pudendal blocks. Labor can be initiated by infusions of exogenous oxytocin. It may be used in connection with slow onset of labor or simply because the mother or the doctor wants to control the timing of labor. Oxytocin may also be given to augment slowly progressing labor. When oxytocin is administered, the uterine contractions often become very painful, and to relieve the pain, an epidural analgesia is often given. Since administration of epidural analgesia is by itself often followed by weakened contractions, oxytocin is often administered to compensate for this. Therefore, oxytocin infusions and epidural analgesia are almost always given together. In addition, oxytocin is often given as an intravenous or intramuscular injection after birth or, in the case of Cesarean sections, as an infusion to prevent loss of blood in the period by reinforcing uterine contractions.

These technical and medical interventions are extremely positive and effective in the sense that problematic births can be avoided, pain during labor may be reduced, the duration of labor may be shortened, and bleeding may be reduced. On the other hand, important psychological and physiological adaptations occur during labor and in the period that are dependent on the mother's own oxytocin being released into the circulation and into the brain. Therefore, an important question to ask is whether Cesarean section or different types of pain relief interfere with the release of oxytocin or with the effects of oxytocin normally induced during labor and in the period. Another important question that needs to be explored is what happens to the maternal oxytocin release and oxytocin-related adaptations when exogenous oxytocin is infused during labor or in the period.

The effects of medical interventions during birth on oxytocin levels and oxytocin-related effects in human mothers giving birth by Cesarean section, and those receiving pain relief and administration of exogenous oxytocin during vaginal birth will be described in the following three chapters.

Oxytocin Release During Labor

The effects of oxytocin in connection with labor are well conserved. Oxytocin is involved in the control of labor in all mammalian species, including humans. It also exerts an important control on maternal behavior in all mammalian

species, and even human mothers express some aspects of oxytocin-related behavioral and physiological maternal adaptations as described in a previous chapter.

During labor the fetus is "ejected" from the uterus. The contractions in the uterine wall help bring the fetus down to the birth canal, but a relaxation of the cervix is equally important.

Oxytocin is released during labor to stimulate uterine contractions and to help relax the cervix of the uterus and the birth canal. Without the preceding and concomitant relaxation process, the contractions are not efficient. The situation is very similar to that of milk ejection. Oxytocin contracts the myoepithelial cells to induce milk ejection, but it also helps relax the sphincters of the milk ducts.

Oxytocin Acts Together With the Autonomic Nervous System During Labor

The autonomic nervous system also contributes to the uterine contractions. The uterus is innervated by both sympathetic and parasympathetic nerves. The parasympathetic fibers stimulate uterine contractions and uterine blood flow. The sympathetic nerves also give rise to uterine contractions, but these are more long lasting than the ones caused by parasympathetic stimulation and lack the concomitant stimulation of blood flow (Sato et al., 1996). The parasympathetic sacral plexa are innervated by long oxytocinergic fibers that project from the PVN (Puder & Papka, 2001). As discussed in detail before, oxytocinergic fibers also innervate the DMX, the vagal parasympathetic nucleus.

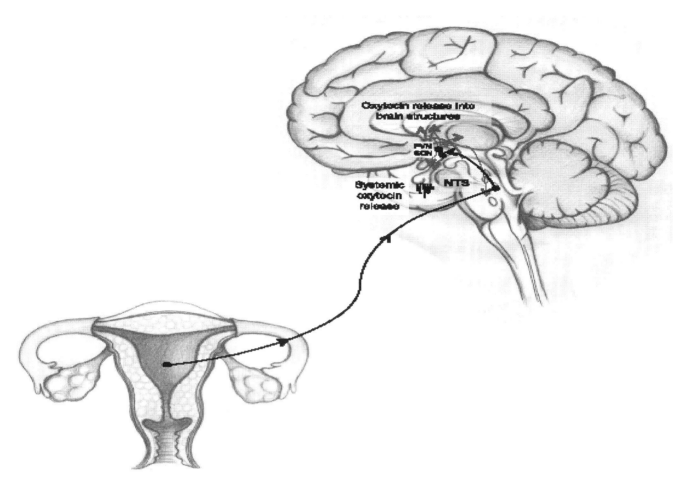

Figure 25.1. Brain – Uterus Connection

Source: Adapted from Uvnäs-Moberg & Prime, 2013. Used with permission.

The Ferguson Reflex

It is not known what actually starts labor and oxytocin release. During the first phase of labor, oxytocin is released in pulses that occur in irregular intervals. During the second phase of labor, the oxytocin pulses are more frequent and may occur at 90-second intervals (Fuchs et al., 1991). During labor the fetus is moved downward in the uterus, and its head (most often) presses against the cervix of the uterus. Sensory fibers traveling in the hypogastric and pelvic nerves are activated, and information travels via the spinal cord and the NTS to activate oxytocin release from the SON and PVN. In this way, more oxytocin is released and the pressure on the cervix increases even more, which results in even more oxytocin being released into the circulation, and so on (Figure 25.1; Ferguson, 1941).

The Extended Ferguson Reflex

When oxytocin release into the circulation is stimulated, e.g., in response to activation of the Ferguson reflex, oxytocinergic fibers emanating in the PVN and projecting to other areas in the brain are activated in parallel. In this way, oxytocin may increase the threshold for pain by actions in the PAG and in the spinal cord. Oxytocin influences

areas, such as the amygdala, to decrease anxiety and increase social interactive behaviors—the maternal adaptations—as will be described below. The autonomic nervous system is influenced by oxytocinergic function, and the function of parasympathetic fibers to the sacral plexa are increased. In this way, the effects on labor by circulating oxytocin are reinforced by the oxytocinergic nerves involved in parasympathetic nervous function.

Again, this extended function of oxytocin is analogous to the situation during breastfeeding. Oxytocin is not only released into the circulation to induce milk ejection, it is also released into the brain to induce the various behavioral and physiological adaptations, which have been described in detail in previous chapters.

Cesarean Section

Increased Frequency of Cesarean Section

Cesarean sections are, for a variety of reasons, becoming increasingly common as a way of giving birth. Originally, emergency c-sections were performed when labor did not advance as it should, or if the life of mother and baby were in danger. Today, emergency c-sections are performed more often and elective sections may be performed if the mother and/or the obstetrician so decide. The rate of Cesarean sections has increased from 12% to 18% in Sweden during the last ten years (The Swedish National Board of Health and Welfare) and is still increasing. In other countries, the frequency of Cesarean sections is even greater.

The risk of the surgical interventions for the mothers who deliver by Cesarean section has decreased dramatically, as the surgical techniques have developed and become refined (Stark & Finkel, 1994). On the other hand, mothers giving birth by Cesarean section have, according to some studies, more problems breastfeeding and bonding to their infants than mothers giving birth vaginally (Rowe-Murray & Fisher, 2001, 2002; Tulman, 1986).

There is also increased literature showing that children born by Cesarean section have an increased risk of developing diseases, such as asthma. An important factor behind this effect is the sterile environment in which the infant is born. Normally, the bacteria transferred from the mother to the newborn colonizes its gut and helps activate the immune system (Bager, Wohlfahrt, & Westergaard, 2008; Renz-Polster et al., 2005; Roduit et al., 2009; Thavagnanam, Fleming, Bromley, Shields, & Cardwell, 2008; Weng & Walker, 2013).

Clinical Studies

Studies have been performed in which the effect of Cesarean section on oxytocin levels and some oxytocin-linked behaviors were explored.

1. Twenty-four blood samples were collected in 37 primiparous women in connection with breastfeeding two days after birth; 20 women were delivered by Cesarean section and 17 had a vaginal delivery. The amount of milk ejected in connection with the breastfeed and the duration of breastfeeding were recorded. Oxytocin and prolactin levels were measured and were related to other breastfeeding variables. Oxytocin levels were measured with RIA. The women filled in the Karolinska Scales of Personality (KSP). The results of the KSP formula were related to the oxytocin levels (Nissen et al., 1998; Nissen et al., 1996).

2. Forty-two infants born via Cesarean section were randomized to have skin-to-skin contact with either their mother or father for a 25-minute period after birth. The interactive behavior of the parents and their infants during the first two hours after birth was observed and recorded on videotape, allowing for recording of sounds. The infants' breast-seeking and breastfeeding behaviors were also recorded.

    Fifty percent of the mothers received oxytocin as an infusion during the observation period. Seventeen blood samples were collected at five- or

15-minute intervals in both mothers and fathers during a 90-minute period. Oxytocin levels were analyzed by RIA.

The influence of infusion of exogenous oxytocin on endogenous oxytocin levels was explored. The Karolinska Scales of Personality was filled in by the mothers two days after birth. The effect of skin-to-skin contact and/or infusion of oxytocin on the KSP levels were investigated (Velandia, Uvnäs-Moberg, et al., 2014b).

Main Results

*   No rise of oxytocin levels was observed in response to skin-to-skin contact and suckling immediately after birth in mothers having had an elective Cesarean section (Velandia, Uvnäs-Moberg, et al., 2014b).

*   The number of oxytocin peaks induced by breastfeeding was significantly reduced in mothers having had a Cesarean section two days after birth (Nissen et al., 1996).

*   Cesarean section was associated with reduced milk ejection during a breastfeed two days after birth (Nissen et al., 1996).

*   Suckling failed to release prolactin in the women who delivered by Cesarean section two days after birth (Nissen et al., 1996).

*   The approach behavior of Cesarean-delivered newborns and start of suckling were delayed when compared with the breast-seeking behavior observed in vaginally delivered newborns (Velandia, Uvnäs-Moberg, et al., 2014b).

*   The reduction of anxiety levels and the increase of social skills normally seen in breastfeeding mothers two days after birth, were less developed in the Cesarean section group (Nissen et al., 1998; Velandia, Uvnäs-Moberg, et al., 2014b).

*   The number of oxytocin peaks induced by breastfeeding was related to the level of socialization according to the KSP (Nissen et al., 1998).

Cesarean Section and Lack of Oxytocin

Absence of or Reduced Oxytocin Release During Labor

The labor-related oxytocin release may be completely absent in women having an elective Cesarean section, whereas women having an emergency Cesarean section may have some release of oxytocin, depending on how long the mother had contractions before surgical intervention. The absence of labor may explain the well-known fact that both mothers and infants have lower oxytocin levels after Cesarean section birth than after vaginal birth, which is consistent with the absence of oxytocin release and contractions (Marchini et al., 1988).

No Oxytocin Release by Skin-to-Skin Contact and Suckling After Cesarean Section

Skin-to-skin contact and suckling failed to release oxytocin during the first two hours postpartum in mothers' giving birth via Cesarean section. The lack of oxytocin release in response to the sensory stimulation caused by skin-to-skin contact or suckling may be a consequence of the absent or low oxytocin secretion during labor. As described previously, oxytocin increases the sensitivity of, e.g., the skin and the nipple, by facilitating the transmission in the somatosensory nerves, which are linked to oxytocin release in the NTS. The higher the oxytocin levels in the NTS, the better the effect of sensory stimulation on oxytocin release.

The Breast-Seeking Behavior of the Newborn Not Adequately Stimulated

In addition, the newborn's breast-seeking behavior and first sucking is delayed after Cesarean section (Velandia, Uvans-Moberg, et al., 2014a). The lack of maternal oxytocin release during labor, resulting in a lack of oxytocin release in response to skin-to-skin contact and suckling might have contributed to the delay in the infant's approach and breastfeeding (Velandia et al., 2010). The mothers' handling of the infants is reduced (Rowe-Murray & Fisher, 2001; Tulman, 1986), and maternal cues, e.g., giving of warmth and secretion of pheromones, may have been incompletely developed as a consequence of the reduced release of oxytocin.

Reduced Levels of Oxytocin in the Infants

It is, of course, also possible that infants having been born by Cesarean section are less active by themselves than those born vaginally. Assuming that oxytocin also promotes approach behaviors in the newborns, their lower oxytocin levels may lie behind the delayed approach behavior of the newborns.

The reason for the lower levels of oxytocin after birth could be that the uterine contractions also stimulate oxytocin release in the infants via activation of somatosensory nerves, and as infants born by Cesarean section have not been exposed to this stimulation, their oxytocin levels are lower.

Role of Spinal Anesthesia

Another important factor behind the low levels of oxytocin in both mothers and infants may be the spinal anesthesia given to the mothers in connection with Cesarean section. Both the local anesthetic and the opioid component of the spinal anesthesia diffuse into the maternal circulation and pass the placental barrier to reach the circulation of the fetus. Marcaine may reduce oxytocin release not only in the spinal cord of the mother, but also by inhibiting

the transmission in somatosensory nerves and opioids by inhibiting oxytocin release directly from the oxytocin-producing neurons. In support of this hypothesis, the sensitivity of the skin in the mother's breasts was extremely low during the first hour after Cesarean section with spinal analgesia. Also, the sensitivity of the infants' skin may have been decreased by marcaine, and thereby their oxytocin release.

Reduced Number of Oxytocin Peaks in Response to Breastfeeding Two Days After Birth

The oxytocin pattern in response to breastfeeding two days after Cesarean birth was different from that of vaginally delivered women, as the number of oxytocin pulses was reduced. The statistical analysis of the data indicated that the lack of the second stage of labor, and delayed skin-to-skin contact after birth, were responsible for the absence of oxytocin peaks in the Cesarean-delivered women (Nissen et al., 1996). The reduced number of oxytocin peaks caused by breastfeeding was probably related to an incomplete stimulation of oxytocin release during labor and in the period due to absent or low levels of oxytocin during birth. This effect might have been sustained, as it occurred during the early sensitive period.

Perhaps the insensitivity to sensory stimuli is not only present directly after birth, but also several days after birth in mothers giving birth by Cesarean section.

Contribution of Pain

The post-operative pain and stress may have also contributed to the decreased release of oxytocin in the Cesarean section mothers (Karlstrom, Engstrom-Olofsson, Norbergh, Sjoling, & Hildingsson, 2007), as certain types of stress, as described in detail previously, inhibit oxytocin release.

Early skin-to-skin contact after birth was associated with a relatively more pulsatile oxytocin pattern in the Cesarean section mothers, probably by reducing their stress levels, which may have contributed to the normalization of oxytocin release in response to breastfeeding two days later (Nissen et al., 1996). However, it cannot be excluded that the mothers who responded with more oxytocin pulses two days after birth, already had relatively higher oxytocin levels in connection with the birth, and therefore, were in skin-to-skin contact with their infants at an earlier age.

Link Between Low Levels of Oxytocin and Prolactin and Breastfeeding Problems

The decrease in breastfeeding-related oxytocin pulsatility observed in the women having a Cesarean delivery was related to a reduction in the amount of milk ejected during the breastfeed. The amount of milk ejected in response to the breastfeed two days after birth correlated with the number of oxytocin peaks. This finding is in agreement with the fact that milk ejection is caused by rising plasma levels of oxytocin. Since the number of oxytocin peaks during breastfeeding is reduced in women having a Cesarean section, less milk is secreted by the mother and ingested by the infant (Nissen et al., 1998).

The compromised oxytocin release observed in women having a Cesarean delivery and the reduced amount of milk ejected may be behind breastfeeding problems sometimes observed in women having a Cesarean section. The absence of breastfeeding-related prolactin release may be another factor behind the reduced milk production/breastfeeding problems observed in the mothers having a Cesarean section (Nissen, et al., 1996; Jonas et al., 1996). The lack of oxytocin during labor and in the early period, as well as in connection with the breastfeeding episode two days after birth, may lie behind the low prolactin levels, since oxytocin promotes the release of prolactin (Samson et al., 1986).

Decreased Oxytocin Release in the Brain May Explain the Lack of KSP Changes

Oxytocin is released in parallel into the circulation and into the brain in response to suckling (Kendrick et al., 1986). A decrease or lack of release of oxytocin into the brain during labor in women having a Cesarean section may explain why the psychological maternal adaptations normally seen in women two days after birth were not fully developed in these women. The results from the KSP showed that the changes characterized by decreased levels of anxiety and increased levels of socialization were not as well developed in the women having a Cesarean section (Nissen et al., 1998; Velandia, Uvnäs-Moberg, et al., 2014b).

The suggestion that oxytocin lies behind the absence of changes in the KSP is supported by previous studies showing correlations between oxytocin levels and scores obtained in the Karolinska Scales of Personality Profile (Uvnäs Moberg et al., 1990; Nissen et al., 1998). Mothers' basal levels of oxytocin were inversely correlated with the scores obtained for anxiety, and the number of oxytocin pulses correlated positively with the scores of items indicating interest in social interaction. Together, these results support the role of oxytocin in decreasing the level of anxiety and increasing the level of social interactive behavior (Nissen et al., 1998).

Obviously, the maternal behavioral adaptations normally seen in breastfeeding women were not seen after Cesarean section, suggesting that not only the oxytocin-dependent milk ejection/production, but also the oxytocin-linked maternal behavioral adaptations were not as well developed in the first days after a Cesarean section.

Summary

- Women giving birth by elective Cesarean section did not respond with oxytocin release following skin-to-skin contact and suckling immediately after birth.

- The number of oxytocin peaks induced by breastfeeding two days after birth was reduced after Cesarean section, and thereby the amount of milk ejected.

- No prolactin was released in response to breastfeeding two days after Cesarean section.

- The newborns' breastfeeding behaviors and suckling were also delayed after Cesarean section.

- The absence of oxytocin release in connection with Cesarean section may lie behind the absence of oxytocin release in response to skin-to-skin contact and suckling immediately after birth, as oxytocin release facilitates the sensory input from the skin, which results in oxytocin release.

- The delayed-approach behavior of infants seen after Cesarean section may be related to a lack of oxytocin in infants.

- In addition to the absence of labor, the local anesthetic marcaine from the spinal anesthesia may have contributed to the insensitivity of the skin in both mothers and infants after birth, and thereby to the low levels of oxytocin.

- The adaptations of the KSP profile towards reduced anxiety and increased socialization normally seen two days after birth, had not developed in mothers who had given birth by Cesarean section.

- The lack of prolactin release and of maternal adaptations in the KSP profile two days after birth may be related to the lack of oxytocin released into the brain during labor and in the period.

Chapter 26

Interventions During Labor: Epidural Analgesia and Other Types of Pain Relief

Extreme pain during labor is not only a subjective, negative experience, it is also linked to fear and increased levels of stress hormones. In addition, it may reduce oxytocin secretion or antagonize the effects of oxytocin and prolong labor. It is, therefore, sometimes necessary to reduce pain during labor. In Sweden, every woman is by law guaranteed pain relief during labor if she so wishes.

Pethidine and Pudendal Block

Substances that decrease pain, such as pethidine, and local anesthetics given to block the transmission of pain from the cervix of the uterus, have been used for decades to alleviate pain during labor.

Drugs given during labor to reduce pain may influence mother/infant interaction after birth, as they cross the placenta by passive diffusion, and the concentration of drugs in infant and mother equilibrate (Belfrage, Berlin, Raabe, & Thalme, 1975; Yurth, 1982). Suckling is delayed in infants exposed to pethidine in utero, and infants exposed to pethidine during labor had delayed breast-seeking and sucking behavior, particularly if the drug was given shortly before delivery (Belsey et al., 1981; Nissen, Lilja, Matthiesen, et al., 1995; Righard & Alade, 1990). The effect on the developing breastfeeding behavior caused by pethidine is likely to be exerted in the brain (Nissen, Lilja, Matthiesen, et al., 1995; Nissen et al., 1997). Local anesthetics, such as bupivacaine, disturbed and reduced mother and infant interactions after birth (Rosenblatt et al., 1981; Sepkoski, Lester, Ostheimer, & Brazelton, 1992). The mechanism behind these effects will be described later on in this chapter.

Epidural Analgesia

Today, epidural analgesia has become the most common intervention to prevent pain during labor, and its use is continually increasing. Fifty percent of all primiparas in Sweden received an epidural analgesia for pain relief during labor in 2003 (Swedish National Board of Health and Welfare). Similar figures can be obtained for other countries.

Reduction of Pain, But Also Prolonged Labor and Delayed Breastfeeding

In addition to providing pain relief, epidural analgesia reduced fear and reduced levels of stress hormones, such as cortisol and catecholamines (Alehagen, Wijma, Lundberg, & Wijma, 2005). Administration of epidural

analgesia has also been linked to negative consequences, such as prolonged labor, particularly second-stage labor, increased risk of instrumental vaginal birth, and oxytocin augmentation (Anim-Somuah, Smyth, & Howell, 2005; Anim-Somuah, Smyth, & Jones, 2011; Leighton & Halpern, 2002; Lieberman & O'Donoghue, 2002).

Some studies, but not all, suggest that epidural analgesia may be linked to problems with breastfeeding. For example, one study suggested that newborns were less likely to breastfeed within the first hours of life if the mother received an epidural analgesia, and that they breastfed for a shorter time (Beilin et al., 2005; Chang & Heaman, 2005; Henderson, Dickinson, Evans, McDonald, & Paech, 2003; Torvaldsen, Roberts, Simpson, Thompson, & Ellwood, 2006; Wiklund, Norman, Uvnäs-Moberg, Ransjo-Arvidson, & Andolf, 2009).

Clinical Studies

The effect of maternal analgesia on mother/infant interaction on the developing breast-seeking behavior has been investigated by comparing results from mothers with and without administration of maternal analgesia. Also, the effect of epidural analgesia on breastfeeding-related variables was studied in response to breastfeeding two days after birth. The role of these interventions on oxytocin release and oxytocin-related effect patterns was explored.

1. Twenty-eight women and their newborns participated in the study and were placed in skin-to-skin contact after birth. Ten of the women did not receive any pain relief during labor, whereas the rest of the women received pain relief, such as injections of meperidine, an epidural, or a pudendal block. Blood samples were collected in 15-minute intervals and oxytocin levels were measured. The mother/infant interaction was videotaped and analyzed. Scores of behaviors and oxytocin levels were related to the different treatments (Ransjo-Arvidson et al., 2001; Matthiesen et al., 2001a; Matthiesen et al., 2001b).

2. Sixty-nine breastfeeding primiparas participated in the study. All had a vaginal delivery and skin-to-skin contact after birth, and all were exclusively breastfeeding. Some of them had been exposed to different medical interventions during labor, such as epidural analgesia, oxytocin infusions, epidural analgesia and oxytocin infusion, or intramuscular administration of oxytocin after birth. Twenty-

four blood samples were collected during a breastfeeding session two days after birth, and oxytocin, prolactin, ACTH, and cortisol levels in plasma were measured. Oxytocin levels were measured with Elisa.

Blood pressure was measured before and after breastfeeding two days after birth, and in a subgroup of mothers for a six-month period.

The Karolinska Scales of Personality were filled in two days, two months, and six months postpartum.

Skin temperature was measured in the newborns during breastfeeding two days after birth (Handlin et al., 2009; Jonas et al., 2009; Jonas, Nissen, Ransjo-Arvidson, Matthiesen, et al., 2008; Jonas, Nissen, Ransjo-Arvidson, Wiklund, et al., 2008; Jonas et al., 2007; Handlin et al., 2012).

Main Results

- The local anesthetic, marcaine, given alone or in combination with pethidine, disturbed infants' breast-seeking behavior after birth (Ransjo-Arvidson et al., 2001).

- The infants of mothers receiving pethidine and/or marcaine during labor performed less hand massage postpartum, and less oxytocin was released in these mothers (Ransjo-Arvidson et al., 2001; Matthiesen et al., 2001b).

- The mothers' capacity to release oxytocin was also influenced. Infants needed to give more massage in mothers given marcaine and pethidine to induce the same amount of oxytocin released in mothers who had not received any analgesia (Matthiesen et al., 2001b).

- Administration of epidural analgesia did not influence the normal peak-shaped oxytocin pattern in response to breastfeeding two days after birth (Jonas et al., 2009).

- No prolactin release was observed in response to breastfeeding two days after birth in mothers having received epidural analgesia (Jonas et al., 2009).

- Basal blood pressure, in particular diastolic blood pressure, was decreased in women having had an epidural analgesia, and no decrease of blood pressure was observed in response to breastfeeding two days after birth (Handlin et al., 2012; Jonas, Nissen, Ransjo-Arvidson, Wiklund, et al., 2008).

- Epidural analgesia attenuated the changes of the KSP profile towards decreased anxiety and increased levels of socialization normally observed after vaginal delivery two days after birth. The effect was, however, restored after six weeks and six months of exclusive breastfeeding (Jonas, Nissen,

Ransjo-Arvidson, Matthiesen, et al., 2008).

- The rise in skin temperature seen in the infants in response to suckling was blocked two days after birth if the mother had epidural analgesia during birth (Jonas et al., 2007).

Effects of Marcaine and Pethidine

Disturbed Breast-Seeking Behavior in Newborns by Local Anesthetics and Pethidine Given During Labor

The local anesthetic, marcaine, given alone or in combination with pethidine, disturbed infants' breast-seeking behavior after birth. The infants of mothers who had received pethidine, local anesthetics, or a combination of the two, performed less hand-to-mouth movements, touched the areola and the nipple less, performed less hand massage of the breast, and sucked less than infants born to mothers who did not receive such pain relief (Ransjo-Arvidson et al., 2001).

Decreased Oxytocin Release

Infants stimulate their mothers' oxytocin release in a dose-dependent way by massaging their breasts if allowed skin-to-skin contact after birth (Matthiesen et al., 2001a). The infants of mothers receiving pethidine and/or marcaine during labor performed less hand massage postpartum. Consequently, less oxytocin was released in these mothers (Matthiesen et al., 2001b). Interestingly, the mothers' capacity to release oxytocin was also influenced. Infants needed to give more massage in mothers given marcaine and pethidine to induce the same amount of oxytocin released in mothers who had not received any analgesia (Matthiesen et al., 2001b).

Role of Oxytocin

The mothers having received marcaine or pethidine released less oxytocin into the circulation than those without these interventions in response to infants' hand massage after birth. They were also less sensitive to the stimulation. Whether this inability to release oxytocin is due to a decreased sensitivity of the touch receptors in the breast in mothers who had received marcaine is not known, but is probable, as marcaine acts as a local anesthetic.

In fact, oxytocin release might have already been inhibited during birth as a consequence of the elevated levels of marcaine in the circulation, which may have decreased the activity in the pelvic and hypogastric nerves, as well as in somatosensory nerves. The already low levels of oxytocin may have contributed to the insensitivity of the mothers to the infants' hand massage.

As described in previous chapters, oxytocin released from oxytocinergic neurons projecting from the paraventricular nucleus in the PVN to the NTS is important for the ability of skin-to-skin contact and suckling to induce oxytocin release, or in other words, oxytocin increases the sensitivity to oxytocin-releasing stimuli of the skin. Therefore, the decreased oxytocin secretion to the NTS must have resulted in a decreased maternal sensitivity to the infants' breast massage.

As opioids inhibit oxytocin release, administration of pethidine may have reduced oxytocin secretion in mothers who had received pethidine.

Similar Oxytocin-Linked Mechanisms Operate in Newborns

Both marcaine and pethidine pass the placental barrier and reach the circulation of the children (Belfrage et al., 1982). Therefore, similar mechanisms are likely to operate in newborns as in mothers. Their oxytocin levels might have already been decreased by the interventions during labor. As marcaine renders the skin insensitive, the somatosensory stimulation caused by labor may not have resulted in any oxytocin release. After birth, the skin remains insensitive due to the presence of marcaine and low oxytocin levels. As previously described, oxytocin increases the sensitivity to sensory stimulation and, therefore, for oxytocin release in response to sensory stimulation. This may explain the insensitivy to touch and suckling in the infants born to mothers who had received marcaine.

A low oxytocin level in infants may also lie behind the decreased infant hand massage, the decreased sucking capacity of the infant, and the delay of the first breastfeeding in the period, as all of these behaviors are expressions of the newborn's approach to the mother. As also repeatedly stated previously, oxytocin stimulates various types of social approach behaviors (Ransjö Arvidsson et al., 2001).

Effects of Epidural Analgesia

Epidural analgesia is given in order to inhibit or reduce the pain of labor. It contains a mixture of local anesthetics (e.g., marcaine) and pain-relieving opioids (e.g., sufentanil). It is administered into the epidural cavity. In this way, the transmission in nerve fibers that mediate the sensation of pain from the paracervical region and mediated by the pelvic and hypogastric nerves is blocked (Eltzschig, Lieberman, & Camann, 2003).

Inhibition of the Ferguson Reflex

It should be remembered that not only sensory nerves mediating the modality of pain, but also other types of nerve fibers enter the spinal cord at this level to transmit information to the central nervous system. The pelvic and hypogastric nerves also contain nerve fibers that mediate the Ferguson reflex.

When the fetus is pushing against the cervix during uterine contractions, muscles in the cervix dilate, and as a consequence of this, sensory nerves emanating from the uterine cervix are activated. Activation of these nerves, via transmission in the spinal cord, leads to a release of oxytocin from the paraventricular and the supraoptical nucleus in the

hypothalamus, the Ferguson reflex. As oxytocin is released into the circulation, the frequency of uterine contractions increases and, consequently, the pressure of the head of the fetus on the cervix becomes stronger. The sensory nerves mediating the Ferguson reflex become even more activated and more oxytocin is released, and so on. The positive circle continues, creating a feed-forward process (Ferguson, 1941).

If the transmission of nerve impulses emanating from the cervix and transmitted to the spinal cord is blocked, e.g., by administration of epidural analgesia, the function of the Ferguson reflex might be expected to be blocked or at least reduced. It has been shown that oxytocin levels in the circulation are reduced in women having received epidural analgesia (Goodfellow, Hull, Swaab, Dogterom, & Buijs, 1983; Rahm, Hallgren, Hogberg, Hurtig, & Odlind, 2002; Stocche, Klamt, Antunes-Rodrigues, Garcia, & Moreira, 2001).

As mentioned previously, the stimuli that trigger oxytocin release are most often of lower intensity than those that induce pain. Therefore, it follows that epidural analgesia containing marcaine will block the transmission in nerves linked to oxytocin release at lower concentrations than needed to block pain impulses, and that transmission in the Fergusson reflex may be blocked before the nerve fibers mediating pain.

Inhibition of Uterine Contractions

A reduced function of the Ferguson reflex and a consequent decrease of circulating oxytocin levels should be followed by decreased frequency of uterine contractions during the second stage of labor. In women receiving an epidural analgesia, the second stage of labor is prolonged. This prolongation is likely to be a consequence of the inhibited activity of the Ferguson reflex, decreasing oxytocin levels and uterine contractions. This may also explain why synthetic oxytocin often needs to be administered to women receiving epidural analgesia to augment uterine contractions (Anim-Somuah et al., 2005; Leighton & Halpern, 2002; Lieberman & O'Donoghue, 2002). The effects of the combined use of epidural analgesia and infusion of oxytocin will be discussed in the next chapter.

Inhibition of Parasympathetic Stimulation

The role of the autonomic nervous system and, in particular, the role of the parasympathetic nerves in the control of uterine contractions were described in the previous chapter. A reduction in the function of the oxytocinergic nerves projecting to the sacral plexa must also have contributed to the inhibition of uterine contractions in women receiving epidural analgesia.

Delayed Breastfeeding

As oxytocin levels during birth are lowered by the epidural analgesia during birth, oxytocin levels are likely to also be low immediately after birth. Low oxytocin levels during the period may be one factor behind the delayed onset of breastfeeding sometimes seen in women receiving epidural analgesia during labor, as oxytocin stimulates the interaction between mother and infant.

Breastfeeding failed to release prolactin into the circulation two days after birth in women who had received epidural analgesia during labor (Jonas et al., 2009). Prolactin is important for stimulation of milk production, particularly in the beginning of the breastfeeding period. The low levels of prolactin may partly explain why women who have an epidural analgesia, according to some studies, have problems with breastfeeding (Henderson et al., 2003; Torvaldsen et al., 2006; Wiklund et al., 2009). As oxytocin stimulates prolactin release, the low levels of oxytocin in connection with birth may be responsible for the reduced prolactin levels observed in connection with breastfeeding two days later.

Delayed Development of Maternal Adaptations

The inhibition of oxytocin release during labor caused by epidural analgesia may partly explain why mothers who have received this type of pain relief did not develop the maternal psychological adaptations demonstrated to occur after vaginal delivery (Jonas, Nissen, Ransjo-Arvidson, Matthiesen, et al., 2008). Breastfeeding mothers are less anxious and more social two or four days after birth in comparison to women who are not pregnant or breastfeeding, according to the Karolinska Scales of Personality. Obviously, the changes observed in these previous studies are not only related to oxytocin released into the brain in response to breastfeeding, but also to oxytocin flooding the brain during labor. These results are consistent with the finding that administration of epidural anesthesia during labor in ewes is linked to an inhibition of maternal behavior and bonding to the young, which can be restored by administration of oxytocin to the brain (Keverne & Kendrick, 1994).

As oxytocin levels in response to breastfeeding two days after birth appeared to be normal, the lack of effects on maternal psychological adaptations seen in the mothers with epidural analgesia must be a consequence of low oxytocin levels during labor and right after birth.

Memory of Pain Not Relieved

One aspect of the oxytocin-mediated effects is pain relief by actions in the periaqueductal grey (PAG) and the dorsal column of the spinal cord. Since the activity of the oxytocinergic system is reduced in women having received epidural analgesia, the endogenous oxytocinergic inhibition of pain is not fully activated in these women. Interestingly, the memory of the pain of labor is more intense after three months in women who had epidural analgesia (Waldenström & Schutt, 2009). Perhaps the amnesic effect of oxytocin is also lost after epidural analgesia.

The Infants of Breastfeeding Mothers Are Also Affected by Epidural Analgesia

Surprisingly, the infants of mothers receiving epidural analgesia were affected during breastfeeding two days after birth. Normally, the infant's skin temperature increases when placed in skin-to-skin contact with the mother and during breastfeeding (Bystrova et al., 2003). No such rise in skin temperature was observed in the infants whose mothers had epidural analgesia during labor two days earlier, whereas it did rise in the infants of mothers who had not received epidural analgesia (Jonas et al., 2007).

Whether the lack of temperature response is a consequence of a change in infant skin temperature regulation caused by the epidural analgesia in connection with birth, or whether it is secondary to a change in the maternal/infant interaction is not known.

Study mothers receiving epidural analgesia during birth failed to release prolactin during breastfeeding, and their psychological maternal adaptations were not fully developed immediately after birth (Jonas, Nissen, Ransjo-Arvidson, Matthiesen, et al., 2008). It is, therefore, possible that the infants failed to respond because they did not get the appropriate signals from the mothers.

Reduced Activity in the Infant's Oxytocinergic System?

As shown in the study reported above, marcaine administered to the mothers during birth was shown to decrease the spontaneous breast-seeking behavior in the newborn infants, suggesting that their oxytocin levels were decreased after birth as a consequence of exposure to marcaine. As also discussed in detail above, low oxytocin levels are associated with insensitivity in the skin to further oxytocin release. It is, therefore, tempting to suggest that the infant's oxytocin system remains at a low functional level two days after birth, rendering the skin insensitive to the contact with the mother. Whether the effect of skin sensitivity was imprinted during the sensitive period around birth, or is caused by low oxytocin levels two days later, remains to be established.

Both Cesarean Section and Epidural Analgesia Linked to Low Levels of Oxytocin During Birth

Both Cesarean section and epidural analgesia were associated with less developed maternal psychological adaptations and prolactin release in connection with breastfeeding two days after birth, which are caused by levels of oxytocin too low during birth. Both Cesarean section and epidural anesthesia decrease the release of oxytocin during labor, but in different ways. If elective Cesarean sections are performed before labor has started, no labor-associated oxytocin release occurs. If an emergency c-section is performed, oxytocin release during the second stage of labor is often reduced. In women receiving epidural

Oxytocin: The Biological Guide To Motherhood 155

analgesia, oxytocin release is also diminished, as the activity in the Ferguson reflex is blocked and less oxytocin is released during labor, both in the brain and into the circulation.

Cesarean Section Induces Stress Whereas Epidural Analgesia Reduces Stress

The surgical intervention linked to Cesarean section naturally imposes severe stress to the organism. In women having a Cesarean section, the oxytocin release caused by breastfeeding was less pulsatile. A lower number of oxytocin pulses was associated with both a reduction of the mother's ability for social interaction and a reduction in the amount of milk ejected during the breastfeed studied. As oxytocin release is very sensitive to stress, the decreased number of oxytocin peaks might reflect the consequences of stress to the organism caused by the surgical intervention when the baby was born, which was still present two days after birth.

A more likely explanation is that these sustained effects on oxytocin release, milk production, and psychological adaptations are, in fact, due to the absence of oxytocin secretion during birth. Oxytocin release might be hampered in a long-term way, as the function of the oxytocin system is not adequately stimulated. As oxytocin also stimulates the sensitivity to sensory stimulation, and thereby the responsiveness to stimuli that release oxytocin, a sustained decrease in sensitivity of the skin may also contribute to the faulty oxytocin release and absence of prolactin release in response to breastfeeding two days after birth.

Effects Caused Both by Inhibition of Pain and Oxytocin Release in Epidural Analgesia

Mothers receiving epidural analgesia did not display the development of increased social interaction and decreased levels of anxiety seen in vaginally delivered women, as a consequence of the lack of oxytocin released during labor. Additionaly, they did not release prolactin in response to breastfeeding two days after birth. Still, these mothers had a normal pulsatile release of oxytocin in connection with labor two days after birth. In fact, the mothers' giving birth with epidural analgesia experienced less fear and pain during labor and had lower levels of cortisol and catecholamines during labor (Alehagen et al., 2005). These effects are consistent with the finding of lower blood pressure in the mothers having received epidural analgesia two days after birth. This "double" effect may be due to the fact that epidural analgesia, via its effects in the spinal cord, blocks both fibers associated with oxytocin release and fibers associated with pain, and consequent activation of the sympathetic nervous system and the HPA axis.

Summary

- Administration of marcaine or pethidine as pain relief during labor is associated with a disturbed and delayed breast-seeking behavior, hand massage, and suckling in the newborns.

- Administration of marcaine and pethidine are also linked to a reduced release of oxytocin in response to breast massage in the mothers, which is partly due to the reduction of the infants' hand massage and also to an insensitivity to the infants' hand massage.

- Marcaine and pethidine may have reduced oxytocin secretion in both infants and mothers, and thereby reduced the infants' spontaneous breast-seeking behavior and the mothers' sensitivity to breast massage.

- As a consequence of low oxytocin levels, the sensitivity to sensory input is decreased in both mothers and infants, and thereby the release of oxytocin in response to sensory stimulation is further antagonized.

- Epidural analgesia decreases the perception of pain during labor and also dampens stress reactions, as evidenced by lower activity in the sympathetic nervous system and the HPA activity.

- Epidural analgesia blocks the Ferguson reflex, thereby decreasing the release of oxytocin. Epidural analgesia may result in prolonged labor, as a result of a reduction of oxytocin release and stimulation of uterine contractions.

- Epidural analgesia is associated with decreased prolactin release in connection with breastfeeding two days after birth, and the maternal psychological adaptations recorded by the KSP are not developed. These effects are likely to be secondary to the decreased oxytocin release from oxytocinergic projections in the brain in connection with labor.

- In addition, skin temperature of the infants fails to rise in response to breastfeeding two days after birth. This may be due to a sustained insensitivity of the skin due to low oxytocin levels caused by marcaine during birth.

Chapter 27

Interventions During Labor: Administration of Exogenous Oxytocin

Oxytocin was the first hormone to be isolated, sequenced, and synthesized. It has been used clinically to stimulate labor and milk ejection and to reduce bleeding postpartum since the 1950s (Engstrom, 1958; Holmes, 1954).

Infusion of Oxytocin During Labor

Many mothers receive oxytocin as an intravenous infusion to initiate labor when spontaneous onset is delayed or if the mother and obstetrician decide to induce labor for other reasons.

Intravenous oxytocin infusions are also given to augment labor in prolonged deliveries. Today, about 50% of primiparas receive extra oxytocin during labor in most clinics in Sweden, and the use of oxytocin is increasing.

Oxytocin Needed When Deliveries Are Prolonged

Women requiring oxytocin to stimulate contractions have a more protracted labor than those not receiving oxytocin (Bugg, Stanley, Baker, Taggart, & Johnston, 2006; Svärdby, Nordstrom, & Sellstrom, 2007).

Oxytocin Infusions Give Rise to Painful Contractions and Subsequent Use of Epidural Analgesia

The contractions caused by administration of exogenous oxytocin are often very strong, protracted, and connected to severe, sometimes unbearable pain. For this reason, epidural analgesia is often given to mothers receiving oxytocin to relieve the pain. In this way, the use of infusions of exogenous oxytocin increases the need for epidural analgesia.

Epidural Analgesia Gives Rise to Prolonged Labor and Subsequent Need for Oxytocin Infusions

As was discussed in the previous chapter, many women receive pain relief during labor, e.g., epidural analgesia. The use of epidural analgesia is often linked to a slow progression of labor, as a consequence of decreased uterine contractions. The reason for this is that epidural analgesia causes an inhibition of the Ferguson reflex, and thereby a decreased endogenous oxytocin release (Anim-Somuah et al., 2011; Beilin et al., 2005; Leighton & Halpern, 2002).

In these cases, infusions of exogenous oxytocin are given in an attempt to increase contractions and normalize labor. As the use of epidural analgesia has increased, the demand for infusions of exogenous oxytocin to stimulate uterine contractions has increased.

As infusions of oxytocin increase the need for epidural analgesia, and since epidural analgesia increases the need for oxytocin infusions, the use of these two medical interventions often occur together.

Women receiving oxytocin stimulation during labor are more likely to have instrumental deliveries, such as Cesarean section and/or use of forceps (Bugg et al., 2006; Svardby et al., 2007).

Consequences to the Fetus

Oxytocin may, if used in an uncautious way, induce hyperstimulation of the uterine contractions, and fetal asphyxia and metabolic acidosis, with lower pH in the umbilical cord, may ensue (Berglund, Grunewald, Pettersson, & Cnattingius, 2008; Berglund, Pettersson, Cnattingius, & Grunewald, 2010; Jonsson, Norden, & Hanson, 2007; Jonsson, Norden-Lindeberg, Ostlund, & Hanson, 2008).

Endogenous Versus Exogenous Oxytocin

When oxytocin is administered as an intravenous infusion, injection, or nasal spray, the nine-amino-acid oxytocin molecule is used. The exogenous oxytocin is produced chemically (synthesized) by linking individual amino acids together. It is often believed that synthetic (exogenous) oxytocin differs from natural (endogenous) oxytocin, but the chemical structure of exogenous and endogenous oxytocin is identical. They both contain the same nine amino acids, which are linked to each other in the same order.

Still, there are some differences between administration of exogenous oxytocin and release of endogenous oxytocin:

- When endogenous oxytocin is released from the pituitary, several extended or longer forms of oxytocin are released from the posterior pituitary, in addition to the nine-amino-acid oxytocin molecule. Oxytocin is produced as a result of a gradual breakdown from longer precursor molecules, and part of this degradation occurs in the circulation (Amico & Hempel, 1990; Burbach et al., 2006). These longer oxytocin molecules may have effects, which, in part, differ from the nine-amino-acid oxytocin molecule. Therefore, the effects of administration of synthetic oxytocin may differ from the effects induced by the cocktail released from the posterior pituitary. The longer precursor molecules of oxytocin are, e.g., linked to stronger stimulation of growth than the shorter ones.

- A second important difference between endogenous release of oxytocin and infusion of synthetic oxytocin is that endogenous oxytocin is released in a pulsatile fashion during labor (Fuchs et al., 1991), whereas oxytocin infusions give rise to stable or flat oxytocin levels. This difference in oxytocin pattern may be associated with important differences in the effect patterns induced by endogenous and exogenous oxytocin. Often, physiological processes are better stimulated by pulses than stable hormone levels, and this is why many hormones, in particular peptides like oxytocin, are released in a pulsatile pattern.

- Thirdly, endogenous oxytocin is normally released in parallel into the circulation and into the brain to exert peripheral and central effects. In contrast, intravenously administered oxytocin only penetrates into the brain to a minor extent, because the blood-brain barrier stops the passage of oxytocin into the brain (Jones & Robinson, 1982). Oxytocin, like other peptides (molecules that are built up by chains of amino acids), are electrically charged substances that penetrate biological membranes, such as the blood-brain barrier, poorly, whereas electrically uncharged or lipophilic substances, such as the steroid hormones and cortisol, easily pass biological membranes. Less than 1% of oxytocin administered into the circulation passes into the brain (Jones & Robinson, 1982). Since the concentrations of oxytocin obtained in response to infusions of exogenous oxytocin are relatively low, intravenous infusion of oxytocin should not be expected to give rise to an elevation of oxytocin levels in the brain.

Still, exogenous oxytocin may, to a certain extent, influence oxytocin levels in the brain. This effect is indirect and due to the ability of circulating oxytocin to activate oxytocin receptors on peripheral sensory neurons, e.g., on the pelvic and hypogastric nerves, and also on somatosensory nerves, e.g., the CT fibers, which gives rise to an increased secretion of oxytocin from oxytocin-producing neurons in the SON and PVN (Jonas et al., 2009).

- Uterine contractions, and thereby the progression of labor, are not only stimulated by circulating oxytocin. As was described in the previous chapters,

the Ferguson reflex also involves activation of the parasympathetic nerves, which innervate the uterus (Sato et al., 1996). Oxytocinergic neurons, which project to the parasympathetic sacral plexa, stimulate uterine contractions and the relaxation of the cervix, thereby facilitating the effect of circulating oxytocin (Puder & Papka, 2001). These nerves are activated at the same time as oxytocin is released into the circulation, as they also emanate from the PVN, one of the main sources of oxytocin release into the circulation.

Obviously, administration of exogenous oxytocin into the circulation can increase circulating oxytocin levels, but it cannot substitute for the oxytocin-mediated stimulation of the parasympathetic nerves, which facilitates the effects of circulating oxytocin on uterine contractions.

It is even possible that the rise in circulating oxytocin levels caused by infusion of exogenous oxytocin may influence the activity of the autonomic nervous system in a negative way, causing a shift from parasympathetic to sympathetic dominance. As contractions induced by the sympathetic nerves are longer and linked to less uterine blood flow, an increased sympathetic nerve activity may explain why oxytocin-induced contractions are more long lasting and painful than contractions in the absence of oxytocin infusions. This effect may be a negative consequence of the lack of pulsatility in the oxytocin levels following infusion of exogenous oxytocin.

Amounts of Oxytocin May Be Expressed in International Units (IU) or Micrograms

It is a confusing fact that amounts of synthesized oxytocin are often given as international units and not as weight units. This is a remnant from the time when oxytocin was extracted and produced from the pituitaries of dead animals. Since the pituitaries from different animals contained different amounts of oxytocin, it was important to assess how much oxytocin was actually produced from the different animal pituitaries. Therefore, the biological activity of the unknown sample was assessed by its ability to contract uterine muscles and compared with a standard sample with a known activity expressed in international units. Today, oxytocin is synthesized—the different amino acids are linked in machines to form chains of amino acids and polypeptides, like oxytocin. The amount of oxytocin produced in this way can be expressed in normal weight units, such as micrograms or milligrams. The corresponding amount of 1.67 micrograms of oxytocin would be one international unit (IU).

Effects of Exogenous Oxytocin on Endogenous Oxytocin and Oxytocin-Related Effects

Little is known of the effects caused by administration of exogenous oxytocin on the release of endogenous oxytocin and oxytocin-mediated effects. The effects of intravenous infusion of exogenous oxytocin during labor and intramuscular injection, or intravenous infusion of exogenous oxytocin postpartum on the release of oxytocin and prolactin in response to breastfeeding and other breastfeeding-related variables two days after birth were explored in clinical studies described in the previous chapters. In addition, the combined effects of infusions of oxytocin and epidural analgesia were investigated.

Main Results

- Infusion of exogenous oxytocin did not influence or tended to increase oxytocin levels in response to suckling two days after birh (Jonas et al., 2009).

- The prolactin release in response to breastfeeding two days after birth was reinforced (Jonas et al., 2009).

- Infusion of oxytocin reinforced the changes of the KSP profile normally occurring after birth toward decreased anxiety and increased socialization (Jonas, Nissen, Ransjo-Arvidson, Matthiesen, et al., 2008).

- The rise of skin temperature in infants in response to suckling was reinforced if the mothers had received an infusion of oxytocin during labor (Jonas et al., 2007).

- Oxytocin levels were significantly lower in connection with breastfeeding two days postpartum in women having received both epidural analgesia and oxytocin, than in women having received epidural analgesia or oxytocin infusion alone, and mean endogenous oxytocin levels were dose-dependently decreased following administration of exogenous oxytocin in connection with breastfeeding two days after birth (Jonas et al., 2009).

- Diastolic blood pressure was higher in the women having received both oxytocin and epidural analgesia than oxytocin infusion alone in connection with breastfeeding two days after birth (Handlin et al., 2012; Jonas, Nissen, Ransjo-Arvidson, Wiklund, et al., 2008).

- Cortisol levels in response to breastfeeding two days after birth were significantly higher in the group receiving both epidural analgesia and oxytocin than in the group receiving epidural analgesia alone (Handlin et al., 2009).

- The lack of prolactin release in women having had epidural analgesia in response to breastfeeding two days after birth was restored by infusions of exogenous oxytocin.

- The lack of change in the KSP pattern observed in women having had an epidural analgesia two days postpartum was partly restored by oxytocin infusions (Jonas, Nissen, Ransjo-Arvidson, Matthiesen, et al., 2008).

- Infusion of exogenous oxytocin after birth restored the release of oxytocin in response to skin-to-skin contact and suckling, which was absent in women giving birth by elective Cesarean section.

- Infusion of exogenous oxytocin after birth restored the changes in the KSP profile, which were absent in women giving birth by elective Cesarean section.

Infusion of Oxytocin Alone During Labor Does Not Influence Endogenous Oxytocin Release, But Oxytocin in Combination with Epidural Analgesia Does

Oxytocin infusions alone during labor were not influenced or tended to increase endogenous oxytocin levels in connection with breastfeeding two days after birth. In contrast, endogenous oxytocin levels were significantly decreased if oxytocin infusion was combined with epidural analgesia. In fact, oxytocin levels were dose-dependently decreased (Jonas, Nissen, Ransjo-Arvidson, Matthiesen, et al., 2008).

Infusions of Exogenous Oxytocin May Stimulate Endogenous Release of Oxytocin

As mentioned above, infusion of exogenous oxytocin alone, if anything, increased endogenous oxytocin levels two days after birth. This effect may be a consequence of an increased oxytocin-mediated activation of the Ferguson reflex in connection with birth. This effect may be induced indirectly by an increased activity in the Ferguson reflex due to enhanced uterine contractions, or directly due to stimulation of oxytocin receptors on the pelvic or the hypogastric nerves, or even on other somatosensory nerves.

When the release of endogenous oxytocin is stimulated, oxytocin is released not only into the circulation, but also from nerves within the brain, e.g., in the NTS. When oxytocin levels are high in the NTS, the transmission in somatosensory nerves, which are involved in oxytocin release, are reinforced. In this way, the sensitivity of the nervous mechanisms involved in oxytocin release is increased, and sensory stimulation results in more release of oxytocin.

Epidural Analgesia Inhibits Oxytocin Release

The dose-dependent decrease of endogenous oxytocin levels caused by infusions of exogenous oxytocin in combination with epidural analgesia may, at first sight, suggest that an inhibitory feedback mechanism was activated by the release of exogenous oxytocin under these circumstances.

However, a more reasonable explanation to the finding of decreased levels of endogenous oxytocin in mothers who had received both exogenous oxytocin and epidural analgesia in connection with birth is that the epidural analgesia blocked the stimulation of endogenous-oxytocin release caused by oxytocin infusions by interfering with the transmission in the spinal cord (Jonas et al., 2009). The most reasonable explanation is, therefore, that the epidural analgesia inhibited the Ferguson reflex.

In fact, the amount of oxytocin and epidural analgesia given to the mothers increased in parallel—the longer the duration of oxytocin infusions, the longer the duration of epidural analgesia. Therefore, the seemingly dose-dependent-inhibitory effect of oxytocin infusions on oxytocin levels two days postpartum reflects a dose-dependent-inhibitory effect on oxytocin release of epidural analgesia. In fact, the correlation between the amount of oxytocin and epidural analgesia given was very high (Jonas, Nissen, Handlin, Ransjo-Arvidsson, & Uvnäs-Moberg, 2005).

This interpretation is in agreement with the data presented in the previous chapter, where epidural analgesia or other ways of administration of marcaine was shown to decrease maternal oxytocin release in connection with birth.

As mentioned above, oxytocin infusions resulting in a non-pulsatile elevation of oxytocin levels changes the pattern of uterine contractions. The long and painful contractions may be linked to an increased sympathetic nervous tone. The oxytocin release caused by activation of the Ferguson reflex may be counteracted more easily by the epidural analgesia than the nervous mechanisms mediating pain. Such an imbalance in the effects on oxytocin release and pain transmission may contribute to the lower oxytocin levels seen following prolonged adminstration of epidural analgesia or adminstration of larger amounts of epidural analgesia.

In Summary:

- Infusions of exogenous oxytocin stimulate the release of endogenous oxytocin into the circulation and into the brain by augmenting the effect of the Ferguson reflex.
- Infusions of epidural analgesia dose-dependently counteract the release of oxytocin in response to activation of the Ferguson reflex.

Other Expressions of Increased Release of Oxytocin in Response to Exogenous Administration of Oxytocin During Labor

Increased Prolactin Levels

The release of prolactin in response to breastfeeding two days after birth was significantly increased in mothers who had received oxytocin infusion in connection with birth in relation to the prolactin release observed in mothers who had not received exogenous oxytocin. As oxytocin, via neurogenic actions in the anterior pituitary, facilitates prolactin release, the oxytocin infusion during labor may have increased the activity in those oxytocinergic neurons that stimulate prolactin release (Jonas et al., 2009).

Reinforced Maternal Adaptations

The scores obtained for social interaction and anxiety in the KSP were dose-dependently influenced two days after birth in the women receiving oxytocin infusion during labor. The more oxytocin the mothers received during labor, the higher their scores in items reflecting social interactive skills, and the lower their scores in items reflecting anxiety. Thus, the adaptive pattern of psychological changes that normally occurs during labor, was reinforced by the extra oxytocin infused during labor (Jonas, Nissen, Ransjo-Arvidson, Matthiesen, et al., 2008).

Long-Term Effects

The Early Sensitive Period

Exposure to skin-to-skin contact in the immediate period gave rise to long-lasting, positive effects on social interaction and the stress-buffering capacity in both mothers and infants (Bystrova et al., 2009; Bystrova et al., 2003). These effects were most likely mediated by a release of endogenous oxytocin in the brain in response to activation of sensory nerves caused by skin-to-skin contact and suckling.

As infusions of oxytocin give rise to some of these effects, the effects of exogenous oxytocin infusions must have exerted similar effects in the brain. As infused oxytocin does not penetrate into the brain because the blood-brain barrier is impermeable to peptides, the effects of exogenously infused oxytocin on maternal adaptations and prolactin release must have been primarily induced outside the brain. As discussed above, exogenous oxytocin may have caused a transient release of endogenous oxytocin in the brain indirectly by reinforcing the activity in sensory nerves involved in the Ferguson reflex. In this way, the release of oxytocin in the anterior pituitary and areas in the brain involved in the maternal adaptations may have been increased during the early sensitive period, which may include not only the first hours after birth, but also labor. The extra oxytocin infusion also released oxytocin into the NTS, and thereby increased the sensitivity of the skin to the stimulation of skin-to-skin contact and suckling after birth. As also described in previous chapters, the release of oxytocin occurring in response to these stimuli is dependent on oxytocin levels.

Increased Rise of Skin Temperature in the Suckling Infant

The rise in skin temperature observed in the infants during a breastfeed two days after birth was more clearly expressed in infants whose mothers had received oxytocin infusions after birth. These data suggest that the mothers who had received oxytocin infusions during birth might have been more maternal, as supported by the reinforced changes in the KSP, i.e., more socially interactive and less anxious, and they somehow transmitted this to their infants. Perhaps their chest temperatures were higher. This, in turn, gave rise to a better expression of relaxation in the infant during breastfeeding, including a lowered sympathetic nervous tone and increased skin temperature (Jonas et al., 2007). Alternatively, the release of oxytocin was stimulated in infants of mothers receiving extra oxytocin infusion.

Oxytocin Infusion During Labor Counteracts Some of the Negative Effects of Epidural Analgesia

Some of the negative consequences of epidural analgesia are at least partially reversed by concomitant infusion of exogenous oxytocin during labor. The blunted effect on prolactin release and the maternal adaptations induced by epidural analgesia were, in part, counteracted in mothers who received oxytocin during labor. The oxytocin infusions seemed to facilitate the breastfeeding-related influence on maternal-behavioral adaptations.

Competition Between Oxytocin and Inhibitory Effects of Epidural Analgesia

These findings are consistent with the fact that epidural analgesia reduces the production of endogenous oxytocin secretion. The infused oxytocin can, to a certain extent, compensate for the lowered secretion of endogenous oxytocin caused by epidural analgesia alone during birth.

Infused Oxytocin Influences Brain Function Via the Ferguson Reflex

The positive effects of oxytocin may be exerted by an increased contractile activity in the uterine muscles and increased pressure on the cervix by the head of the infant, or by activation of oxytocin receptors on the nervous pathways involved in the Ferguson reflex, e.g., on the pelvic or hypogastric nerves. In this way, the infused oxytocin may, to a certain extent, overcome the blockade of nervous transmission caused by epidural analgesia in the spinal cord in connection with labor, and thereby activate the oxytocin nerves in the brain involved in the control of social interaction, anxiety, and milk production (Jonas et al., 2009; Jonas, Nissen, Ransjo-Arvidson, Matthiesen, et al., 2008).

Oxytocin Release in Connection With Breastfeeding Can Restore Oxytocin Effects

In addition, the mothers who received oxytocin and epidural analgesia caught up after six weeks and were no longer different from the mothers who did not have any medical interventions during birth. These results show that repeated exposure to oxytocin brought about by breastfeeding can compensate for the lack of stimulation in connection with birth.

Increased Stress Levels

In addition to reducing oxytocin levels two days postpartum, oxytocin infusion in combination with epidural analgesia during labor was associated with an increase in basal blood pressure and cortisol levels. These data suggest that the low circulating oxytocin levels two days after birth are linked to an elevated sympathetic nervous tone and increased function in the HPA axis. Blood pressure is increased by an elevated sympathetic nervous tone. Cortisol levels can be increased by an elevation of sympathetic nervous tone, as it influences the sensitivity to ACTH, the hormone that stimulates cortisol secretion from the adrenal cortex. The elevated cortisol levels observed two days after birth in mothers who had received oxytocin infusions during labor are, therefore, likely due to the increased sympathetic nervous tone (Handlin et al., 2009).

As sympathetic nervous activity is decreased by oxytocinergic activity in the brain, the lowered circulating levels of oxytocin observed in connection with breastfeeding two days after birth may reflect the lowered activity in the oxytocinergic nerves that innervate areas in the brain involved in the control of sympathetic nervous tone and of the HPA axis.

Differential Regulation of Oxytocin Neurons Involved in Social Interaction and Decreased Levels of Anxiety and Those Involved in Anti-stress Effects

The present data demonstrating that the effects induced by oxytocin infusions in connection with epidural analgesia stimulate and inhibit some of the oxytocin-related effects suggest that several different mechanisms are involved. The activity of the oxytocin neurons that give rise to increased social interaction, decreased levels of anxiety, and stimulation of prolactin are facilitated by infusions of oxytocin, whereas the oxytocin neurons linked to anti-stress effects, such as decreased levels of cortisol and low blood pressure, are counteracted by infusions of oxytocin during labor. These seemingly opposite effects depend on when and where in the brain they were initiated.

The effects on prolactin levels and maternal psychological adaptations are most likely induced during labor or during skin-to-skin contact immediately after birth. As they are induced during the early sensitive period, they become sustained and can be recorded two days after birth.

The lowered oxytocin secretion develops gradually as the amount of epidural analgesia given to the mothers increases. Oxytocin secretion is increased initially in response to infusion of exogenous infusions of oxytocin. As the duration and thereby the amount of epidural analgesia increases, the endogenous oxytocin released, induced by the infusion of exogenous oxytocin, is counteracted, and after a while, the oxytocin released, induced by the Ferguson reflex, is also blunted. As the effect of oxytocin release occurs during the early sensitive period, the effects become sustained.

As oxytocin levels in the circulation and, therefore, also in the brain are reduced in mothers having had an epidural analgesia, the inhibitory effect of oxytocinergic nerves involved in stress regulation is reduced and, consequently, blood pressure and cortisol levels rise in connection with breastfeeding two days after birth.

However, it can't be ruled out that infusion of exogenous oxytocin influences autonomic balance in a more direct way. The disturbed pattern of uterine contractions, with longer and more painful contractions, are indicative of an increased sympathetic nervous tone during labor. This increase in sympathetic nervous tone may be reflected by the higher blood pressure and cortisol seen in mothers who received oxytocin infusions during labor, observed in connection with breastfeeding two days after birth.

Effects of Administration of Oxytocin Postpartum

Oxytocin may be given as an intravenous or intramuscular injection after birth to contract the uterus to stop bleeding. In Sweden, all women receive 10 IU of oxytocin immediately postpartum, and oxytocin, often in higher doses, is often given as an intravenous infusion in women having a Cesarean section (Maughan, Heim, & Galazka, 2006; Murphy, MacGregor, Munishankar, & McLeod, 2009).

If oxytocin is given as an intravenous bolus postpartum in women having a Cesarean section, cardiovascular side effects, such as tachycardia, hypotension, and myocardial ischemia, may be induced. These side effects are reduced if lower doses or a reduced rate of administration is used (Jonsson, Hanson, Lidell, & Norden-Lindeberg, 2010; Svanstrom et al., 2008; Thomas, Koh, & Cooper, 2007). In addition, oxytocin given postpartum has been associated with lower breastfeeding rates 48 hours postpartum (Jordan et al., 2009).

Effects of Intramuscular Administration of Exogenous Oxytocin Postpartum

Very little is known about the effects of administration of oxytocin on the endogenous oxytocin system. The effect of intramuscular administration of oxytocin was part of the study described in the beginning of this chapter, in which the effects of various medical interventions during labor were studied.

Oxytocin given as an intramuscular or intravenous bolus injection after birth does not induce the same effect pattern as is observed following infusions of oxytocin during labor. No effect was observed on oxytocin or prolactin levels, and the maternal adaptations as measured by the KSP (social interaction and anxiety) were not influenced.

In contrast, oxytocin administered as a bolus postpartum seemed to facilitate the lowering of blood pressure and cortisol levels induced by skin-to-skin contact in connection with breastfeeding two days after birth. The effect of oxytocin in decreasing blood pressure and cortisol involves activation of alpha-2 adrenoceptors located in the hypothalamus and the NTS. In order to create this effect, oxytocin has to penetrate the blood-brain barrier (Handlin et al., 2012).

When 10 IU of oxytocin is given as a bolus, very high concentrations of oxytocin are obtained for a short period of time. It is possible that such high concentrations of oxytocin allow oxytocin to penetrate the blood-brain barrier in order to influence blood pressure and cortisol levels by bolus injections of oxytocin given after birth.

Effects of Intravenous Administration of Oxytocin Postpartum

The effects of intravenous infusion of oxytocin after birth were studied in women giving birth by elective Cesarean section. When oxytocin was infused postpartum (50 IU were infused during approximately two hours) in mothers who had a Cesarean Section, oxytocin levels rose in response to skin-to-skin contact between mother and infant, and in response to infant suckling. As described in chapter 25, no effect of skin-to-skin contact or suckling was seen in the absence of oxytocin infusion (Velandia, Uvnäs-Moberg, et al., 2014a).

The results showing that skin-to-skin contact and suckling induced a release of oxytocin in mothers having received a infusion of oxytocin, indicate that the inhibition of the response to touch and suckling induced by Cesarean section was, in part, reversed by the infusion of oxytocin after birth. The finding that infusions of oxytocin restored the sensitivity of the nervous mechanisms activated by skin-to-skin contact and suckling suggests that the infused oxytocin facilitated the effects of sensory stimulation of the skin by actions in the NTS.

Of course, it is also possible that the infused oxytocin

acted by facilitating the effect of the nervous transmission from the skin. The high levels of marcaine from the spinal anesthesia might have rendered the receptors in the skin insensitive, an effect which was reversed by the exogenous oxytocin.

A further consequence of intravenous infusions of oxytocin postpartum was the changes in the KSP, showing that administration of oxytocin increased social interactive skills and decreased the levels of anxiety in the mothers two days after birth (Velandia, Uvnäs-Moberg, et al., 2014b). A similar effect was observed two days after birth in the mothers who received oxytocin during labor (Jonas, Nissen, Ransjo-Arvidson, Matthiesen, et al., 2008).

As discussed before, the effect of exogenous oxytocin infusions on skin sensitivity and the KSP pattern must have been exerted in the brain. As oxytocin does not penetrate the blood-brain barrier, the effects of oxytocin must have been exerted in the periphery by activation of oxytocin receptors probably located on sensory nerves (e.g., the hypogastric and pelvic nerves, but also others), which, in turn, led to stimulation of the release of oxytocin from nerves emanating from the paraventricular nucleus of the hypothalamus to brain areas involved in regulation of skin sensitivity to stimuli that release oxytocin (NTS), anxiety, and social interaction.

Do Infusions of Oxytocin During Labor or in the Period Induce Long-Term Effects?

Skin-to-skin contact between mother and infant immediately after birth (the early sensitive period) may induce immediate effects in the infant. It may also exert long-term, positive effects on the relationship between the mother and infant, and make the infant more tolerant to stress. Such effects can be detected one year after birth (Bystrova et al., 2009; Bystrova et al., 2003).

As these effects are linked to oxytocin release and the release of oxytocin is influenced by Cesarean section (reduction or complete absence) and by epidural analgesia (reduction as a consequence of blockade of the Ferguson reflex), it is necessary to ask whether the effects of Cesarean section and epidural analgesia will also have long-term effects. The data obtained in our studies suggest that the KSP profile of mothers who had a Cesarean section or epidural analgesia during labor differed from that of vaginally delivered women two days after birth in the sense that they did not differ from the non-lactating control group (Jonas, et al., 2009; Jonas, Nissen, Ransjo-Arvidson, Matthiesen, et al., 2008; Nissen et al., 1998; Nissen et al., 1996).

Infusions of exogenous oxytocin during labor and after birth were demonstrated to induce effects that could be observed in connection with breastfeeding two days later, but in an opposite direction, i.e., the maternal adaptations observed after vaginal delivery in women were reinforced.

Taken together, any intervention that influences spontaneous oxytocin release during labor or in the early period may cause changes that last for at least two days. Just as positive interventions during the early sensitive period, such as skin-to-skin contact, may induce effects that can be observed after a year in both mothers and infants, medical interventions (Cesarean section, epidural analgesia, infusion of oxytocin) applied during labor or immediately postpartum (the early sensitive period around birth), might also have the potential to induce effects of similar long-term duration. No studies have yet been performed to study these effects.

Does Oxytocin Administered to the Mother During Labor or in the Period Influence the Fetus or the Newborn?

Administration of exogenous oxytocin during labor is bound to influence the fetus. Too much oxytocin may in rare cases induce hyperstimulation of the uterus and induce fetal asphyxia.

Even milder changes in the pattern of contractions may influence the fetus. Depending on the pattern of contractions, either painful or noxious stimulation or non-noxious stimulation will be induced.

Maternal Oxytocin Not Likely to Pass into the Circulation of the Fetus During Labor

It has been suggested that oxytocin infused into the maternal circulation would pass into the fetus via the placenta. It is unlikely that this is the case for several reasons.

High amounts of oxytocin are produced in the fetus. At birth, the circulating levels of oxytocin in the fetal circulation are higher than the oxytocin levels in the mother (Marchini et al., 1988). This difference suggests that if oxytocin diffuses freely between the circulation of the mother and the infant, the direction would be from the fetus to the mother. However, this balance would be different when the mother received infusions of oxytocin, which resulted in a marked elevation of maternal circulating oxytocin levels. Infusions of oxytocin have been demonstrated to raise the levels of oxytocin dose-dependently in men (Legros, Chiodera, Geenen, Smitz, & von Frenckell, 1984). However, it does not seem as if infusions of oxytocin in the doses normally given during labor give rise to very high oxytocin levels, and the levels induced are several-fold lower than those obtained in response to the same doses in other situations (Fuchs et al., 1991).

The placental barrier, like the blood-brain barrier, should be relatively impermeable to peptides, as electrically charged polypeptides, like oxytocin, do not easily pass biological membranes, and thereby inhibit the transfer of peptides between mother and infant. In addition, placental oxytocinases are present in the circulation and in the placenta at the site of interaction between the mother and the fetus, which will lead to degradation of biologically active peptide hormones at the site of transfer (Ito et al., 2003; Naruki et al., 1996).

Oxytocin Ingested Via Milk Does Not Contribute to Circulating Oxytocin Levels in Infants

After birth, synthetic oxytocin might hypothetically reach the infant via ingested milk if the infants are allowed to breastfeed after birth. Some oxytocin is secreted into milk under normal circumstances, but the concentrations are relatively low (Ito et al., 2003). Even if more oxytocin were secreted into milk during infusion of oxytocin after birth, the total amount would be very small regarding the small volumes of colostrum/milk that are produced by the mothers immediately after birth (Uvnäs-Moberg & Prime, 2013).

Surprisingly, ingested oxytocin via the milk survives in the stomach of the newborn, in spite of already functioning endocrine and exocrine secretion in the gastrointestinal tract at birth (Ito et al., 2003; Widstrom, Christensson, et al., 1988). If the small amounts of oxytocin were absorbed from the gastrointestinal tract, it would be diluted in the blood and would not be sufficient to elevate the circulating levels of oxytocin in the infant. Still, ingested oxytocin might exert local effects on the mucosa of the gastrointestinal tract.

Oxytocin Spray Stimulates the Milk Ejection Reflex

Breastfeeding women may be given oxytocin as a nasal spray in order to facilitate milk ejection—5-10 IU of oxytocin is administered intranasally before breastfeeding in order to raise oxytocin levels enough to induce milk ejection. The reason for administering oxytocin as a nasal spray is that the blood-brain barrier is relatively weak in the nasal mucosa and, therefore, permeable to oxytocin. Oxytocin penetrates the nasal mucosa into the blood vessels and reaches the mammary gland via the circulation, where it contracts the myoepithelial cells and causes ejection of milk. The effects of administration of oxytocin to stimulate milk ejection has, however, been questioned in some studies (Anderson & Valdes, 2007; Fewtrell, Loh, Blake, Ridout, & Hawdon, 2006).

Recently, intranasal administration of oxytocin to men (slightly higher doses than those used in connection with breastfeeding) has been demonstrated to reduce anxiety, increase social interaction, and increase trust (Domes et al., 2007; Heinrichs et al., 2003; Kosfeld et al., 2005). It is, therefore, very likely that some of the positive effects caused by intranasal spray on milk ejection may, in part, be attributed to decreased anxiety by effects in the amygdala. When the levels of anxiety decrease, the activity in the sympathetic nervous system is reduced, which may facilitate milk letdown by opening the milk ducts.

Oxytocin Analogues

Oxytocin-like drugs (oxytocin analogues) have been created

to substitute for the use of synthetic "natural" oxytocin. These drugs have been chemically modified to become more long lasting and more effective, or to penetrate the blood-brain barrier more easily than the original oxytocin. Carbetocin is a chemically modified oxytocin molecule, which has a considerably longer half-life than oxytocin. It is currently used to stop bleeding and to prevent uterine atony during Cesarean section in some countries (Su, Chong, & Samuel, 2012; Triopon et al., 2010).

Carbetocin has been demonstrated to reduce the perception of pain in women giving birth via Cesarean section and to decrease the use of analgesic drugs (De Bonis et al., 2011). These data suggest that carbetocin induces effects in the brain. As oxytocin induces different types of effects in the brain, e.g., it stimulates social interaction, reduces anxiety and stress, and induces anti-stress effects at different locations in the brain and by different types of oxytocin receptors, it is important to explore how carbetocin acts at these other sites. This is of particular importance, as it is given during the early sensitive period, when long-term effects may be induced. Other oxytocin agonists, peptidergic and non-peptidergic, are being developed, but most of them are not yet used clinically.

Oxytocin Antagonists

As oxytocin stimulates labor, it should be possible to use drugs that block the activity of oxytocin receptors to antagonize labor. Atosiban is an oxytocin antagonist used clinically to inhibit premature labor (Vrachnis et al., 2011). The inhibitory effects on premature labor are as good as those induced by beta blockers. In some studies, atosiban has been demonstrated to exert fewer cardiovascular side effects than beta blockers when used to inhibit preterm labor (Fabry, De Paepe, Kips, & Van Bortel, 2011; Wex, Abou-Setta, Clerici, & Di Renzo, 2011). Whether atosiban also inhibits other effects of oxytocin is not known.

Summary

- Infusion of exogenous oxytocin in connection with labor reinforces maternal behavioral adaptations and prolactin release in connection with suckling two days after birth.

- These effects are induced by an increased release of endogenous oxytocin during labor caused by an enhanced, direct or indirect, activation of the Ferguson reflex by the exogenous oxytocin.

- When oxytocin infusions are combined with epidural analgesia, a dose-dependent decrease of oxytocin levels is observed two days after birth. This seemingly oxytocin-dependent effect is most likely due to a dose-dependent inhibition of oxytocin release caused by epidural analgesia during birth.

- Intramuscular injections of oxytocin postpartum do not give rise to the effect pattern described above.

- Intravenous infusion of oxytocin postpartum after Cesarean section restores oxytocin release caused by skin-to-skin contact and suckling.

- Intravenous infusion of oxytocin postpartum after Cesarean section restores maternal psychological adaptations seen after vaginal delivery.

Chapter 28

Closeness and Support: The Gateway to Oxytocin

Routines around birth are changing. We easily forget that the era during which birth has taken place in hospitals is short. Before that, babies were born at home, with the assistance of midwives and/or other competent women. Routines around birth are still changing, and today, at least in the Western civilization, more and more technical and medical interventions are being used in connection with birth.

Towards Increased Technicalization and Medicalization

The use of Cesarean section is increasing, and if performed according to modern techniques, it is almost without risk for the mother's life. In Sweden, 20% of all deliveries are performed by Cesarean section. In some areas of the world, the use of Cesarean sections is even larger.

If mothers do give birth vaginally, they may be offered different kinds of medical pain relief, since it is considered important for women to give birth without pain. In Sweden, pain relief during birth is a right by law, and today 50% of all primiparas in Sweden receive epidural analgesia to decrease pain during birth. In addition, infusions of oxytocin may be given to induce or augment labor. Since epidural analgesia reduces uterine contractions and slows down the progress of labor, and since infusions of oxytocin give rise to painful contractions, epidural analgesia and infusions of oxytocin are very often given together.

As a consequence of moving birth from home to hospitals, mothers and infants were separated after birth. Instead of the infants being brought to the mothers immediately after birth and staying close to them during the first days of life, babies were separated from their mothers after birth and moved to nurseries, to be brought back to the mothers only for breastfeeding. Otherwise, nurses cared for the newborns.

Today, these routines are changing in some parts of the world. In Sweden, most women routinely have their babies placed in skin-to-skin contact immediately after birth, and the practice of rooming-in is becoming more common, i.e., infants are allowed to stay with their mothers during the entire stay in the maternity ward, not in a nursery.

In other countries, mothers and infants are still often separated from each other, i.e., they are not receiving skin-to-skin contact during the early sensitive period or during rooming-in. A new emerging problem is that the positive effects of skin-to-skin contact may not reach their full potential, due to the consequences of medical interventions.

Breastfeeding was originally absolutely necessary for mothers to feed their babies. Mothers who lived in cultures of hunters and gatherers (which still some do) often breastfed their children for several years, and they breastfed very frequently, particularly at night. If problems emerged, another woman, perhaps the mother of the mother or a sister, could help with breastfeeding.

Later on, women found out that cows' milk might be used to feed infants, and in some cultures, rich women did not breastfeed their children, but left them to a wet nurse.

Today, it is possible for everybody to avoid breastfeeding, since high-quality milk formula is available. In Sweden, the rate of breastfeeding has been high for the last 20 years, but is on the decline again. Presently, 60% of Swedish mothers breastfeed their infants exclusively for six months, whereas in many other Western countries, women breastfeed only for a short time. In some parts of the world, women use breastpumps and give their own milk to the infants by bottle. In other areas of the world, breastfeeding has been more or less replaced by bottle feeding.

Does It Really Matter?

An important question to ask is does it really matter if mothers have a normal vaginal birth or give birth by Cesarean section, whether they have a vaginal birth with or without medical interventions, if they have skin-to-skin contact with their babies after birth or are separated from them, or whether they breastfeed or bottle-feed their infants?

Obviously, with modern techniques, it is not dangerous to have a Cesarean section. Children that are separated from their mothers after birth survive, as do children who are given formula by bottle.

Cesarean sections are often necessary and may save the lives of both mother and baby if something goes wrong during pregnancy or labor. In addition, many mothers find it easier and more practical to give birth by Cesarean section, since they don't need to be afraid of labor, they have more control, and they can plan when the birth is going to take place. Other women want to avoid any tearing or physical damage that can be an unfortunate consequence of vaginal birth, perhaps particularly in unnatural settings. A tired mother may feel relieved when the newborn is taken care of by midwives and nurses at the maternity and labor ward. To breastfeed is not necessarily easy, and some mothers may find it to be animalistic. Bottle feeding may seem an easier and more practical solution. They might think that bottle feeding will give them more freedom to leave the care of the infants to others, and also that fathers will be involved in the care of the infant in a more natural way.

Loss of Oxytocin-Related Adaptations on Interactive Social Skills

Why, then, advocate for natural birth and breastfeeding? Because the most important consequence of all these "unnatural solutions" has been overlooked, i.e., the loss of the oxytocin release and oxytocin-related adaptations in both mother and infant, which are associated with normal birth, skin-to-skin contact in the period, and breastfeeding.

The positive effects of oxytocin release induced during birth, skin-to-skin contact, and breastfeeding, and the negative consequences of medical interventions are summarized below.

Oxytocin Release and Maternal Adaptations in Connection with Vaginal Delivery

Oxytocin is not only released into the circulation during labor to stimulate uterine contractions, it is also released into the brain, where it induces maternal adaptations. Mothers become less anxious and more interactive or "social" from the oxytocin released during labor. These conclusions were drawn based on the fact that the scores in items reflecting interest in social interaction and levels of anxiety in the personality inventory, the Karolinska Scales of Personality, were more pronounced two days after birth in women who had a normal vaginal delivery than in a similar-aged group of women who were not pregnant or breastfeeding. In addition, oxytocin exerts pain-relieving effects during labor and changes the memory of the often very painful labor into a more positive and forgiving one. Some women experience labor as pleasurable, particularly if they give birth in a familiar place, as, e.g., during home birth. Women who have had a normal birth may feel very proud of what they have achieved, and in this way, giving birth is an empowering experience for women.

Cesarean Section and Epidural Analgesia Counteract the Maternal Adaptations by Inhibition of Oxytocin Release

Both women who gave birth by Cesarean section and

those who received epidural analgesia with vaginal delivery failed to develop the maternal adaptations described above. In addition, the release of prolactin in response to breastfeeding two days after birth was reduced.

The mechanisms behind the negative consequences of Cesarean section and epidural analgesia on the development of maternal adaptations are, in part, the same, since they both reflect the lack of oxytocin during labor. Both Cesarean section and epidural analgesia decrease the release of oxytocin during labor, but in different ways. If elective Cesarean sections are performed before labor has started, no labor-associated oxytocin release occurs. If an emergency c-section is performed, oxytocin released during the second stage of labor is often substantially reduced. In women receiving epidural analgesia, oxytocin release is also diminished, as the activity in the Ferguson reflex is counteracted as a consequence of the diminished transmission in the spinal cord, and less oxytocin is released during labor, both in the brain and into the circulation.

Infusion of Exogenous Oxytocin During Labor Promotes Some Maternal Adaptations and Inhibits Some Maternal Adaptations

Infusions of exogenous oxytocin increase circulating oxytocin levels, and thereby reinforce uterine contractions. Infusions of exogenous oxytocin also enhance the effect of the Ferguson reflex in connection with birth, and, therefore, increase the release of oxytocin in the brain, and consequently, some maternal adaptations are reinforced. The inclination for social interaction is increased and the levels of anxiety are decreased. In addition, prolactin levels in response to suckling are increased.

If infusions of oxytocin are given in women who have also received epidural analgesia, the levels of oxytocin are decreased during breastfeeding two days later. The more oxytocin that has been given, i.e., the longer the duration of oxytocin infusion, the lower the levels of oxytocin two days later. This relationship is most likely indirect, as the duration of administration of epidural analgesia is increased at the same time. The infusion of epidural analgesia most likely inhibits the stimulation of endogenous oxytocin that occurs in response to exogenous oxytocin. The longer the period of oxytocin infusion, the longer the period of administration of epidural analgesia.

Stimulation of Labor and Natural Pain Relief by a Doula

Moving birth from homes to hospitals brought about beneficial effects, sometimes even lifesaving effects, for mother and infant, but some positive effects of home births were lost. In the natural home setting, women from the family or other experienced women were often present during the birth. They may have facilitated the birth process merely by their presence, through touching and being emotionally supportive.

There is a natural way of creating a quicker, less painful birth and a more positive outcome of birth in our society—the presence of a supportive woman, a doula, during labor. Several studies indicate that if a woman giving birth is physically and mentally supported by another women, both short-term and long-term effects of a beneficial nature are induced. The duration of labor is shortened and the experience of pain is reduced. The need for medical interventions, such as Cesarean section, administration of exogenous oxytocin, and the use of medical pain relief, such as epidurals, is decreased. The support during labor also results in long-term effects—the mother has a more positive memory of labor, she is in a better mood, and she has a better relationship with her infant and her partner several weeks later (Campbell, Scott, Klaus, & Falk, 2007; Chalmers & Wolman, 1993; Paterno, Van Zandt, Murphy, & Jordan, 2012; Scott, Berkowitz, & Klaus, 1999; Scott, Klaus, & Klaus, 1999; Sosa, Kennell, Klaus, Robertson, & Urrutia, 1980).

Mechanisms by Which the Doula Facilitates Labor

The doula promotes labor by touching the mother and by being mentally supportive. The doula facilitates oxytocin release by activation of sensory nerves and thereby labor. In addition, the stimulation of sensory nerves also decreases stress reactions and promotes parasympathetic nerve activity, which further facilitates labor via activation of the parasympathetic innervation of the uterus. The support and warmth given by the doula also decrease fear and anxiety, and stimulate oxytocin release by mental actions. By these positive actions, less exogenous oxytocin is needed to stimulate labor, and less medical interventions are needed, such as Cesarean sections. In addition, the facilitated oxytocin release acts to relieve the pain of the mother by stimulation of endogenous opioidergic mechanisms and, therefore, the need for pain relief.

The doula promotes not only the mother's experience of labor and birth, but also increases the interaction between the mother and the infant, and enhances the mother's mood in a more long-term perspective. These effects are linked to oxytocin's ability to enhance the stimulation of dopamine and serotonin, and other transmitter systems involved in reward and wellbeing.

Oxytocin Release and Maternal and Infant Adaptations in Connection with Skin-to-Skin Contact After Birth

Oxytocin is released both into the circulation and into the brain of mothers (and fathers) having skin-to-skin contact with their infants immediately after birth. A parallel increase of oxytocin release occurs in the infant. While in skin-to-skin contact, the social interaction, tactile and vocal, between mother and infant is facilitated and synchronized in several ways, and they become calm and relaxed.

The calming and relaxing effects caused by skin-to-skin contact may play a special role in infants after vaginal delivery, since it may help counteract the stress of being born. A high stress level in infants is of great physiological importance for a short while after birth, e.g., for the maturation of lung function, but in a more long-term perspective, a high stress level is detrimental. Skin-to-skin contact exerts powerful anti-stress effects by lowering levels of cortisol, adrenaline, and noradrenaline, and activating growth-promoting effects. The fight-or-flight system is inhibited, while the calm and connection system is reinforced.

There seems to be a period immediately after birth, the early sensitive period, during which the oxytocin-related increase in social skills and calm in both mother and infant caused by skin-to-skin contact turns into a more long-lasting effect. Positive effects on social interactive skills and the ability to regulate stress may indeed be observed after one year in mother and infants having been allowed skin-to-skin contact immediately after birth.

This biological window is not absolute in the sense that the possibility to induce long-term positive effects on interaction and stress levels by skin-to-skin contact is completely lost later on. Similar positive effects can be obtained by closeness later on, but it takes more time to induce the long-term effects.

Mothers allowed to have their children close to them in the maternity ward, the practice of rooming-in, has demonstrated some interesting effects that may be related to a more continuous release of oxytocin. For example, the rate of child neglect and abuse is diminished. If rooming-in is combined with skin-to-skin contact and suckling in the immediate period, infant abandonment is significantly reduced. In addition, breastfeeding is facilitated and stimulated by rooming-in.

Separation of Mother and Infant After Birth Counteracts the Adaptations in Mothers and Infants, Since No Oxytocin Released

It has long been known that if infants are separated from their mothers after birth, they cry more and have a higher heart and respiratory rate than infants not separated from their mothers. Separated infants also have higher cortisol values. Mothers of infants exposed to nursery care in the maternity ward have reduced milk production and a shorter duration of breastfeeding. Separation of mother and infant after birth and in the maternity ward is linked to a lack of stimulation of oxytocin release and oxytocin-related stimulation of social interaction and increased stress levels.

The interaction between mother and infant may be disturbed in more subtle ways. For example, the positive effects of early skin-to-skin contact are decreased when babies are dressed in baby clothes. Obviously, the clothes act like an insulator, which, to a certain extent, hinders the positive effects of skin-to-skin contact.

Administration of Marcaine Disturbs the Interaction Between Mothers and Infant After Birth

The interaction between mother and infant after birth may also be disturbed in mothers who received analgesic drugs or local anesthetic agents during labor. This is obvious after birth, as these drugs make both mothers and infants numb and disturb motor activity. As infants' breast-seeking behavior, including the massage of the breast, is reduced in infants exposed to marcaine and/or pethidine in connection with labor, it is likely that newborns' oxytocin levels are decreased. As oxytocin increases the sensitivity of the skin, then the sensitivity of the exposed infants' skin is also decreased. This insensitivity explains why infants fail to react with increased skin temperature during a breastfeeding session two days after birth.

Oxytocin Release and Maternal Adaptations in Connection With Breastfeeding

Each time a mother breastfeeds, oxytocin is released into the circulation to cause milk ejection. At the same time, oxytocin is released into the brain. As a result of this, breastfeeding mothers are more social and less stressed, and more tolerant to monotonous tasks when compared to women who do not breastfeed. The higher the mother's oxytocin levels during breastfeeding, the more social, less anxious, and more tolerant to monotonous tasks she is. In addition, the mother's stress hormones and her blood pressure fall, and the activity in her gastrointestinal tract increases in response to a breastfeed. Sympathetic nervous tone is decreased and parasympathetic nervous tone is increased during breastfeeding. In the long term, maternal health is promoted by breastfeeding. The more children a mother breastfeeds and the longer she breastfeeds them, the more she is protected from cardiovascular disease later in life.

The suckling child profits from oxytocin release and oxytocin-mediated effects, both as a consequence of the suckling stimulus and from the closeness associated with it. The infant's digestion and growth processes are stimulated. In addition, their social capacity is stimulated and their stress reactions are modified. Recently, it has been shown that the frequency of overweight is reduced in breastfeeding infants.

Perhaps the repeated suckling stimulus and consequent oxytocin release in breastfed infants optimize regulation of food intake and metabolism.

Bottle Feeding

It is obvious that women who do not breastfeed and children who are not breastfed are not exposed to the same intensity of oxytocin-mediated changes. Even if mother and infant spend a lot of the time being close to each other, they will not be exposed to the oxytocin release and consequences of the suckling stimulus, which, in certain aspects, induce effects that are different from the effects caused by closeness. Bottle-feeding mothers smile and interact less with their infants when they are feeding them compared to breastfeeding mothers. The bottle-feeding mothers also have higher blood pressure and other signs of elevated sympathetic nervous tone.

Continuous Exposure to Oxytocin During Labor, the Period, and Breastfeeding

It is obvious that natural vaginal birth, skin-to-skin contact immediately after birth, and breastfeeding all give rise to oxytocin release via different kinds of sensory stimulation. During birth, the pressure on the cervix of the uterus caused by the head of the fetus stimulates oxytocin release by increasing the activity in the Ferguson reflex. At the same time, oxytocin levels in the fetus are activated by the contractions. In the immediate period, the sensory interaction induced by warmth, light pressure, stroking, and massage of the skin stimulate oxytocin release. During breastfeeding, both skin-to-skin contact and suckling stimulate oxytocin release. At the same time, the infant's oxytocin is released in response to skin-to-skin contact or by sucking.

As oxytocin is released in all these different situations, similar oxytocin-effect patterns are induced, and the activity of the calm and connection response is stimulated. Still, there is a difference between the different situations in the sense that skin-to-skin contact and breastfeeding involve touch, and, therefore, the anti-stress effects are more strongly expressed. It also seems that the effects induced during and directly after birth give rise to particularly long-lasting effects.

Perhaps birth, postpartum skin-to-skin contact, and breastfeeding should be regarded as an entity, as they all induce maternal adaptations that are very important for the development of the future interaction between the mother and child. Any intervention that counteracts these effects should be avoided.

Since oxytocin is released during labor, in response to close contact after labor, and during breastfeeding to induce oxytocin-related effects, an important question is whether lack of oxytocin release during one of these phases can be compensated for by the exposure to oxytocin occurring during one of the other phases? It seems that this is the case, and some examples will be given below.

Skin-to-Skin Contact After Birth May Alleviate Some of the Consequences of Cesarean Section

Oxytocin release in response to skin-to-skin contact in the period to a certain extent compensates for lack of oxytocin in women having had an elective Cesarean section. As mentioned above, women who had a Cesarean section didn't express the psychological maternal adaptations recorded two days after birth according to the Karolinska Scales of Personality, and they released less oxytocin in connection with a breastfeed. This may be due to the fact that women who gave birth by Cesarean section had no or a decreased release of oxytocin during birth. Early skin-to-skin contact, in part, compensated for the lack of oxytocin release following Cesarean section in the sense that more oxytocin was released in response to breastfeeding two days after birth. However, these results should be regarded with some caution because infants who breastfed early might have had higher oxytocin levels.

However, the first interpretation is in line with findings showing that women who had an elective Cesarean section and were allowed skin-to-skin contact after completion of the Cesarean section expressed more caretaking maternal behavior during the days following birth and when the infant was one month old compared to mothers who had Cesarean sections and did not have skin-to-skin contact (McClellan & Cabianca, 1980).

Breastfeeding Compensates for Lack of Development of Maternal Adaptations Caused by Epidural Analgesia During Birth

As mentioned above, breastfeeding women differed in their personality profile as measured by the Karolinska Scales of Personality (KSP) from non-pregnant/non-breastfeeding women of the same age in the sense that they had lower scores on items reflecting anxiety and higher scores on items reflecting social interaction. Mothers who received epidural analgesia in connection with birth did not express this pattern two days after birth (Jonas et al., 2008). This deviation was most likely caused by an inhibition of the Ferguson reflex and a consequent reduced amount of oxytocin released in the brain during labor.

In contrast, there was no difference between the scores on the KSP at two and six months in mothers who had received epidural analgesia and those who had not. One possible explanation for this is that the repeated release of oxytocin occurring during breastfeeding compensated for the lack of effect occurring during labor, since all the women who participated in the study breastfed exclusively (Jonas et al., 2008).

Long-Term Positive Effects of Oxytocin Release During Labor, in the Period, and During Breastfeeding

Vaginal birth, particularly without medical interventions, skin-to-skin contact after birth, and breastfeeding are all associated with oxytocin release in the mother and in the fetus or child. As oxytocin stimulates interactive behavior and reduces anxiety, the effects caused during birth, in the period, and during breastfeeding are added to each other and may be of long duration.

Oxytocin and Attachment

Oxytocin has been documented to promote the establishment of a bond between a mother and her young postpartum in several mammalian species. Olfactory, auditory, and visual cues take part in this learning process. Oxytocin has been shown to promote the formation of this bond.

Oxytocin and Secure Attachment

An interesting question to ask is whether oxytocin also promotes the formation of bonding between a human mother and her infant and vice versa in the period, and in a more long-term perspective, is early bonding linked to the formation of secure attachment also seen in humans?

The long-term effects of skin-to-skin contact, i.e., increased social interaction and enhanced ability to handle stress, display some similarities with the expressions of secure attachment, as reflected in the strange situations test. An intriguing question is, therefore, if secure attachment is associated with a well-functioning oxytocinergic system?

It might be assumed that skin-to-skin contact, especially if induced repeatedly and early in life, could be an important mechanism through which secure attachment is developed. The oxytocin release and the positive effects of skin-to-skin contact, originally triggered by the cutaneous sensory stimulation in connection with skin-to-skin contact, over time may be developed into a "conditioned reflex." After a while, just seeing, hearing, or smelling the mother may trigger oxytocin release in the infant in a Pavlovian manner. Further more, just the thought or the mental image of the mother may be enough to trigger oxytocin release in the child. The more closeness a child receives, the more the function of the oxytocin system will be stimulated. In the end, individuals who have a well-developed oxytocin system will interact with others in a secure and trustful way, and their ability to handle stressful situations will be optimized.

Findings of higher oxytocin levels in individuals with secure attachment than in those with insecure attachment support the role of a well-functioning oxytocin system in individuals with secure attachment.

Routines Linked to Oxytocin Release Should Be Promoted

Assuming that oxytocin is advantageous for the mother and helps her in her role as a mother, some of her innate or competence is lost if she does not give birth vaginally, have the child on her chest after birth, or breastfeed, since oxytocin as her inner guide to motherhood has not come into play. It is possible that she will find it more difficult to develop interaction with the child and more boring and tedious to take care of the baby, and her anxiety may be enhanced.

The routine separation of mother and infant after birth should be avoided since the communication between the two that takes place during the early sensitive period might have important positive effects on future interaction between mother and infant, both short and long term. The child will also be influenced. If the infant receives skin-to-skin contact, it might become more interactive and more capable of tolerating stress. This means that it is not only a question of the mother's ability to interact with her child, it is also a question of the child's future—its ability to communicate with other individuals, its ability to handle stress, and perhaps a question of its health in the long run.

Health-Promoting Effects

Breastfeeding is dose-dependently linked to positive health effects in the mother. The risk of developing cardiovascular disease, such as stroke, hypertension, diabetes type 2, and heart infarction, is diminished, as is the risk of developing certain types of cancer. The repetitive exposure to endogenous oxytocin may lie behind these long-term health-promoting effects.

Also, the infant's health may be linked to high oxytocin levels and secure attachment, which may be a consequence of close interaction between mother and child. Individuals with secure attachment have less anxiety and depression than those with insecure attachment. In addition, they also have less pain and inflammation.

Can a Lack of Oxytocin Be Transmitted to Other Generations?

There is an even larger question built into the loss of oxytocin if normal birth and breastfeeding is abandoned. Rats exposed to extrasensory stimulation during the first week of life became less anxious and more socially interactive as adults, and also less easily stressed (Caldji et al., 2011). The first week of life in rats might, in this respect, correspond to the first hour after birth in humans.

From the perspective of this chapter, the most important effect described by Caldji and his collaborators was that the female rat pups exposed to extrasensory stimulation became more interactive as mothers when they gave birth to their own litters. It is very likely that a similar transition of certain competencies also occurs in humans between generations. Perhaps human mothers who received more interaction when they were small interact more with their infants as grown ups. Perhaps the early learning is an epigenetic phenomenon also found in humans.

If a mother transfers her "oxytocin competence" to her baby, her baby is likely to transfer it to her baby, and so forth. This means that a reduced "oxytocin competence" may also be transferred to the next generation. What happens after ten, 100, or 1,000 generations? Will the human competence of loving and caring for others become attenuated? Do the next generations become like aliens?

Medical and technical interventions during birth and ward routines after birth a society chooses to support is not only important for mothers and babies, but may have much more important consequences as to the competence of communicative skills and the ability to love in future generations, and thereby might affect society as a whole.

Can Administration of Exogenous Oxytocin Substitute for Loss of Endogenous Oxytocin?

If technical and medical interventions during birth and ward routines which allow separation between mother and infant lead to a decreased release of oxytocin, some people may argue that these deficiencies could be restored by administration of exogenous oxytocin.

In fact, administration of oxytocin during labor dose-dependently enhanced the maternal adaptations towards increased social interaction and decreased levels of anxiety observed in connection with breastfeeding two days after birth. Infusion of oxytocin postpartum enhanced the release of endogenous oxytocin in mothers in response to skin-to-skin contact and suckling immediately postpartum in mothers delivered by Cesarean section, and promoted maternal psychological adaptations two days later. These effects were promoted both in mothers who had skin-to-skin contact with their infants after birth and in those who were not allowed to have skin-to-skin contact. These effects are likely to have been induced by an increased release of endogenous oxytocin into the brain and into the circulation, as a result of an enhanced activation of peripheral sensory nerves by the infused exogenous oxytocin.

On the other hand, infusion of exogenous oxytocin in combination with epidural analgesia was also related to a dose-dependent decrease of endogenous oxytocin secretion and increased stress reactivity, as evidenced by increased cortisol levels and blood pressure in the mothers two days after birth. This means that exogenous oxytocin administered via the circulation does not give rise to the same oxytocin-release pattern and effect pattern, as does the release of endogenous oxytocin, because it induces a feedback inhibition of oxytocin release.

The findings that oxytocin infusions during birth and in the period influence the psychological and physiological reaction patterns of mothers must be taken seriously and should be investigated in detail. The fact that such subtle, but yet vital things as trust, loyalty, love, bonding, and attachment are influenced by oxytocin raises a red flag. Do mothers want to be exposed to chemicals that influence the very core of life? Or should administration of exogenous oxytocin be considered a valuable tool in compensating for endogenous oxytocin that is not released in mothers being exposed to medical interventions that block the release of oxytocin, such as Cesarean section and epidural analgesia?

Recently, more long-lasting oxytocin-like drugs (oxytocin analogues) have been introduced to stop bleedings in some countries. These drugs have been demonstrated to exert pain-relieving effects and are, therefore, likely to mimic centrally induced oxytocin-linked effect, to a larger or lesser degree. All chemical modifications change activity patterns of a given substance. Unexpected effects could be induced as a result of administration of such drugs. Functional changes induced during the early sensitive period might alter brain function for a long period, if not for life. Therefore, the effect profile of such substances should be investigated in great detail before being given to large numbers of women.

The Best Solution Is to Promote Mother's Own Abilities

Obviously, Cesarean section, epidural analgesia, and oxytocin infusions influence maternal psychological and physiological adaptations that normally occur during birth. Since the effects are induced during the early sensitive period, the effects persist after two days, and it is possible that they are even more long lasting.

These data lead to the conclusion that medical interventions during birth should be avoided if not necessary for medical reasons.

During labor, emotional and physiological support by doulas (or husbands, other relatives, and friends) should be provided and used as much as possible.

Skin-to-skin contact after birth should be allowed in order to use the strong potential for strengthening of social interactive skills and capacity to handle stress during this period.

Breastfeeding should be encouraged, since it strengthens the oxytocin-induced effects initiated in connection with birth. Both should be supported in the maternity ward and by the healthcare system.

It is also important to recognize that as the use of medical interventions during birth and bottle feeding increase, there is a large group of women with a growing awareness of the importance of natural birth and breastfeeding. Many women want to give birth vaginally, with as little medical intervention as possible. They explicitly want to have their baby in skin-to-skin contact after birth. They want to have their children with them in the maternity ward and to breastfeed on demand for as long as possible.

Conclusion

From a Mother's Point of View

Mothers have their own free will. They, themselves, have to decide what type of birth they want, if they want to have skin-to-skin contact with their babies after birth, and if they want to breastfeed. To be able to make their own decisions, they need to be informed about all aspects of giving birth and breastfeeding, both good and bad.

All mothers want to do whatever is best for their children, which is one aspect of the adaptation to motherhood. This attitude is probably the reason why mothers so easily have given up their own intuitive knowledge when exposed to people from the medical establishment who advise them. Without this openness, which is actually in its deepest sense meant to allow mothers to be open to their newborns' needs and to advice from older women and relatives, mothers would probably never have agreed to give birth in hospitals in a very unnatural way.

But this openness to positive information can also be used to make mothers understand that natural birth, skin-to-skin contact, and breastfeeding might help them and their infants develop their oxytocin competence. If women are informed about the effects of oxytocin, how they can get access to it, and how they can become carriers of oxytocin, the inner guide to motherhood, they may choose more natural birth routines

From the Physician's and the Scientist's Point of View

Medical staff, including doctors, involved in the care of women around childbirth and breastfeeding should be taught about the beneficial effects of oxytocin. They should be informed about the many positive effects of oxytocin and about how it is released to help mother and baby during labor and birth, during skin-to-skin contact, particularly after birth, and also during breastfeeding. They should also be taught about the early sensitive period and that the function of the endogenous-oxytocin system can be positively influenced during natural birth and in the period.

The techniques for medical interventions during birth have developed dramatically and so has the use of these techniques in connection with birth. The intention is, of course, always good, i.e., to help mothers who can't give birth in a natural way for different reasons to give birth by Cesarean section, to give pain relief during birth for mothers who find the pain of labor too frightening or unbearable, or to give infusions of oxytocin when labor does not progress.

When new drugs are introduced, they are exposed to rigorous tests before being registered by medical authorities to be used clinically. All side effects should, of course, be noted. When drugs for severe diseases are registered, side effects can sometimes be accepted, but when drugs are developed for minor illnesses or for preventive purposes, the acceptance of side effects is much lower.

Medical interventions, e.g., Cesarean section, can be lifesaving, and pain relief may have very positive effects for some mothers' mental health. Minor negative consequences of the interventions can, of course, be accepted. But is this the case when the use of medical interventions, such as Cesarean sections, epidural analgesia, and infusions of exogenous oxytocin, are given without such indications? Today, the use of medical interventions has increased dramatically and the indications for their use have expanded.

As presented and discussed in this book, several of the medical interventions presently used seem to influence the function of endogenous oxytocin on both mothers and infants, not only in connection with birth, but for days and perhaps much longer, as they are given during the early sensitive period. In particular, the use of Cesarean section and epidural analgesia in connection with infusions of exogenous oxytocin seem to influence oxytocin levels and some of the oxytocin-related effects negatively. These are preliminary studies, but they all point in the same direction.

Epidemiological studies point to possible relationships between medical interventions during birth and development of certain types of disease.

It is, therefore, the responsibility not only of the medical society, but also of society in general to allocate resources for high-quality studies to investigate if certain ward routines and medical interventions in connection with birth are associated with "side effects." As giving birth per se is not a disease, side effects should not be accepted unless in the presence of real indications for the interventions.

New drugs based on the oxytocin principle are being developed and used to stop uterine bleeding after birth, which may be lifesaving. However, it should be explored if these substances also induce other oxytocin-linked effects on behavior and physiology, and if so, to what extent.

Women have the right to know what will happen to them and their children if they are exposed to unnecessary medical interventions.

Appendix

Clinical Studies

Study 1

Seventy-two primiparous women were consecutively recruited in connection with birth to be studied in connection with breastfeeding two days after birth. Some had received medical interventions, such as intravenous administration of oxytocin, epidural analgesia, or both during labor. Some received intramuscular and administration of oxytocin postpartum.

The infants were put in skin-to-skin contact on the mothers' chest before breastfeeding, and they initiated breastfeeding themselves.

Twenty-four blood samples were collected in 63 mothers. Oxytocin and prolactin levels were determined in all mothers. Cortisol levels were measured in eight samples and adrenocorticotrophic hormone (ACTH) levels in nine samples.

The duration of skin-to-skin contact before suckling and the duration of suckling were measured.

Blood pressure was measured four times before and after breastfeeding in 66 of the women. In a subgroup of these mothers (33), blood pressure was measured repeatedly before and after breastfeeding during a six-month period.

Sixty-nine of the breastfeeding mothers filled in the KSP formula two days after birth, at two months, and at six months after birth.

Skin temperature was measured in the newborns during breastfeeding two days after birth.

Jonas, K., Johansson, L. M., Nissen, E., Ejdeback, M., Ransjo-Arvidson, A. B., & Uvnäs-Moberg, K. (2009). Effects of intrapartum oxytocin administration and epidural analgesia on the concentration of plasma oxytocin and prolactin, in response to suckling during the second day postpartum. *Breastfeed Med, 4*(2), 71-82.

Jonas, W., Nissen, E., Ransjo-Arvidson, A. B., Matthiesen, A. S., & Uvnäs-Moberg, K. (2008). Influence of oxytocin or epidural analgesia on personality profile in breastfeeding women: a comparative study. *Arch Womens Ment Health, 11*(5-6), 335-345.

Jonas, W., Nissen, E., Ransjo-Arvidson, A. B., Wiklund, I., Henriksson, P., & Uvnäs-Moberg, K. (2008). Short- and long-term decrease of blood pressure in women during breastfeeding. *Breastfeed Med, 3*(2), 103-109.

Jonas, W., Wiklund, I., Nissen, E., Ransjo-Arvidson, A. B., & Uvnäs-Moberg, K. (2007). Newborn skin temperature two days postpartum during breastfeeding related to different labour ward practices. *Early Hum Dev, 83*(1), 55-62.

Handlin, L., Jonas, W., Petersson, M., Ejdeback, M., Ransjo-Arvidson, A. B., Nissen, E., Uvnäs-Moberg, K. (2009). Effects of sucking and skin-to-skin contact on maternal ACTH and cortisol levels during the second day postpartum-influence of epidural analgesia and oxytocin in the perinatal period. *Breastfeeding Medicine, 4*(4), 207-220.

Study 2

Seventeen mothers with emergency c-sections and 20 mothers with normal vaginal deliveries (37 primiparous women) participated in the study.

The infants were put directly to the breast after a period of separation and helped to initiate breastfeeding by the midwife.

Twenty-four blood samples were collected before, during, and after breastfeeding two days after birth. Oxytocin, prolactin, and cortisol levels were measured.

The amount of milk ejected in connection with the breastfeed and the duration of breastfeeding was recorded.

Blood pressure was measured before breastfeeding and 60 minutes after breastfeeding.

The women filled in the KSP inventory two days after birth.

Nissen, E., Uvnäs-Moberg, K., Svensson, K., Stock, S., Widstrom, A. M., & Winberg, J. (1996). Different patterns of oxytocin, prolactin but not cortisol release during breastfeeding in women delivered by caesarean section or by the vaginal route. *Early Hum Dev, 45*(1-2), 103-118.

Nissen, E., Gustavsson, P., Widstrom, A. M., Uvnäs-Moberg, K. (1998). Oxytocin,prolactin, milk production and their relationship with personality traits in women after vaginal delivery or Cesarean section. *J Psychosom Obstet Gynaecol, 19*(1), 49-58.

Study 3

Eighteen blood samples were collected before, during, and after breastfeeding four days after birth and during established breastfeeding (three to four months after birth) in 55 and 36 primiparous women, respectively. Oxytocin, prolactin, and somatostatin levels were measured and were related to other breastfeeding variables, such as milk yield, duration of suckling, duration of breastfeeding, and weaning.

The women's smoking habits were recorded. The weight of the infant at birth, as well as placental weight were noted.

Fifty-two of the mothers filled in the KSP formula four days after giving birth. They were all primiparas and had undergone a normal vaginal birth.

Uvnäs-Moberg, K., Widstrom, A. M., Werner, S., Matthiesen, A. S., & Winberg, J. (1990). Oxytocin and prolactin levels in breast-feeding women. Correlation with milk yield and duration of breastfeeding. *Acta Obstet Gynecol Scand, 69*(4), 301-306.

Uvnäs-Moberg K, W. A.-M., Nissen E, Björvell H. (1990). Personality traits in women 4 days postpartum and their correlation with plasma levels of oxytocin and prolactin. *J Psychosom Obstet Gynaecol, 11*, 261-273.

Widstrom, A. M., Matthiesen, A. S., Winberg, J., & Uvnäs-Moberg, K. (1989).Maternal somatostatin levels and their correlation with infant birth weight. *Early Hum Dev, 20*(3-4), 165-174.

Widstrom, A. M., Werner, S., Matthiesen, A. S., Svensson, K., & Uvnäs-Moberg, K. (1991). Somatostatin levels in plasma in nonsmoking and smoking breast-feeding women. *Acta Paediatr Scand, 80*(1), 13-21.

Study 4

Six blood samples were collected in connection with breastfeeding in six women during established lactation. The mothers' experiences of the milk ejection reflex was noted. The third blood sample was collected one minute after the occurrence of the milk ejection reflex. Gastrin, insulin, and prolactin levels were measured with RIA (Widstrom, et al., 1984).

The occurrence of the milk ejection reflex during breastfeeding was recorded by an observed flow of milk from the contra-lateral nipple, by swallowing sounds from the infant, or by a sensation of tingling or pressure in the mother's breast.

Widstrom, A. M., Winberg, J., Werner, S., Hamberger, B., Eneroth, P., & UvnäsMoberg, K. (1984). Suckling in lactating women stimulates the secretion of insulin and prolactin without concomitant effects on gastrin, growth hormone, calcitonin, vasopressin or catecholamines. *Early Hum Dev, 10*(1-2), 115-122.

Study 5

This study was performed on 15 multiparous women in connection with a breastfeed. Gastrin and somatostatin levels were measured in 11 blood samples collected during the breastfeeding session. The amount of milk received by the infants during the breastfeed was recorded.

Widstrom, A. M., Winberg, J., Werner, S., Svensson, K., Posloncec, B., & Uvnäs-Moberg, K. (1988). Breast feeding-induced effects on plasma gastrin and somatostatin levels and their correlation with milk yield in lactating females. *Early Hum Dev, 16*(2-3), 293-301.

Study 6

Repeated blood samples were collected during pregnancy and breastfeeding. Oxytocin, somatostatin, gastrin, and insulin levels were measured and linked to the outcome of breastfeeding.

Silber, M., Larsson, B., & Uvnäs-Moberg, K. (1991). Oxytocin, somatostatin, insulin and gastrin concentrations vis-a-vis late pregnancy, breastfeeding and oral contraceptives. *Acta Obstet Gynecol Scand, 70*(4-5), 283-289.

Study 7

Gastric aspirates were collected from 25 newborns immediately after birth. The volume and pH of the contents were analyzed. Gastrin and somatostatin levels were also analyzed in the aspirates.

Widstrom, A. M., Christensson, K., Ransjo-Arvidson, A. B., Matthiesen, A. S., Winberg, J., & Uvnäs-Moberg, K. (1988). Gastric aspirates of newborn infants: pH, volume and levels of gastrin- and somatostatin-like immunoreactivity. *Acta Paediatr Scand, 77*(4), 502-508.

Study 8

Eight preterm infants were tube-fed twice with maternal milk—once without and once with sucking on a pacifier 15 minutes before, during, and after tube feeding. Gastric aspirates were withdrawn. Volume and pH, as well as gastrin and somatostatin levels of the aspirates were measured.

Widstrom, A. M., Marchini, G., Matthiesen, A. S., Werner, S., Winberg, J., & Uvnäs-Moberg, K. (1988). Nonnutritive sucking in tube-fed preterm infants: effects on gastric motility and gastric contents of somatostatin. *J Pediatr Gastroenterol Nutr, 7*(4), 517-523.

Study 9

Blood samples were collected from an umbilical catheter from premature and full-term newborns in response to suckling of a pacifier. Insulin, gastrin, and somatostatin levels were measured with radioimmunoassay.

Marchini, G., Lagercrantz, H., Feuerberg, Y., Winberg, J., & Uvnäs-Moberg, K. (1987). The effect of non-nutritive sucking on plasma insulin, gastrin, and somatostatin levels in infants. *Acta Paediatr Scand, 76*(4), 573-578.

Study 10

Blood samples were collected in 58 newborn infants. Each child contributed with one blood sample collected before, just after, or at ten, 30, and 60 minutes after breastfeeding. Determination of plasma levels of cholecystokinin (CCK) was performed by HPLC and radioimmunoassay.

Uvnäs-Moberg, K., Marchini, G., & Winberg, J. (1993). Plasma cholecystokinin concentrations after breast feeding in healthy 4 day old infants. *Arch Dis Child, 68*(1 Spec No), 46-48.

Study 11

The Karolinska Scales of Personality (KSP) formula was filled in by 161 women on three different occasions—in the third trimester of pregnancy, and during breastfeeding at three and six months after delivery.

Sjogren, B., Widstrom, A. M., Edman, G., & Uvnäs-Moberg, K. (2000). Changes in personality pattern during the first pregnancy and lactation. *J Psychosom Obstet Gynaecol, 21*(1), 31-38.

Study 12

Thirteen primiparas and 16 multiparas having undergone normal vaginal deliveries filled in the KSP formula two days postpartum. Eight blood samples were collected in the postpartum period and oxytocin, gastrin, somatostatin, and cholecystokinin levels were analyzed.

Uvnäs Moberg, K. & Nissen, E. (2005). Hormonal regulation of maternal behavior during breastfeeding. In B. Sjogren (Ed.). *Psychosocial aspects on birth and obstetrics.* Studentlitteratur, pp. 181-196.

Study 13

Twenty-one newborn infants were placed on their mothers' chests immediately after birth, and the interaction between mothers and infants was recorded for a 120-minute period. Detailed observations of mothers' and infants' behaviors were analyzed. Some of the infants were subjected to gastric suction and the effect of this procedure was studied.

Widstrom, A. M., Ransjo-Arvidson, A. B., Christensson, K., Matthiesen, A. S., Winberg, J., & Uvnäs-Moberg, K. (1987). Gastric suction in healthy newborn infants. Effects on circulation and developing feeding behaviour. *Acta Paediatr Scand, 76*(4), 566-572.

Study 14

Fifty mother infant dyads were randomized to either skin-to-skin contact alone or to skin-to-skin contact in addition to suckling of the breast immediately after birth.

Four days after birth, the mothers were observed during a breastfeeding session and their interactions with the child were recorded. Milk production was measured and blood samples, which were analyzed for prolactin and gastrin, were collected before and after a breastfeed. The mothers were asked to describe how anxious they were and how close they felt to their children. They were also asked to fill in a diary regarding the amount of time they spent with their infants four days after birth. At this time, the infants were kept in a nursery in the maternity ward and the mothers fetched them when they were supposed to breastfeed or just when they wanted to be with them.

Widstrom, A. M., Wahlberg, V., Matthiesen, A. S., Eneroth, P., Uvnäs-Moberg, K., Werner, S., et al. (1990). Short-term effects of early suckling and touch of the nipple on maternal behaviour. *Early Hum Dev, 21*(3), 153-163.

Study 15

Fourteen newborn infants were placed in skin-to-skin contact with the mother, fifteen in a cot, and fifteen in a cot and thereafter in skin-to-skin contact with the mother. The newborns' cries was recorded by a tape recorder for 90 minutes after birth).

Christensson, K., Cabrera, T., Christensson, E., Uvnäs-Moberg, K., & Winberg, J. (1995). Separation distress call in the human neonate in the absence of maternal body contact. *Acta Paediatr, 84*(5), 468-473.

Study 16

Eighteen healthy women were allowed skin-to-skin contact after birth. Ten blood samples were collected at 15-minute intervals. Oxytocin levels were measured with RIA.

Nissen, E., Lilja, G., Matthiesen, A. S., Ransjo-Arvidsson, A. B., Uvnäs-Moberg, K., & Widstrom, A. M. (1995). Effects of maternal pethidine on infants' developing breast feeding behaviour. *Acta Paediatr, 84*(2), 140-145.

Study 17

The behavior of 28 mother and infant dyads was video recorded during a two-hour period of skin-to-skin contact after birth. Ten of the women did not receive any pain relief during labor, whereas 18 women had received one or two types of analgesia, such as injections of meperidine, an epidural, or a pudendal block. Ten blood samples were collected at 15-minute intervals for a two-hour period after birth. Plasma levels of oxytocin were analyzed by RIA.

A detailed study of the infants' hand movements and sucking activity was performed based on analyses of the video recordings. The amount of hand massage and suckling were related to oxytocin levels. Scores of behaviors and oxytocin levels were related to the use of different types of analgesia. The efficiency of infants' hand massage on mothers' oxytocin release was calculated.

Matthiesen, A. S., Ransjo-Arvidson, A. B., Nissen, E., & Uvnäs-Moberg, K. (2001). Postpartum maternal oxytocin release by newborns: effects of infant hand massage and sucking. *Birth, 28*(1), 13-19.

Ransjo-Arvidson, A. B., Matthiesen, A. S., Lilja, G., Nissen, E., Widstrom, A. M., & Uvnäs-Moberg, K. 2001). Maternal analgesia during labor disturbs newborn behavior: effects on breastfeeding, temperature, and crying. *Birth, 28*(1), 5-12.

Study 18

Forty-two infants born with Cesarean section were randomized to have skin-to-skin contact with either their mother or father for a 25-minute period after birth. The interaction between parents and their infants during the first two hours after birth was observed and recorded on videotape, also allowing recording of sounds. Detailed observations of motor behavior, tactile interaction, and vocal communication were performed from the video recordings. Differences between mothers and fathers, and between boys and girls were noted.

The amount of oxytocin the mothers received postpartum was recorded. Seventeen blood samples were collected at 5- or 15-minute intervals in mothers and fathers during a 90-minute period. Oxytocin levels were analyzed by RIA.

Behavior and oxytocin levels in mothers and fathers who had skin-to-skin contact or not were compared. The influence of infusion of exogenous oxytocin on endogenous oxytocin levels was explored.

Velandia, M., Matthisen, A. S., Uvnäs-Moberg, K., & Nissen, E. (2010). Onset of vocal interaction between parents and newborns in skin-to-skin contact immediately after elective cesarean section. *Birth, 37*(3), 192-201.

Velandia, M., Uvnäs-Moberg, K., & Nissen, E. (2011). Sex differences in newborn interaction with mother or father during skin-to-skin contact after Caesarean section. *Acta Paediatr, 101*(4), 360-367.

Study 19

One hundred seventy-six mothers and their infants participated in the study. The mothers were randomized to have skin-to-skin contact with their infants (group 1), to hold their dressed infants (group 2), or to be separated from their infants, who were placed in a cot in a nursery in the labor ward (groups 3 and 4) during a two-hour period after birth. After that, the mother/infant dyads in groups 1, 2, and 4 were assigned to a four-day period of rooming-in in the maternity ward, whereas the infants of mothers in group 3 were placed in a nursery in the maternity ward. The mother/infant dyads in group 4 were only separated between 25 and 120 minutes after birth in the labor ward, whereas the mothers in group 3 were separated from their infants both during the stay in the labor ward and in the maternity ward.

During the four-day stay in the maternity ward, the infants were either dressed in clothes or were swaddled according to the Russian tradition, irrespective of being together with their mothers or staying in the nursery.

The number and duration of breastfeeds, the amount of milk ingested by the infant in connection with a breastfeed on day four postpartum, and the duration of nearly exclusive breastfeeding were recorded. The occurrence of whether the infant sucked immediately after birth was noted.

Maternal breast temperature and the infants' axillar, scapular, thigh, and foot skin temperatures were recorded at 15-minute intervals from 30 minutes until two hours after birth. The skin temperatures recorded in the different treatment groups were compared.

When the children were one year old, behavioral observations were performed on both mother and infant. The interaction between mothers and infants was studied in two different situations, during free play, i.e., the mothers and children played with whatever they wanted, or during a structured play, when the mothers and infants played after receiving certain instructions. Both interactions were recorded on videotape. The tapes were analyzed by psychologists according to a standardized schedule (the PCERA). According to this method, certain aspects of the interaction between mother and infant and the behavior of mothers and infants were studied.

Bystrova, K., Ivanova, V., Edhborg, M., Matthiesen, A. S., Ransjo-Arvidson, A. B., Mukhamedrakhimov, R., Uvnäs-Moberg, K. (2009). Early contact versus separation: effects on mother-infant interaction one year later. *Birth, 36*(2), 97-109.

Bystrova, K., Matthiesen, A. S., Vorontsov, I., Widstrom, A. M., Ransjo-Arvidson, A. B., & Uvnäs-Moberg, K. (2007). Maternal axillar and breast temperature after giving birth: effects of delivery ward practices and relation to infant temperature. *Birth, 34*(4), 291-300.

Bystrova, K., Matthiesen, A. S., Widstrom, A. M., Ransjo-Arvidson, A. B., Welles-Nystrom, B., Vorontsov, Uvnäs-Moberg, K (2007). The effect of Russian Maternity Home routines on breastfeeding and neonatal weight loss with special reference to swaddling. *Early Hum Dev, 83*(1), 29-39.

Bystrova, K., Widstrom, A. M., Matthiesen, A. S., Ransjo-Arvidson, A. B., Welles-Nystrom, B., Vorontsov, Uvnäs-Moberg, K, (2007). Early lactation performance in primiparous and multiparous women in relation to different maternity home practices. A randomised trial in St. Petersburg. *Int Breastfeed J, 2*, 9.

Bystrova, K., Widstrom, A. M., Matthiesen, A. S., Ransjo-Arvidson, A. B., Welles-Nystrom, B., Wassberg, C., Vorontsov, I., Uvnäs-Moberg, K. (2003). Skin-to-skin contact may reduce negative consequences of "the stress of being born": a study on temperature in newborn infants, subjected to different ward routines in St. Petersburg. *Acta Paediatr, 92*(3), 320-326.

Study 20

A standard dose of pethidine was given to 13 healthy primiparae during labor.

The infants developing breastfeeding behavior were investigated and were related to dose delivery time and to concentration of pethidine and pethidine metabolites in cord blood at birth.

Nissen, E., Widstrom, A. M., Lilja, G., Matthiesen, A. S., Uvnäs-Moberg, K., Jacobsson, G., et al. (1997). Effects of routinely given pethidine during labour on infants' developing breastfeeding behaviour. Effects of dose-delivery time interval and various concentrations of pethidine/norpethidine in cord plasma. *Acta Paediatr, 86*(2), 201-208.

Study 21

Forty-four healthy mother infant dyads were observed immediately after birth. Eighteen of the mothers had received pethidine during labor. The infants were placed in skin-to-skin contact. The development of infants' mouth and suckling movements, as well as rooting behavior was studied and differences between infants whose mothers had received pethidine or those who had not during labor were noted.

Nissen, E., Lilja, G., Matthiesen, A. S., Ransjo-Arvidsson, A. B., Uvnäs-Moberg, K., & Widstrom, A. M. (1995). Effects of maternal pethidine on infants' developing breast feeding behaviour. *Acta Paediatr, 84*(2), 140-145.

Study 22

Eighteen infants, median 24 weeks and birth weight 1230g received kangaroo care (KC) for 60 minutes at three days of age. Blood samples were collected before KC and at 5, 30, and 60 minutes. Eight infants receiving KC and 68 infants not receiving KC were fed by nasogastric tube. Blood samples were taken before and 30 minutes after the end of feeding. All blood samples were analyzed for somatostatin and cholecystokinin.

Törnhage, C. J., Serenius, F., Uvnäs-Moberg, K., & Lindberg, T. (1998). Plasma somatostatin and cholecystokinin levels in preterm infants during kangaroo care with and without nasogastric tube-feeding. *J Pediatr Endocrinol Metab, 11*(5), 645-651.

Study 23

Thirty-three healthy women with an uncomplicated pregnancy and their healthy newborns delivered at term participated in the study. Maternal venous samples and samples from the umbilical artery were collected after vaginal delivery and Cesarean section. Gastrin, somatostatin and oxytocin levels were measured with RIA.

Marchini, G., Lagercrantz, H., Winberg, J., & Uvnäs-Moberg, K. (1988). Fetal and maternal plasma levels of gastrin, somatostatin and oxytocin after vaginal delivery and elective cesarean section. *Early Hum Dev, 18*(1), 73-79.

References

Abdulkader, H.M., Freer, Y., Fleetwood-Walker, S.M., & McIntosh, N. (2007). Effect of suckling on the peripheral sensitivity of full-term newborn infants. *Arch Dis Child Fetal Neonatal Ed, 92*(2), F130-131.

Acher, A., Chauvet, J. and Chauvet, M.T. (1995). Man and the Chimaera: Selective verus neutral oxytocin evolution. In R. I. a. J. A. Russel). (Ed.), *Oxytocin, Cellular and Molecular Approaches in Medicine and Research*. New York: Plenum Press.

Adams, E.J., Grummer-Strawn, L., & Chavez, G. (2003). Food insecurity is associated with increased risk of obesity in California women. *J Nutr, 133*(4), 1070-1074.

Adan, R.A., Van Leeuwen, F.W., Sonnemans, M.A., Brouns, M., Hoffman, G., Verbalis, J.G., et al. (1995). Rat oxytocin receptor in brain, pituitary, mammary gland, and uterus: partial sequence and immunocytochemical localization. *Endocrinology, 136*(9), 4022-4028.

Agren, G., Lundeberg, T., & Uvnäs-Moberg, K. (1997). Pheromones released following administration of exogenous oxytocin to rats induces release of endogenous oxytocin in cagemates. Unpublished data.

Agren, G., Lundeberg, T., Uvnäs-Moberg, K., & Sato, A. (1995). The oxytocin antagonist 1-deamino-2-D-Tyr-(Oet)-4-Thr-8-Orn-oxytocin reverses the increase in the withdrawal response latency to thermal, but not mechanical nociceptive stimuli following oxytocin administration or massage-like stroking in rats. *Neurosci Lett, 187*(1), 49-52.

Agren, G., Olsson, C., Uvnäs-Moberg, K., & Lundeberg, T. (1997). Olfactory cues from an oxytocin-injected male rat can reduce energy loss in its cagemates. *Neuroreport, 8*(11), 2551-2555.

Alehagen, S., Wijma, B., Lundberg, U., & Wijma, K. (2005). Fear, pain and stress hormones during childbirth. *J Psychosom Obstet Gynaecol, 26*(3), 153-165.

Alfvén, G., de la Torre, B., & Uvnäs-Moberg, K. (1994). Depressed concentrations of oxytocin and cortisol in children with recurrent abdominal pain of non-organic origin. *Acta Paediatr, 83*(10), 1076-1080.

Algers, B., Madej, A., Rojanasthien, S., & Uvnäs-Moberg, K. (1991). Quantitative relationships between suckling-induced teat stimulation and the release of prolactin, gastrin, somatostatin, insulin, glucagon and vasoactive intestinal polypeptide in sows. *Vet Res Commun, 15*(5), 395-407.

Algers, B., & Uvnäs-Moberg, K. (2007). Maternal behavior in pigs. *Horm Behav, 52*(1), 78-85.

Almay, B.G., von Knorring, L., & Oreland, L. (1987). Platelet MAO in patients with idiopathic pain disorders. *J Neural Transm, 69*(3-4), 243-253.

Altemus, M. (1995). Neuropeptides in anxiety disorders. Effects of lactation. *Ann N Y Acad Sci, 771*, 697-707.

Altemus, M., Deuster, P.A., Galliven, E., Carter, C.S., & Gold, P.W. (1995). Suppression of hypothalmic-pituitary-adrenal axis responses to stress in lactating women. *J Clin Endocrinol Metab, 80*(10), 2954-2959.

Altemus, M., Redwine, L.S., Leong, Y.M., Frye, C.A., Porges, S.W., & Carter, C.S. (2001). Responses to laboratory psychosocial stress in postpartum women. *Psychosom Med, 63*(5), 814-821.

Amico, J.A., & Hempel, J. (1990). An oxytocin precursor intermediate circulates in the plasma of humans and rhesus monkeys administered estrogen. *Neuroendocrinology, 51*(4), 437-443.

Amico, J.A., Johnston, J.M., & Vagnucci, A.H. (1994). Suckling-induced attenuation of plasma cortisol concentrations in postpartum lactating women. *Endocr Res, 20*(1), 79-87.

Amico, J.A., Mantella, R.C., Vollmer, R.R., Li, X. (2004). Anxiety and stress responses in female oxytocin deficient mice. *Journal of Neuroendocrinology, 16*(4), 319-324.

Amico, J.A., Miedlar, J.A., Cai, H.M., & Vollmer, R.R. (2008). Oxytocin knockout mice: a model for studying stress-related and ingestive behaviours. *Prog Brain Res, 170*, 53-64.

Amico, J.A., Seif, S.M., & Robinson, A.G. (1981). Elevation of oxytocin and the oxytocin-associated neurophysin in the plasma of normal women during midcycle. *J Clin Endocrinol Metab, 53*(6), 1229-1232.

Anderberg, U.M., & Uvnäs-Moberg, K. (2000). Plasma oxytocin levels in female fibromyalgia syndrome patients. *Z Rheumatol, 59*(6), 373-379.

Anderson, P.O., & Valdes, V. (2007). A critical review of pharmaceutical galactagogues. *Breastfeed Med, 2*(4), 229-242.

Anim-Somuah, M., Smyth, R., & Howell, C. (2005). Epidural versus non-epidural or no analgesia in labour. *Cochrane Database Syst Rev*(4), CD000331.

Anim-Somuah, M., Smyth, R.M., & Jones, L. (2011). Epidural versus non-epidural or no analgesia in labour. *Cochrane Database Syst Rev, 12*, CD000331.

Araki, T., Ito, K., Kurosawa, M., & Sato, A. (1984). Responses of adrenal sympathetic nerve activity and catecholamine secretion to cutaneous stimulation in anesthetized rats. *Neuroscience, 12*(1), 289-299.

Argiolas, A., & Gessa, G.L. (1991). Central functions of oxytocin. *Neurosci Biobehav Rev, 15*(2), 217-231.

Bager, P., Wohlfahrt, J., & Westergaard, T. (2008). Caesarean delivery and risk of atopy and allergic disease: meta-analyses. *Clin Exp Allergy, 38*(4), 634-42. doi: 10.1111/j.1365-2222.2008.02939.x.

Bartels, A., & Zeki, S. (2004). The neural correlates of maternal and romantic love. *Neuroimage, 21*(3), 1155-1166.

Bartz, J., Simeon, D., Hamilton, H., Kim, S., Crystal, S., Braun, A., Vicens, V., & Hollander, E. (2011). Oxytocin can hinder trust and cooperation in borderline personality disorder. *Soc Cogn Affect Neurosci, 6*(5):556-63. doi: 10.1093/scan/nsq085.

Battin, D.A., Marrs, R.P., Fleiss, P.M., & Mishell, D.R., Jr. (1985). Effect of suckling on serum prolactin, luteinizing hormone, follicle-stimulating hormone, and estradiol during prolonged lactation. *Obstet Gynecol, 65*(6), 785-788.

Beilin, Y., Bodian, C.A., Weiser, J., Hossain, S., Arnold, I., Feierman, D.E., et al. (2005). Effect of labor epidural analgesia with and without fentanyl on infant breast-feeding: a prospective, randomized, double-blind study. *Anesthesiology, 103*(6), 1211-1217.

Belfrage, P., Berlin, A., Raabe, N., & Thalme, B. (1975). Lumbar epidural analgesia with bupivacaine in labor. Drug concentration in maternal and neonatal blood at birth and during the first day of life. *Am J Obstet Gynecol, 123*(8), 839-844.

Belsey, E.M., Rosenblatt, D.B., Lieberman, B.A., Redshaw, M., Caldwell, J., Notarianni, L., et al. (1981). The influence of maternal analgesia on neonatal behaviour: I. Pethidine. *Br J Obstet Gynaecol, 88*(4), 398-406.

Berglund, S., Grunewald, C., Pettersson, H., & Cnattingius, S. (2008). Severe asphyxia due to delivery-related malpractice in Sweden 1990-2005. *BJOG, 115*(3), 316-323.

Berglund, S., Pettersson, H., Cnattingius, S., & Grunewald, C. (2010). How often is a low Apgar score the result of substandard care during labour? *BJOG, 117*(8), 968-978.

Bergman, N. (2005). More than a cuddle: skin-to-skin contact is key. *Pract Midwife, 8*(9), 44.

Bergman, N.J., Linley, L.L., & Fawcus, S.R. (2004). Randomized controlled trial of skin-to-skin contact from birth versus conventional incubator for physiological stabilization in 1200- to 2199-gram newborns. Acta Paediatr, 93(6), 779-785.

Bernbaum, J.C., Pereira, G.R., Watkins, J.B., & Peckham, G.J. (1983). Nonnutritive sucking during gavage feeding enhances growth and maturation in premature infants. *Pediatrics, 71*(1), 41-45.

Bertsch, K., Schmidinger, I., Neumann, I.D., & Herpertz, S.C. (2013). Reduced plasma oxytocin levels in female patients with borderline personality disorder. *Horm Behav, 63*(3), 424-9. doi: 10.1016/j.yhbeh.2012.11.013.

Björklund, A., Hökfelt, T. and Owman, C. (1988). The peripheral nervous system *Handbook of Chemical Neuroanatomy* (Vol. 6). Amsterdam: Elsevier.

Bjorkstrand, E., Ahlenius, S., Smedh, U., & Uvnäs-Moberg, K. (1996). The oxytocin receptor antagonist 1-deamino-2-D-Tyr-(OEt)-4-Thr-8-Orn-oxytocin inhibits effects of the 5-HT1A receptor agonist 8-OH-DPAT on plasma levels of insulin, cholecystokinin and somatostatin. *Regul Pept, 63*(1), 47-52.

Bjorkstrand, E., Eriksson, M., & Uvnäs-Moberg, K. (1992). Plasma levels of oxytocin after food deprivation and hypoglycaemia, and effects of 1-deamino-2-D-Tyr-(OEt)-4-Thr-8-Orn-oxytocin on blood glucose in rats. *Acta Physiol Scand, 144*(3), 355-359.

Bjorkstrand, E., Eriksson, M., & Uvnäs-Moberg, K. (1996). Evidence of a peripheral and a central effect of oxytocin on pancreatic hormone release in rats. *Neuroendocrinology, 63*(4), 377-383.

Björkstrand, E., Hulting, A.L., & Uvnäs-Moberg, K. (1997). Evidence for a dual function of oxytocin in the control of growth hormone secretion in rats. *Regul Pept, 69*(1), 1-5.

Bjorkstrand, E., & Uvnäs-Moberg, K. (1996). Central oxytocin increases food intake and daily weight gain in rats. *Physiol Behav, 59*(4-5), 947-952.

Blevins, J.E., Eakin, T.J., Murphy, J.A., Schwartz, M.W., & Baskin, D.G. (2003). Oxytocin innervation of caudal brainstem nuclei activated by cholecystokinin. *Brain Res, 993*(1-2), 30-41.

Bolander, F.F., Jr., Nicholas, K.R., Van Wyk, J.J., & Topper, Y.J. (1981). Insulin is essential for accumulation of casein mRNA in mouse mammary epithelial cells. *Proc Natl Acad Sci U S A, 78*(9), 5682-5684.

Bonetto, V., Andersson, M., Bergman, T., Sillard, R., Norberg, A., Mutt, V., et al. (1999). Spleen antibacterial peptides: high levels of PR-39 and presence of two forms of NK-lysin. *Cell Mol Life Sci, 56*(1-2), 174-178.

Borg, J., Melander, O., Johansson, L., Uvnäs-Moberg, K., Rehfeld, J.F., & Ohlsson, B. (2010). Gastroparesis is associated with oxytocin deficiency, oesophageal dysmotility with hyperCCKemia, and autonomic neuropathy with hypergastrinemia. *BMC Gastroenterol.* 2009 9, 17. doi: 10.1186/1471-230X-9-17.

Bosch, O.J., & Neumann, I.D. (2011). Both oxytocin and vasopressin are mediators of maternal care and aggression in rodents: From central release to sites of action. *Horm Behav.*

Broad, K.D., Curley, J.P., & Keverne, E.B. (2006). Mother-infant bonding and the evolution of mammalian social relationships. *Philos Trans R Soc Lond B Biol Sci, 361*(1476), 2199-2214.

Broad, K.D., Curley, J.P., & Keverne E.B. (2009). Increased apoptosis during neonatal brain development underlies the adult behavioral deficits seen in mice lacking a functional paternally expressed gene 3 (Peg3). *Dev Neurobiol, 69*(5), 314-325. doi: 10.1002/dneu.20702.

Bruckmaier, R.M., Pfeilsticker, H.U., & Blum, J.W. (1996). Milk yield, oxytocin and beta-endorphin gradually normalize during repeated milking in unfamiliar surroundings. *J Dairy Res, 63*(2), 191-200. Bruckmaier, R.M., Schams, D., Blum, J.W. (1993). Milk removal in familiar and unfamiliar surroundings: concentration of oxytocin, prolacin, cortisol and beta-endorphin. *J.Dairy Res, 60,* 449-456.

Bruckmaier, R.M., Schams, D., Blum, J.W. (1993). Milk removal in familiar and unfamiliar surroundings: concentration of oxytocin, prolacin, cortisol and beta-endorphin. *J.Dairy Res, 60,* 449-456.

Bruckmaier, R.M., Wellnitz, O., & Blum, J.W. (1997). Inhibition of milk ejection in cows by oxytocin receptor blockade, alpha-adrenergic receptor stimulation and in unfamiliar surroundings. *J Dairy Res, 64*(3), 315-325.

Bugg, G.J., Stanley, E., Baker, P.N., Taggart, M.J., & Johnston, T.A. (2006). Outcomes of labours augmented with oxytocin. *Eur J Obstet Gynecol Reprod Biol, 124*(1), 37-41.

Buijs, R.M. (1983). Vasopressin and oxytocin--their role in neurotransmission. *Pharmacol Ther, 22*(1), 127-141.

Buijs, R.M., De Vries, G.J., & Van Leeuwen, F.W. (1985). *The distribution and synaptic release of oxytocin in the central nervous system.* Amsterdam: Elsevier Science Publishers BV.

Buijs, R.M., & Swaab, D.F. (1979). Immuno-electron microscopical demonstration of vasopressin and oxytocin synapses in the limbic system of the rat. *Cell Tissue Res, 204*(3), 355-365.

Buller, K.M., & Day, T.A. (1996). Involvement of medullary catecholamine cells in neuroendocrine responses to systemic cholecystokinin. *J Neuroendocrinol, 8*(11), 819-824.

Buma, P., & Nieuwenhuys, R. (1988). Ultrastructural characterization of exocytotic release sites in different layers of the median eminence of the rat. *Cell Tissue Res, 252*(1), 107-114.

Burbach, J.P., & Lebouille, J.L. (1983). Proteolytic conversion of arginine-vasopressin and oxytocin by brain synaptic membranes. Characterization of formed peptides and mechanisms of proteolysis. *J Biol Chem, 258*(3), 1487-1494.

Burbach, J.P.H., Young, L.J., & Russell, J.A. (2006). Oxytocin: Synthesis, secretion and reproductive functions. In: *Knobil and Neill´s Physiology of Reproduction* (3 ed.): Elsevier.

Bystrova, K., Ivanova, V., Edhborg, M., Matthiesen, A.S., Ransjo-Arvidson, A.B., Mukhamedrakhimov, R., et al. (2009). Early contact versus separation: Effects on mother-infant interaction one year later. *Birth, 36*(2), 97-109.

Bystrova, K., Matthiesen, A.S., Vorontsov, I., Widstrom, A.M., Ransjo-Arvidson, A.B., & Uvnäs-Moberg, K. (2007). Maternal axillar and breast temperature after giving birth: Effects of delivery ward practices and relation to infant temperature. *Birth, 34*(4), 291-300.

Bystrova, K., Matthiesen, A.S., Widstrom, A.M., Ransjo-Arvidson, A.B., Welles-Nystrom, B., Vorontsov, I., et al. (2007). The effect of Russian Maternity Home routines on breastfeeding and neonatal weight loss with special reference to swaddling. *Early Hum Dev, 83*(1), 29-39.

Bystrova, K., Widstrom, A.M., Matthiesen, A.S., Ransjo-Arvidson, A.B., Welles-Nystrom, B., Vorontsov, I., et al. (2007). Early lactation performance in primiparous and multiparous women in relation to different maternity home practices. A randomised trial in St. Petersburg. *Int Breastfeed J, 2*, 9.

Bystrova, K., Widstrom, A.M., Matthiesen, A.S., Ransjo-Arvidson, A.B., Welles-Nystrom, B., Wassberg, C., et al. (2003). Skin-to-skin contact may reduce negative consequences of "the stress of being born": A study on temperature in newborn infants, subjected to different ward routines in St. Petersburg. *Acta Paediatr, 92*(3), 320-326.

Bystrova, K., Widström, A.M., Ransjö-Arvidsson, A.B., & Uvnäs-

Moberg, K. (2014). Skin to skin contact immediately after birth increases mother›s concerns for the infant. Unpublished data.

Caldji, C., Diorio, J., & Meaney, M.J. (2000). Variations in maternal care in infancy regulate the development of stress reactivity. *Biol Psychiatry, 48*(12):1164-74.

Caldji, C., Hellstrom, I.C., Zhang, T.Y., Diorio, J., & Meaney, M.J. (2011). Environmental regulation of the neural epigenome. *FEBS Lett, 585*(13), 2049-58. doi: 10.1016/j.febslet.2011.03.032.

Cameron, N.M., Shahrokh, D., Del Corpo, A., Dhir, S.K., Szyf, M., Champagne, F.A., et al. (2008). Epigenetic programming of phenotypic variations in reproductive strategies in the rat through maternal care. *J Neuroendocrinol, 20*(6), 795-801.

Campbell, D., Scott, K.D., Klaus, M.H., & Falk, M. (2007). Female relatives or friends trained as labor doulas: outcomes at 6 to 8 weeks postpartum. *Birth, 34*(3), 220-227.

Cannon, W.B. (1929). *Bodily changes in pain, hunger , fear and rage.* New York: Appleton.

Cao, Y., & Gimpl, G. (2001). A constitutively active pituitary adenylate cyclase activating polypeptide (PACAP) type I receptor shows enhanced photoaffinity labeling of its highly glycosylated form. *Biochim Biophys Acta, 1548*(1), 139-151.

Carfoot, S., Williamson, P.R., & Dickson, R. (2003). A systematic review of randomised controlled trials evaluating the effect of mother/baby skin-to-skin care on successful breast feeding. *Midwifery, 19*(2), 148-155.

Carmichael, M.S., Humbert, R., Dixen, J., Palmisano, G., Greenleaf, W., & Davidson, J. M. (1987). Plasma oxytocin increases in the human sexual response. *J Clin Endocrinol Metab, 64*(1), 27-31.

Carter, C.S. (1998). Neuroendocrine perspectives on social attachment and love. *Psychoneuroendocrinology, 23*(8), 779-818.

Cassoni, P., Sapino, A., Marrocco, T., Chini, B., & Bussolati, G. (2004). Oxytocin and oxytocin receptors in cancer cells and proliferation. *J Neuroendocrinol, 16*(4), 362-4.

Cernadas, J.M., Noceda, G., Barrera, L., Martinez, A.M., & Garsd, A. (2003). Maternal and perinatal factors influencing the duration of exclusive breastfeeding during the first 6 months of life. J Hum Lact 19(2), 136-44.

Chalmers, B., & Wolman, W. (1993). Social support in labor--a selective review. *J Psychosom Obstet Gynaecol, 14*(1), 1-15.

Champagne, F.A., Curley, J.P., Keverne, E.B., & Bateson, P.P. (2007). Natural variations in postpartum maternal care in inbred and outbred mice. *Physiol Behav, 91*(2-3), 325-334.

Champagne, F., & Meaney, M.J. (2001). Like mother, like daughter: evidence for non-genomic transmission of parental behavior and stress responsivity. *Prog Brain Res, 133*, 287-302.

Champagne, F.A., & Meaney, M.J. (2007). Transgenerational effects of social environment on variations in maternal care and behavioral response to novelty. *Behav Neurosci, 121*(6), 1353-1363.

Chang, Z.M., & Heaman, M.I. (2005). Epidural analgesia during labor and delivery: effects on the initiation and continuation of effective breastfeeding. *J Hum Lact, 21*(3), 305-314; quiz 315-309, 326.

Christensson, K., Cabrera, T., Christensson, E., Uvnäs-Moberg, K., & Winberg, J. (1995). Separation distress call in the human neonate in the absence of maternal body contact. *Acta Paediatr, 84*(5), 468-473.

Christensson, K., Siles, C., Moreno, L., Belaustequi, A., De La Fuente, P., Lagercrantz, H., et al. (1992). Temperature, metabolic adaptation and crying in healthy full-term newborns cared for skin-to-skin or in a cot. *Acta Paediatr, 81*(6-7), 488-493.

Clinton, S.M., Bedrosian, T.A., Abraham, A.D., Watson, S.J., & Akil, H. (2010). Neural and environmental factors impacting maternal behavior differences in high- versus low-novelty-seeking rats. *Horm Behav, 57*(4-5), 463-473.

Clodi, M., Vila, G., Geyeregger, R., Riedl, M., Stulnig, T. M., Struck, J., et al. (2008). Oxytocin alleviates the neuroendocrine and cytokine response to bacterial endotoxin in healthy men. *Am J Physiol Endocrinol Metab, 295*(3), E686-691.

Coureaud, G., Charra, R., Datiche, F., Sinding, C., Thomas-Danguin, T., Languille, S., Hars, B., & Schaal, B. (2010). A pheromone to behave, a pheromone to learn: the rabbit mammary pheromone. *J Comp Physiol A Neuroethol Sens Neural Behav Physiol, 196*(10), 779-790. doi: 10.1007/s00359-010-0548-y.

Cowie, A.T. (1974). Proceedings: Overview of the mammary gland. *J Invest Dermatol, 63*(1), 2-9.

Cowie, A.T., , Forsyth, I.A., Hart, I.C. (1980). Hormonal control of lactation. Berlin: Springer Verlag.

Cowie, A.T., Tindal, J.S., & Yokoyama, A. (1966). The induction of mammary growth in the hypophysectomized goat. *J Endocrinol, 34*(2), 185-195.

Craig, A.D. (2003). Pain mechanisms: labeled lines versus convergence in central processing. *Annu Rev Neurosci, 26*, 1-30.

Czank, C., Henderson, J.J., Kent, J.C. , Tat Lai, C., & Hartmann, P. (2007). Hormonal Control of the Lactation Cycle. In T. W. H. a. P. E. Hartmann (Ed.), *Textbook of Human Lactation*. Amarillo: Hale Publishing.

Dale, H.H. (1906). On some physiological actions of ergot. *J Physiol, 34*(3), 163-206.

Dale, H.H. (1909). The Action of Extracts of the Pituitary Body. *Biochem J, 4*(9), 427-447.

De Bonis, M., Torricelli, M., Leoni, L., Berti, P., Ciani, V., Puzzutiello, R., et al. (2011). Carbetocin versus oxytocin after caesarean section: similar efficacy but reduced pain perception in women with high risk of postpartum haemorrhage. *J Matern Fetal Neonatal Med.*

de Chateau, P., Holmberg, H., Jakobsson, K., & Winberg, J. (1977). A study of factors promoting and inhibiting lactation. *Dev Med Child Neurol, 19*(5), 575-584.

De Chateau, P., & Wiberg, B. (1977a). Long-term effect on mother-infant behaviour of extra contact during the first hour post partum.

I. First observations at 36 hours. *Acta Paediatr Scand, 66*(2), 137-143.

De Chateau, P., & Wiberg, B. (1977b). Long-term effect on mother-infant behaviour of extra contact during the first hour post partum. II. A follow-up at three months. *Acta Paediatr Scand, 66*(2), 145-151.

de Chateau, P., & Wiberg, B. (1984). Long-term effect on mother-infant behaviour of extra contact during the first hour post partum. III. Follow-up at one year. *Scand J Soc Med, 12*(2), 91-103.

De Groot, A.N., Vree, T.B., Hekster, Y.A., Pesman, G.J., Sweep, F.C., Van Dongen, P.J., et al. (1995). Bioavailability and pharmacokinetics of sublingual oxytocin in male volunteers. *J Pharm Pharmacol, 47*(7), 571-575.

de Wied, D., Gaffori, O., Burbach, J.P., Kovacs, G.L., & van Ree, J.M. (1987). Structure activity relationship studies with C-terminal fragments of vasopressin and oxytocin on avoidance behaviors of rats. *J Pharmacol Exp Ther, 241*(1), 268-274.

Demitrack, M.A., Lesem, M.D., Listwak, S.J., Brandt, H.A., Jimerson, D.C., & Gold, P.W. (1990). CSF oxytocin in anorexia nervosa and bulimia nervosa: clinical and pathophysiologic considerations. *Am J Psychiatry, 147*(7), 882-886.

Diaz-Cabiale, Z., Olausson, H., Sohlstrom, A., Agnati, L. F., Narvaez, J. A., Uvnäs-Moberg, K., et al. (2004). Long-term modulation by postnatal oxytocin of the alpha 2-adrenoceptor agonist binding sites in central autonomic regions and the role of prenatal stress. *J Neuroendocrinol, 16*(3), 183-190.

Díaz-Cabiale, Z., Petersson, M., Narváez, J.A., Uvnäs-Moberg, K., & Fuxe, K. (2000). Systemic oxytocin treatment modulates alpha 2-adrenoceptors in telencephalic and diencephalic regions of the rat. *Brain Res, 887*(2), 421-425.

DiGirolamo, A.M., Grummer-Strawn, L.M., & Fein, S.B. (2008). Effect of maternity-care practices on breastfeeding. *Pediatrics, 122 Suppl 2*, S43-49.

Domes, G., Heinrichs, M., Glascher, J., Buchel, C., Braus, D.F., & Herpertz, S. C. (2007). Oxytocin attenuates amygdala responses to emotional faces regardless of valence. *Biol Psychiatry, 62*(10), 1187-1190.

Domes, G., Heinrichs, M., Michel, A., Berger, C., Herpertz, S.C. (2007). Oxytocin improves "mind-reading" in humans. *Biol Psychiatry, 61*(6), 731-733.

Doucet, S., Soussignan, R., Sagot, P., & Schaal, B. (2009). The secretion of areolar (Montgomery's) glands from lactating women elicits selective, unconditional responses in neonates. *PLoS One, 4*(10):e7579. doi: 10.1371/journal.pone.0007579.

Dreifuss, J.J., Raggenbass, M., Charpak, S., Dubois-Dauphin, M., & Tribollet, E. (1988). A role of central oxytocin in autonomic functions: its action in the motor nucleus of the vagus nerve. *Brain Res Bull, 20*(6), 765-770.

Drewett, R.F., Bowen-Jones, A., & Dogterom, J. (1982). Oxytocin levels during breast-feeding in established lactation. *Horm Behav, 16*(2), 245-248.

Dunn, J., & Kendrick, C. (1980). Studying temperament and parent-child interaction: comparison of interview and direct observation. *Dev Med Child Neurol, 22*(4), 484-96.

Du Vigneaud, V., Ressler, C., & Trippett, S. (1953). The sequence of amino acids in oxytocin, with a proposal for the structure of oxytocin. *J Biol Chem, 205*(2), 949-957.

Du, Y.C., Yan, Q.W., & Qiao, L.Y. (1998). Function and molecular basis of action of vasopressin 4-8 and its analogues in rat brain. *Prog Brain Res, 119*, 163-175.

Edvinsson, L., Ekblad, E., Håkanson, R., & Wahlestedt C. (1984). Neuropeptide Y potentiates the effect of various vasoconstrictor agents on rabbit blood vessels. *Br J Pharmacol, 83*(2), 519-525.

Eklund, M.B., Johansson, L.M., Uvnäs-Moberg, K., & Arborelius, L. (2009). Differential effects of repeated long and brief maternal separation on behaviour and neuroendocrine parameters in Wistar dams. *Behav Brain Res, 203*(1):69-75. doi: 10.1016/j.bbr.2009.04.017.

Ekstrom, A., Widstrom, A.M., & Nissen, E. (2003). Breastfeeding support from partners and grandmothers: perceptions of Swedish women. *Birth, 30*(4), 261-266.

Eltzschig, H.K., Lieberman, E.S., & Camann, W.R. (2003). Regional anesthesia and analgesia for labor and delivery. *N Engl J Med, 348*(4), 319-332.

Ely, F., & Petersen, W.E. (1941). Factors involved in the ejection of milk. *J Dairy Sci, 24*, 211-223.

Engstrom, L. (1958). Synthetic oxytocin (syntocinon Sandoz) in intravenous drip for induction of labour around full term. *Acta Obstet Gynecol Scand, 37*(3), 303-311.

Eriksson, M., Bjorkstrand, E., Smedh, U., Alster, P., Matthiesen, A.S., & Uvnäs-Moberg, K. (1994). Role of vagal nerve activity during suckling. Effects on plasma levels of oxytocin, prolactin, VIP, somatostatin, insulin, glucagon, glucose and of milk secretion in lactating rats. *Acta Physiol Scand, 151*(4), 453-459.

Eriksson, M., Linden, A., Stock, S. & Uvnäs-Moberg, K. (1987). Increased levels of vasoactive intestinal peptide (VIP) and oxytocin during suckling in lactating dogs. *Peptides, 8*(3):411-413.

Eriksson, M., Linden, A., & Uvnäs-Moberg, K. (1987). Suckling increases insulin and glucagon levels in peripheral venous blood of lactating dogs. *Acta Physiol Scand, 131*(3), 391-396.

Eriksson, M., Lindh, B., Uvnäs-Moberg, K., & Hokfelt, T. (1996). Distribution and origin of peptide-containing nerve fibres in the rat and human mammary gland. *Neuroscience, 70*(1), 227-245.

Eriksson, M., Lundeberg, T., & Uvnäs-Moberg, K. (1996). Studies on cutaneous blood flow in the mammary gland of lactating rats. *Acta Physiol Scand, 158*(1), 1-6.

Eriksson, M., & Uvnäs-Moberg, K. (1990). Plasma levels of vasoactive intestinal polypeptide and oxytocin in response to suckling, electrical stimulation of the mammary nerve and oxytocin infusion in rats. *Neuroendocrinology, 51*(3), 237-240.

Erlandsson, K., Dsilna, A, Fagerberg, I., & Christensson, K. (2007). Skin-to-skin care with the father after cesarean birth and its effect on newborn crying and prefeeding behavior. *Birth, 34*(2), 105-14.

Fabry, I. G., De Paepe, P., Kips, J. G., & Van Bortel, L.M. (2011). The influence of tocolytic drugs on cardiac function, large arteries, and resistance vessels. *Eur J Clin Pharmacol, 67*(6), 573-580.

Febo, M., Numan, M., & Ferris, C.F. (2005). Functional magnetic resonance imaging shows oxytocin activates brain regions associated with mother-pup bonding during suckling. *J Neurosci, 25*(50), 11637-11644.

Feldman, R., Gordon, I., Schneiderman, I., Weisman, O., & Zagoory-Sharon, O. (2010). Natural variations in maternal and paternal care are associated with systematic changes in oxytocin following parent-infant contact. *Psychoneuroendocrinology, 35*(8), 1133-41. doi: 10.1016/j.psyneuen.2010.01.013.

Feldman, R., Gordon, I., & Zagoory-Sharon, O. (2011). Maternal and paternal plasma, salivary, and urinary oxytocin and parent-infant synchrony: considering stress and affiliation components of human bonding. *Dev Sci, 14*(4), 752-61. doi: 10.1111/j.1467-7687.2010.01021.x.

Feldman, R., Weller, A., Zagoory-Sharon, O., & Levine, A. (2007). Evidence for a neuroendocrinological foundation of human affiliation: plasma oxytocin levels across pregnancy and the postpartum period predict mother-infant bonding. *Psychol Sci, 18*(11), 965-70.

Fell, B.F., Smith, K.A., Campbell, R.M. (1963). Hypertrophic and hyperplastic changes in the alimentary canal of the lactating rat. *J Pathol Bacteriol, 85*, 179-188.

Ferguson, J.K. (1941). A study of the motility of the intact uterus at term. *Surgery Gynecol Obstet, 73*, 359-366.

Fewtrell, M.S., Loh, K.L., Blake, A., Ridout, D.A., & Hawdon, J. (2006). Randomised, double blind trial of oxytocin nasal spray in mothers expressing breast milk for preterm infants. *Arch Dis Child Fetal Neonatal Ed, 91*(3), F169-174.

Findlay, A.L.R., & Grosvenor, C.E. (1969). The role of mammary gland innervation in the control of the motor apparatus of the mammary gland. *Dairy Sci Abstr, 31*(3), 109-116.

Fleming, A.S., Kraemer, G.W., Gonzalez, A., Lovic, V., Rees, S., & Melo, A. (2002). Mothering begets mothering: the transmission of behavior and its neurobiology across generations. *Pharmacol Biochem Behav, 73*(1), 61-75.

Ford, E., & Ayers, S. (2009). Stressful events and support during birth: the effect on anxiety, mood and perceived control. *J Anxiety Disord, 23*(2), 260-268.

Ford, E., & Ayers, S. (2011). Support during birth interacts with prior trauma and birth intervention to predict postnatal post-traumatic stress symptoms. *Psychol Health, 26*(12), 1553-1570.

Francis, D.D., Champagne, F.A., Liu, D., & Meaney, M.J. (1999). Maternal care, gene expression, and the development of individual differences in stress reactivity. *Ann N Y Acad Sci, 896*, 66-84.

Francis, D.D., Young, L.J., Meaney, M.J., & Insel, T.R. (2002). Naturally occurring differences in maternal care are associated with the expression of oxytocin and vasopressin (V1a) receptors: gender differences. *Journal of Neuroendocrinology, 14*(5), 349-353.

Frantz, A.G. (1977). The assay and regulation of prolactin in humans. *Adv Exp Med Biol, 80*, 95-133.

Freeman, M.E., Kanyicska, B., Lerant, A., & Nagy, G. (2000). Prolactin: structure, function, and regulation of secretion. *Physiol Rev, 80*(4), 1523-1631.

Freund-Mercier, M.J., Stoeckel, M.E., Palacios, J.M., Pazos, A., Reichhart, J.M., Porte, A., et al. (1987). Pharmacological characteristics and anatomical distribution of [3H]oxytocin-binding sites in the Wistar rat brain studied by autoradiography. *Neuroscience, 20*(2), 599-614.

Frick, G., Bremme, K., Sjogren, C., Linden, A., & Uvnäs-Moberg, K. (1990). Plasma levels of cholecystokinin and gastrin during the menstrual cycle and pregnancy. *Acta Obstet Gynecol Scand, 69*(4), 317-320.

Fuchs, A.R., Romero, R., Keefe, D., Parra, M., Oyarzun, E., & Behnke, E. (1991). Oxytocin secretion and human parturition: pulse frequency and duration increase during spontaneous labor in women. *Am J Obstet Gynecol, 165*(5 Pt 1), 1515-1523.

Gaffori, O.J., & De Wied, D. (1988). Bimodal effect of oxytocin on avoidance behavior may be caused by the presence of two peptide sequences with opposite action in the same molecule. *Eur J Pharmacol, 147*(2), 157-162.

Gaines, W.L. (1915). A contribution to the physiology of lactation. *Am. J. Physiol., 38*, 447-466.

Geddes, D.T. (2007). Gross anatomy of the lactating breast. In P. E. H. Thomas W. Hale (Ed.), *Textbook of Human Lactation*. Amarillo, Texas: Hale Publishing.

Giacometti, L., & Montagna, W. (1962). The nipple and the areola of the human female breast. *Anat Rec, 144*, 191-197.

Gibson, S.J., Polak, J.M., Bloom, S.R., Sabate, I.M., Mulderry, P.M., Ghatei, M.A., et al. (1984). Calcitonin gene-related peptide immunoreactivity in the spinal cord of man and of eight other species. *J Neurosci, 4*(12), 3101-3111.

Gimpl, G., & Fahrenholz, F. (2001). The oxytocin receptor system: structure, function, and regulation. *Physiol Rev, 81*(2), 629-683.

Gimpl, G., Reitz, J., Brauer, S., & Trossen, C. (2008). Oxytocin receptors: Ligand binding, signalling and cholesterol dependence. *Prog Brain Res, 170*, 193-204.

Glasier, A., McNeilly, A.S., & Howie, P.W. (1988). Hormonal background of lactational infertility. *Int J Fertil, 33 Suppl*, 32-4.

Glover, V., O'Connor, T.G., & O'Donnell, K. (2010). Prenatal stress and the programming of the HPA axis. *Neurosci Biobehav Rev, 35*(1), 17-22.

Goldman, M., Marlow-O'Connor, M., Torres, I., & Carter, C.S. (2008). Diminished plasma oxytocin in schizophrenic patients with neuroendocrine dysfunction and emotional deficits. *Schizophr Res, 98*(1-3), 247-255.

Goodfellow, C.F., Hull, M.G., Swaab, D.F., Dogterom, J., & Buijs, R.M. (1983). Oxytocin deficiency at delivery with epidural analgesia. *Br J Obstet Gynaecol, 90*(3), 214-219.

Gordon, I., Zagoory-Sharon, O., Schneiderman, I., Leckman, J.F., Weller, A., & Feldman, R. (2008). Oxytocin and cortisol in romantically unattached young adults: Associations with bonding and psychological distress. *Psychophysiology, 45*(3), 349-52. doi: 10.1111/j.1469-8986.2008.00649.x.

Gorewit, R.C., Svennersten, K., Butler, W.R., & Uvnäs-Moberg, K. (1992). Endocrine responses in cows milked by hand and machine. *J Dairy Sci, 75*(2), 443-448.

Graff, C.L., & Pollack, G.M. (2005). Nasal drug administration: potential for targeted central nervous system delivery. *J Pharm Sci, 94*(6), 1187-1195.

Gregory, S.G., Connelly, J.J., Towers, A.J., Johnson, J., Biscocho, D., Markunas, C.A., ...Pericak-Vance, M.A. (2009). Genomic and epigenetic evidence for oxytocin receptor deficiency in autism. BMC Med, 7, 62. doi: 10.1186/1741-7015-7-62.

Green, L., Fein, D., Modahl, C., Feinstein, C., Waterhouse, L., & Morris, M. (2001). Oxytocin and autistic disorder: alterations in peptide forms. *Biol Psychiatry, 50*(8), 609-613.

Grewen, K.M., & Light, K.C. (2011). Plasma oxytocin is related to lower cardiovascular and sympathetic reactivity to stress. *Biol Psychol, 87*(3):340-9. doi: 0.1016/j.biopsycho.2011.04.003.

Guastella, A.J., Einfeld, S.L., Gray, K.M., Rinehart, N.J., Tonge, B.J., Lambert, T.J., Hickie, I.B. (2010). Intranasal oxytocin improves emotion recognition for youth with autism spectrum disorders. *Biol Psychiatry, 67*(7), 692-4. doi: 10.1016/j.biopsych.2009.09.020.

Guastella, A.J., Howard, A.L., Dadds, M.R., Mitchell, P., & Carson, D.S. (2009). A randomized controlled trial of intranasal oxytocin as an adjunct to exposure therapy for social anxiety disorder. *Psychoneuroendocrinology, 34*(6):917-923. doi: 10.1016/j.psyneuen.2009.01.005.

Guastella, A.J., Mitchell, P.B., & Dadds, M.R. (2008). Oxytocin increases gaze to the eye region of human faces. *Biol Psychiatry, 63*(1), 3-5.

Gustavsson, P. (1977). *Stability and validity of self-reported personality traits*. Karolinska Institutet Stockholm.

Gutkowska, J., & Jankowski, M. (2008). Oxytocin revisited: It is also a cardiovascular hormone. *J Am Soc Hypertens, 2*(5), 318-325.

Guyton, H. (2002). *Textbook of medical physiology*. Philadelphi: Elsevier, Saunders.

Hadley, M.E. (2000). *Endocrinology* (5th edition ed.). Upper saddle river, NJ, 2000: Prentice-Hall.

Handlin, L., Jonas, W., Petersson, M., Ejdeback, M., Ransjo-Arvidson, A.B., Nissen, E., et al. (2009). Effects of sucking and skin-to-skin contact on maternal ACTH and cortisol levels during the second day postpartum-influence of epidural analgesia and oxytocin in the perinatal period. *Breastfeed Med, 4*(4), 207-220.

Handlin, L., Jonas, W., Ransjö-Arvidson, A.B., Petersson, M., Uvnäs-Moberg, K., & Nissen, E. (2012). Influence of common birth interventions on maternal blood pressure patterns during breastfeeding 2 days after birth. Breastfeed Med, 7(2):93-9. doi: 10.1089/bfm.2010.0099.

Hansen, S., & Ferreira, A. (1986). Food intake, aggression, and fear behavior in the mother rat: control by neural systems concerned with milk ejection and maternal behavior. *Behav Neurosci, 100*(1), 64-70.

Harlow, H.F. (1959). Love in infant monkeys. *Sci Am, 200*(6), 68-74.

Harlow, H.F., & Seay, B. (1964). Affectional Systems in Rhesus Monkeys. *J Ark Med Soc, 61*, 107-110.

Harlow, H.F., & Zimmermann, R.R. (1959). Affectional responses in the infant monkey; orphaned baby monkeys develop a strong and persistent attachment to inanimate surrogate mothers. *Science, 130*(3373), 421-432.

Hartmann, P. (2007). Mammary Gland: Past. Present and Future. In P. Hartmann & T. W. Hale (Ed.), *Textbook of human lactation*. Amarillo, Texas: Hale Publishing.

Hartmann, P.E., Sherriff, J.L., & Mitoulas, L.R. (1998). Homeostatic mechanisms that regulate lactation during energetic stress. *J Nutr, 128*(2 Suppl), 394S-399S.

Hatton, G.I., & Tweedle, C.D. (1982). Magnocellular neuropeptidergic neurons in hypothalamus: increases in membrane apposition and number of specialized synapses from pregnancy to lactation. *Brain Res Bull, 8*(2), 197-204.

Heim, C., Young, L.J., Newport, D.J., Mletzko, T., Miller, A.H., & Nemeroff, C.B. (2009). Lower CSF oxytocin concentrations in women with a history of childhood abuse. *Mol Psychiatry, 14*(10), 954-958. doi: 10.1038/mp.2008.112.

Heinrichs, M., Baumgartner, T., Kirschbaum, C., Ehlert, U. (2003). Social support and oxytocin interact to suppress cortisol and subjective responses to psychosocial stress. *Biol Psychiatry, 54*(12), 1389-1398.

Heinrichs, M., & Domes, G. (2008). Neuropeptides and social behaviour: effects of oxytocin and vasopressin in humans. *Prog Brain Res, 170*, 337-350. doi: 10.1016/S0079-6123(08)00428-7.

Heinrichs, M., Meinlschmidt, G., Neumann, I., Wagner, S., Kirschbaum, C., Ehlert, U., et al. (2001). Effects of suckling on hypothalamic-pituitary-adrenal axis responses to psychosocial stress in postpartum lactating women. *J Clin Endocrinol Metab, 86*(10), 4798-4804.

Heinrichs, M., Meinlschmidt, G., Wippich, W., Ehlert, U., & Hellhammer, D.H. (2004). Selective amnesic effects of oxytocin on human memory. *Physiol Behav, 83*(1), 31-38.

Heinrichs, M., Neumann, I., & Ehlert, U. (2002). Lactation and stress: protective effects of breast-feeding in humans. *Stress, 5*(3), 195-203.

Helena, C.V., Cristancho-Gordo, R., Gonzalez-Iglesias, A.E., Tabak, J., Bertram, R., & Freeman, M.E. (2011). Systemic oxytocin induces a prolactin secretory rhythm via the pelvic nerve in ovariectomized rats. *Am J Physiol Regul Integr Comp Physiol, 301*(3), R676-681.

Henderson, J.J., Dickinson, J.E., Evans, S.F., McDonald, S.J., & Paech, M.J. (2003). Impact of intrapartum epidural analgesia on breast-feeding duration. *Aust N Z J Obstet Gynaecol, 43*(5), 372-377.

Herman, J.P., Ostrander, M.M., Mueller, N.K., & Figueiredo, H. (2005). Limbic system mechanisms of stress regulation: hypothalamo-pituitary-adrenocortical axis. *Prog Neuropsychopharmacol Biol Psychiatry, 29*(8), 1201-1213.

Herman, J.P., Prewitt, C.M., & Cullinan, W.E. (1996). Neuronal circuit regulation of the hypothalamo-pituitary-adrenocortical stress axis. *Crit Rev Neurobiol, 10*(3-4), 371-394.

Hofer, M.A. (1994). Early relationships as regulators of infant physiology and behavior. *Acta Paediatr Suppl, 397*, 9-18.

Hofer, M.A. (1994). Early relationships as regulators of infant physiology and behavior. *Acta Paediatr Suppl, 397*, 9-18.

Hofer, M.A., Brunelli, S.A., & Shair, H.N. (1993). Ultrasonic vocalization responses of rat pups to acute separation and contact comfort do not depend on maternal thermal cues. *Dev Psychobiol, 26*(2), 81-95.

Hoge, E.A., Pollack, M.H., Kaufman, R.E., Zak, P.J., & Simon, N.M. (2008). Oxytocin levels in social anxiety disorder. *CNS Neurosci Ther, 14*(3):165-70. doi: 10.1111/j.1755-5949.2008.00051.x.

Hokfelt, T., Kellerth, J.O., Nilsson, G., & Pernow, B. (1975). Experimental immunohistochemical studies on the localization and distribution of substance P in cat primary sensory neurons. *Brain Res, 100*(2), 235-252.

Hollander, E., Bartz, J., Chaplin, W., Phillips, A., Sumner, J., Soorya, L., Anagnostou, E., Wasserman, S. (2007). Oxytocin increases retention of social cognition in autism. *Biol Psychiatry, 61*(4),498-503.

Holmes, J.M. (1954). The use of continuous intravenous oxytocin in obstetrics. *Lancet, 267*(6850), 1191-1193.

Holst, S., Lund, I., Petersson, M., & Uvnäs-Moberg, K. (2005). Massage-like stroking influences plasma levels of gastrointestinal hormones, including insulin, and increases weight gain in male rats. *Auton Neurosci, 120*(1-2), 73-79.

Holst, S., Uvnäs-Moberg, K., & Petersson, M. (2000). Postnatal oxytocin treatment and postnatal stroking of rats influence the development of dopamine 2 receptors in adulthood. Unpublished data.

Holst, S., Uvnäs-Moberg, K., & Petersson, M. (2002). Postnatal oxytocin treatment and postnatal stroking of rats reduce blood pressure in adulthood. *Auton Neurosci, 99*(2), 85-90.

Holzer, P., Taché, Y., & Rosenfeldt, G.M. (1992). *Calcitonin gene related peptide, Vol 657*. New York: Am N.Y. Acad. Sci.

Houston, M.J, Howie, P.W., & McNeilly, A.S. (1983). Factors affecting the duration of breast feeding: 1. Measurement of breast milk intake in the first week of life. *Early Hum Dev, 8*(1), 49-54.

Houston, M.J., Howie, P.W., Smart, L., McArdle, T., & McNeilly, A.S. (1983). Factors affecting the duration of breast feeding: 2. Early feeding practices and social class. *Early Hum Dev, 8*(1), 55-63.

Humble, M.B., Uvnäs-Moberg, K., Engström, I., & Bejerot, S. (2013). Plasma oxytocin changes and anti-obsessive response during serotonin reuptake inhibitor treatment: a placebo controlled study. *BMC Psychiatry, 13*, 344. doi: 10.1186/1471-244X-13-344.

Insel, T.R. (2003). Is social attachment an addictive disorder? *Physiol Behav, 79*(3), 351-357.

Ito, Y., Kobayashi, T., Kimura, T., Matsuura, N., Wakasugi, E., Takeda, T., ... Monden, M. (1996). Investigation of the oxytocin receptor expression in human breast cancer tissue using newly established monoclonal antibodies. *Endocrinology, 137*(2), 773-779.

Ito, N., Nomura, S., Iwase, A., Ito, T., Ino, K., Nagasaka, T., et al. (2003). Ultrastructural localization of aminopeptidase A/angiotensinase and placental leucine aminopeptidase/oxytocinase in chorionic villi of human placenta. *Early Hum Dev, 71*(1), 29-37.

Johansson, B., Uvnäs-Moberg, K., Knight, C.H., & Svennersten-Sjaunja, K. (1999). Effect of feeding before, during and after milking on milk production and the hormones oxytocin, prolactin, gastrin and somatostatin. *J Dairy Res, 66*(2), 151-63.

Johnston, J.M., & Amico, J.A. (1986). A prospective longitudinal study of the release of oxytocin and prolactin in response to infant suckling in long term lactation. *J Clin Endocrinol Metab, 62*(4), 653-657.

Jokinen, J., Chatzittofis, A., Hellström, C., Nordström, P., Uvnäs-Moberg, K., & Asberg, M. (2012). Low CSF oxytocin reflects high intent in suicide attempters. *Psychoneuroendocrinology, 37*(4):482-90. doi: 10.1016/j.psyneuen.2011.07.016.

Jonas, K., Johansson, L.M., Nissen, E., Ejdeback, M., Ransjo-Arvidson, A.B., & Uvnäs-Moberg, K. (2009). Effects of intrapartum oxytocin administration and epidural analgesia on the concentration of plasma oxytocin and prolactin, in response to suckling during the second day postpartum. *Breastfeed Med, 4*(2), 71-82.

Jonas, W., Mileva-Seitz, V., Girard, A.W., Bisceglia, R., Kennedy, J.L., Sokolowski, M., ...MAVAN Research Team. (2013). Genetic variation in oxytocin rs2740210 and early adversity associated with postpartum depression and breastfeeding duration. *Genes Brain Behav, 12*(7), 681-94. doi: 10.1111/gbb.12069.

Jonas, W. Nissen, E., Handlin, L., Ransjo-Arvidsson, A.B., & Uvnäs-Moberg, K. (2005). Covariation between the amounts of administered exogenous oxytocin and epidural analgesia during labor. Unpublished data.

Jonas, W., Nissen, E., Ransjo-Arvidson, A.B., Matthiesen, A.S., & Uvnäs-Moberg, K. (2008). Influence of oxytocin or epidural analgesia on personality profile in breastfeeding women: a comparative study. *Arch Womens Ment Health, 11*(5-6), 335-345.

Jonas, W., Nissen, E., Ransjo-Arvidson, A.B., Wiklund, I., Henriksson, P., & Uvnäs-Moberg, K. (2008). Short- and long-term decrease of blood pressure in women during breastfeeding. *Breastfeed Med, 3*(2), 103-109.

Jonas, W., Wiklund, I., Nissen, E., Ransjo-Arvidson, A.B., & Uvnäs-Moberg, K. (2007). Newborn skin temperature two days postpartum during breastfeeding related to different labour ward practices. *Early Hum Dev, 83*(1), 55-62.

Jones, P.M., & Robinson, I.C. (1982). Differential clearance of neurophysin and neurohypophysial peptides from the cerebrospinal fluid in conscious guinea pigs. *Neuroendocrinology, 34*(4), 297-302.

Jonsson, M., Hanson, U., Lidell, C., & Norden-Lindeberg, S. (2010). ST depression at caesarean section and the relation to oxytocin dose. A randomised controlled trial. *BJOG, 117*(1), 76-83.

Jonsson, M., Norden, S.L., & Hanson, U. (2007). Analysis of malpractice claims with a focus on oxytocin use in labour. *Acta Obstet Gynecol Scand, 86*(3), 315-319.

Jonsson, M., Norden-Lindeberg, S., Ostlund, I., & Hanson, U. (2008). Acidemia at birth, related to obstetric characteristics and to oxytocin use, during the last two hours of labor. *Acta Obstet Gynecol Scand, 87*(7), 745-750.

Jordan, S., Emery, S., Watkins, A., Evans, J.D., Storey, M., & Morgan, G. (2009). Associations of drugs routinely given in labour with breastfeeding at 48 hours: analysis of the Cardiff Births Survey. *BJOG, 116*(12), 1622-1629; discussion 1630-1622.

Kanwal, J.S., & Rao, P.D. (2002). Oxytocin within auditory nuclei: a neuromodulatory function in sensory processing? *Neuroreport, 13*(17), 2193-2197.

Karlstrom, A., Engstrom-Olofsson, R., Norbergh, K.G., Sjoling, M., & Hildingsson, I. (2007). Postoperative pain after cesarean birth affects breastfeeding and infant care. *J Obstet Gynecol Neonatal Nurs, 36*(5), 430-440.

Kendrick, K.M., Da Costa, A.P., Broad, K.D., Ohkura, S., Guevara, R., Lévy, F., Keverne EB. (1997). Neural control of maternal behaviour and olfactory recognition of offspring. *Brain Res Bull, 44*(4), 383-395.

Kendrick, K.M., Guevara-Guzman, R., Zorrilla, J., Hinton, M.R., Broad, K.D., Mimmack, M., & Ohkura, S. (1997). Formation of olfactory memories mediated by nitric oxide. *Nature, 388*(6643), 670-4.

Kendrick, K.M., Keverne, E.B., & Baldwin, B.A. (1987). Intracerebroventricular oxytocin stimulates maternal behaviour in the sheep. *Neuroendocrinology, 46*(1), 56-61.

Kendrick, K.M., Keverne, E.B., Baldwin, B.A., & Sharman, D.F. (1986). Cerebrospinal fluid levels of acetylcholinesterase, monoamines and oxytocin during labour, parturition, vaginocervical stimulation, lamb separation and suckling in sheep. *Neuroendocrinology, 44*(2), 149-156.

Kendrick, K.M., Levy, F., & Keverne, E.B. (1991). Importance of vaginocervical stimulation for the formation of maternal bonding in primiparous and multiparous parturient ewes. *Physiol Behav, 50*(3), 595-600.

Kennell, J.H., Trause, M.A., & Klaus, M.H. (1975). Evidence for a sensitive period in the human mother. *Ciba Found Symp*(33), 87-101.

Kennett, J.E., Poletini, M.O., Fitch, C.A., & Freeman, M.E. (2009). Antagonism of oxytocin prevents suckling- and estradiol-induced, but not progesterone-induced, secretion of prolactin. *Endocrinology, 150*(5), 2292-2299.

Keverne, E.B., & Kendrick, K.M. (1992). Oxytocin facilitation of maternal behavior in sheep. *Ann N Y Acad Sci, 652*, 83-101.

Keverne, E.B., & Kendrick, K.M. (1994). Maternal behaviour in sheep and its neuroendocrine regulation. *Acta Paediatr Suppl, 397*, 47-56.

Kim, S., Soeken, T.A., Cromer, S.J., Martinez, S.R., Hardy, L.R., & Strathearn, L. (2013). Oxytocin and postpartum depression: Delivering on what's known and what's not. *Brain Res.* Nov 14. pii: S0006-8993(13)01504-7. doi: 10.1016/j.brainres.2013.11.009.

Kimura, C., & Matsuoka, M. (2007). Changes in breast skin temperature during the course of breastfeeding. *J Hum Lact, 23*(1), 60-69.

Kimura, T., Ito, Y., Einspanier, A.,Tohya, K., Nobunaga, T., Tokugawa, Y. (1998). Expression and immunlocalization of the oxytocin receptor in human lactating and nonlactating mammary glands. *Hum Reprod., 13*(9), 26452653.

Kirsch, P., Esslinger, C., Chen, Q., Mier, D., Lis, S., Siddhanti, S., ... Meyer-Lindenberg, A. (2005). Oxytocin modulates neural circuitry for social cognition and fear in humans. *J Neurosci, 25*(49), 11489-11493.

Klaus, M.H., Jerauld, R., Kreger, N.C., McAlpine, W., Steffa, M., & Kennel, J.H. (1972). Maternal attachment. Importance of the first post-partum days. *N Engl J Med, 286*(9), 460-463.

Kleberg, A., Hellstrom-Westas, L., & Widstrom, A.M. (2007). Mothers' perception of Newborn Individualized Developmental Care and Assessment Program (NIDCAP) as compared to conventional care. *Early Hum Dev, 83*(6), 403-411.

Knobloch, H.S., Charlet, A., Hoffmann, L.C., Eliava, M., Khrulev, S., Cetin, A.H., ...Grinevich, V. (2012). Evoked axonal oxytocin release in the central amygdala attenuates fear response. *Neuron, 73*(3), 553-66. doi: 10.1016/j.neuron.2011.11.030.

Komisaruk, B.R., & Sansone, G. (2003). Neural pathways mediating vaginal function: the vagus nerves and spinal cord oxytocin. *Scand J Psychol, 44*(3), 241-250.

Kosfeld, M., Heinrichs, M., Zak, P.J., Fischbacher, U., Fehr, E. (2005). Oxytocin increases trust in humans. *Nature, 435*(7042), 673-676.

Krohn, C.C. (1999). *Consequences of different suckling systems in high producing dairy cows* Paper presented at the International symposium on suckling.

Kurosawa, M., Lundeberg, T., Agren, G., Lund, I., & Uvnäs-Moberg, K. (1995). Massage-like stroking of the abdomen lowers blood pressure in anesthetized rats: influence of oxytocin. *J Auton Nerv Syst, 56*(1-2), 26-30.

Kurosawa, M., Suzuki, A., Utsugi, K., & Araki, T. (1982). Response of adrenal efferent nerve activity to non-noxious mechanical stimulation of the skin in rats. *Neurosci Lett, 34*(3), 295-300.

Labbok, M.H. (2007). Breastfeeding, Birth Spacing, and Family Planning. In P. E. H. Thomas W. Hale (Ed.), *Halen a& Hartmann's Textbook of Lactation.* Amarillo: Hale Publishing.

Lagercrantz, H., & Slotkin, T.A. (1986). The "stress" of being born. *Sci Am, 254*(4), 100-107.

LeDoux, J.E. (2012). Evolution of human emotion: a view through fear. *Prog Brain Res, 195*, 431-442.

Lee, S.Y., Kim, M.T., Jee, S.H., & Yang, H.P. (2005). Does long-term lactation protect premenopausal women against hypertension risk? A Korean women's cohort study. *Prev Med, 41*(2), 433-8.

Lefebvre, D.L., Giaid, A., Bennett, H., Lariviere, R., & Zingg, H.H. (1992). Oxytocin gene expression in rat uterus. *Science, 256*(5063), 1553-1555.

Lefebvre, D.L., Giaid, A., & Zingg, H.H. (1992). Expression of the oxytocin gene in rat placenta. *Endocrinology, 130*(3), 1185-1192.

Lefebvre, D.L., Lariviere, R., & Zingg, H.H. (1993). Rat amnion: a novel site of oxytocin production. *Biol Reprod, 48*(3), 632-639.

Legros, J.J., Chiodera, P., & Geenen, V. (1988). Inhibitory action of exogenous oxytocin on plasma cortisol in normal human subjects: evidence of action at the adrenal level. *Neuroendocrinology, 48*(2), 204-206.

Legros, J.J., Chiodera, P., Geenen, V., Smitz, S., & von Frenckell, R. (1984). Dose-response relationship between plasma oxytocin and cortisol and adrenocorticotropin concentrations during oxytocin infusion in normal men. *J Clin Endocrinol Metab, 58*(1), 105-109.

Leighton, B.L., & Halpern, S.H. (2002). The effects of epidural analgesia on labor, maternal, and neonatal outcomes: a systematic review. *Am J Obstet Gynecol, 186*(5 Suppl Nature), S69-77.

Levine, S., Alpert, M., & Lewis, G.W. (1957). Infantile experience and the maturation of the pituitary adrenal axis. *Science, 126*(3287), 1347.

Levine, A., Zagoory-Sharon, O., Feldman, R., & Weller, A. (2007). Oxytocin during pregnancy and early postpartum: individual patterns and maternal-fetal attachment. *Peptides, 28*(6), 1162-1169.

Levy, F., Kendrick, K.M., Keverne, E.B., Piketty, V., & Poindron, P. (1992). Intracerebral oxytocin is important for the onset of maternal behavior in inexperienced ewes delivered under peridural anesthesia. *Behav Neurosci, 106*(2), 427-432.

Lichtenberger, L.M., & Trier, J.S. (1979). Changes in gastrin levels, food intake, and duodenal mucosal growth during lactation. *Am J Physiol, 237*(1), E98-105.

Lieberman, E., & O'Donoghue, C. (2002). Unintended effects of epidural analgesia during labor: a systematic review. *Am J Obstet Gynecol, 186*(5 Suppl Nature), S31-68.

Light, K.C., Smith, T.E., Johns, J.M., Brownley, K.A., Hofheimer, J.A., & Amico, J.A. (2000). Oxytocin responsivity in mothers of infants: a preliminary study of relationships with blood pressure during laboratory stress and normal ambulatory activity. *Health Psychol, 19*(6), 560-567.

Lightman, S.L., & Young, W.S., 3rd. (1989). Lactation inhibits stress-mediated secretion of corticosterone and oxytocin and hypothalamic accumulation of corticotropin-releasing factor and enkephalin messenger ribonucleic acids. *Endocrinology, 124*(5), 2358-2364.

Lincoln, D.W., Hentzen, K., Hin, T., van der Schoot, P., Clarke, G., & Summerlee, A.J. (1980). Sleep: a prerequisite for reflex milk ejection in the rat. *Exp Brain Res, 38*(2), 151-162.

Linden, A., Carlquist, M., Hansen, S., & Uvnäs-Moberg, K. (1989). Plasma concentrations of cholecystokinin, CCK-8, and CCK-33, 39 in rats, determined by a method based on enzyme digestion of gastrin before HPLC and RIA detection of CCK. *Gut, 30*(2), 213-222.

Linden, A., Eriksson, M., Carlquist, M., & Uvnäs-Moberg, K. (1987). Plasma levels of gastrin, somatostatin, and cholecystokinin immunoreactivity during pregnancy and lactation in dogs. *Gastroenterology, 92*(3), 578-584.

Linden, A., Eriksson, M., Hansen, S., & Uvnäs-Moberg, K. (1990). Suckling-induced release of cholecystokinin into plasma in the lactating rat: effects of abdominal vagotomy and lesions of central pathways concerned with milk ejection. *J Endocrinol, 127*(2), 257-263.

Lindén, A., Uvnäs-Moberg, K., Eneroth, P., & Sodersten, P. (1989). Stimulation of maternal behaviour in rats with cholecystokinin octapeptide. *J Neuroendocrinol, 1*(6):389-92. doi: 10.1111/j.1365-2826.1989.tb00135.x.

Linden, A., Uvnäs-Moberg, K., Forsberg, G., Bednar, I., Enerotht, P., & Sodersten, P. (1990). Involvement of Cholecystokinin in Food Intake: II. Lactational Hyperphagia in the Rat. *J Neuroendocrinol, 2*(6), 791-796.

Linden, A., Uvnäs-Moberg, K., Forsberg, G., Bednar, I., & Sodersten, P. (1989). Plasma concentrations of cholecystokinin octapeptide and food intake in male rats treated with cholecystokinin octapeptide. *J Endocrinol, 121*(1), 59-65.

Linzell, J. (1971). Mammary blood vessels, lymphatics and nerves. In I.R Falconer (Ed.) *Lactation* (pp 41-50). London: Butterworths.

Liu, D., Caldji, C., Sharma, S., Plotsky, P.M., & Meaney, M.J. (2000). Influence of neonatal rearing conditions on stress-induced adrenocorticotropin responses and norepinepherine release in the hypothalamic paraventricular nucleus. *J Neuroendocrinol, 12*(1), 5-12.

Long, C.A. (1969). The origin and evolution of the mammary gland. *Bioscience, 19*, 519-523.

Lonstein, J.S. (2005). Reduced anxiety in postpartum rats requires recent physical interactions with pups, but is independent of suckling and peripheral sources of hormones. *Horm Behav, 47*(3), 241-255.

Lucas, A., Drewett, R.B., & Mitchell, M.D. (1980). Breast-feeding and plasma oxytocin concentrations. *Br Med J, 281*(6244), 834-835.

Luckman, S.M., Hamamura, M., Antonijevic, I., Dye, S., & Leng, G. (1993). Involvement of cholecystokinin receptor types in pathways controlling oxytocin secretion. *Br J Pharmacol, 110*(1), 378-384.

Ludwig, M., & Leng, G. (2006). Dendritic peptide release and peptide-dependent behaviours. *Nat Rev Neurosci, 7*(2), 126-136.

Lund, I., Ge, Y., Yu, L.C., Uvnäs-Moberg, K., Wang, J., Yu, C., et al. (2002). Repeated massage-like stimulation induces long-term effects on nociception: contribution of oxytocinergic mechanisms. *Eur J Neurosci, 16*(2), 330-338.

Lund, I., Lundeberg, T., Kurosawa, M., & Uvnäs-Moberg, K. (1999). Sensory stimulation (massage) reduces blood pressure in unanaesthetized rats. *J Auton Nerv Syst, 78*(1), 0-37.

Lundberg, J.M., Terenius, L., Hokfelt, T., & Goldstein, M. (1983). High levels of neuropeptide Y in peripheral noradrenergic neurons in various mammals including man. *Neurosci Lett, 42*(2), 167-172.

Lundeberg, T., Uvnäs-Moberg, K., Agren, G., & Bruzelius, G. (1994). Anti-nociceptive effects of oxytocin in rats and mice. *Neurosci Lett, 170*(1), 153-157.

Lupoli, B., Johansson, B., Uvnäs-Moberg, K., & Svennersten-Sjaunja, K. (2001). Effect of suckling on the release of oxytocin, prolactin, cortisol, gastrin, cholecystokinin, somatostatin and insulin in dairy cows and their calves. *J Dairy Res, 68*(2), 175-187.

Luppi, P., Levi-Montalcini, R., Bracci-Laudiero, L., Bertolini, A., Arletti, R., Tavernari, D., et al. (1993). NGF is released into plasma during human pregnancy: an oxytocin-mediated response? *Neuroreport, 4*(8), 1063-1065.

Marchini, G., Lagercrantz, H., Feuerberg, Y., Winberg, J., & Uvnäs-Moberg, K. (1987). The effect of non-nutritive sucking on plasma insulin, gastrin, and somatostatin levels in infants. *Acta Paediatr Scand, 76*(4), 573-578.

Marchini, G., Lagercrantz, H., Winberg, J., & Uvnäs-Moberg, K. (1988). Fetal and maternal plasma levels of gastrin, somatostatin and oxytocin after vaginal delivery and elective cesarean section. *Early Hum Dev, 18*(1), 73-79.

Mason, W.T., Ho, Y.W., & Hatton, G.I. (1984). Axon collaterals of supraoptic neurones: anatomical and electrophysiological evidence for their existence in the lateral hypothalamus. *Neuroscience, 11*(1), 169-82.

Matsuguchi, H., Sharabi, F.M., Gordon, F.J., Johnson, A.K., & Schmid, P.G. (1982). Blood pressure and heart rate responses to microinjection of vasopressin into the nucleus tractus solitarius region of the rat. *Neuropharmacology, 21*(7), 687-693.

Matthiesen, A.S., Ransjo-Arvidson, A.B., Nissen, E., & Uvnäs-Moberg, K. (2001a). Postpartum maternal oxytocin release by newborns: Effects of infant hand massage and sucking. *Birth, 28*(1), 13-19.

Matthiesen, A.S., Ransjo-Arvidson, A.B., Nissen, E., & Uvnäs-Moberg, K. (2001b). Maternal analgesia decreases maternal sensitivity to infant breast massage. Unpublished data.

Maughan, K.L., Heim, S.W., & Galazka, S.S. (2006). Preventing postpartum hemorrhage: managing the third stage of labor. *Am Fam Physician, 73*(6), 1025-1028.

Mayer, A.D., & Rosenblatt, J.S. (1987). Hormonal factors influence the onset of maternal aggression in laboratory rats. *Horm Behav, 21*(2), 253-267.

McClellan, M.S., & Cabianca, W.A. (1980). Effects of early mother-infant contact following cesarean birth. *Obstet Gynecol, 56*(1), 52-55.

McKee, D.T., Poletini, M.O., Bertram, R., & Freeman, M.E. (2007). Oxytocin action at the lactotroph is required for prolactin surges in cervically stimulated ovariectomized rats. *Endocrinology*.

McKenna, J.J., Ball, H.L., & Gettler, L.T. (2007). Mother-infant co-sleeping, breastfeeding and sudden infant death syndrome: what biological anthropology has discovered about normal infant sleep and pediatric sleep medicine. *Am J Phys Anthropol Suppl, 45*, 133-61.

McNeilly, A.S., Robinson, I.C., Houston, M.J., & Howie, P.W. (1983). Release of oxytocin and prolactin in response to suckling. *Br Med J (Clin Res Ed), 286*(6361), 257-259.

Mezzacappa, E.S., & Katlin, E.S. (2002). Breast-feeding is associated with reduced perceived stress and negative mood in mothers. *Health Psychol, 21*(2), 187-193.

Mezzacappa, E.S., Kelsey, R.M., & Katkin, E.S. (2005). Breast feeding, bottle feeding, and maternal autonomic responses to stress. *J Psychosom Res, 58*(4), 351-365.

Mezzacappa, E.S., Kelsey, R.M., Myers, M.M., & Katkin, E.S. (2001). Breast-feeding and maternal cardiovascular function. *Psychophysiology, 38*(6), 988-997.

Miranda-Paiva, C.M., Nasello, A.G., Yim, A.J., & Felicio, L.F. (2002). Puerperal blockade of cholecystokinin (CCK1) receptors disrupts maternal behavior in lactating rats. *J Mol Neurosci, 18*(1-2), 97-104.

Modahl, C., Green, L., Fein, D., Morris, M., Waterhouse, L., Feinstein, C., et al. (1998). Plasma oxytocin levels in autistic children. *Biol Psychiatry, 43*(4), 270-277.

Mogg, R.J., & Samson, W.K. (1990). Interactions of dopaminergic and peptidergic factors in the control of prolactin release. *Endocrinology, 126*(2), 728-735.

Moore, E.R., Anderson, G.C., Bergman, N., & Dowswell, T. (2012). Early skin-to-skin contact for mothers and their healthy newborn infants. *Cochrane Database Syst Rev, 5*:CD003519. doi: 10.1002/14651858.CD003519.pub3.

Moos, F., & Richard, P. (1975a). Adrenergic and cholinergic control of oxytocin release evoked by vaginal, vagal and mammary stimulation in lactating rats. *J Physiol (Paris), 70*(3), 315-32.

Moos, F., & Richard P. (1975b). Level of oxytocin release induced by vaginal dilatation (Ferguson reflex) and vagal stimulation (vago-pituitary reflex) in lactating rats. *J Physiol (Paris), 70*(3), 307-14.

Mori, M., Vigh, S., Miyata, A., Yoshihara, T., Oka, S., & Arimura, A. (1990). Oxytocin is the major prolactin releasing factor in the posterior pituitary. *Endocrinology, 126*(2), 1009-1013.

Murphy, D.J., MacGregor, H., Munishankar, B., & McLeod, G. (2009). A randomised controlled trial of oxytocin 5IU and placebo infusion versus oxytocin 5IU and 30IU infusion for the control of blood loss at elective caesarean section--pilot study. RCTN 40302163. *Eur J Obstet Gynecol Reprod Biol, 142*(1), 30-33.

Naruki, M., Mizutani, S., Goto, K., Tsujimoto, M., Nakazato, H.,

Itakura, A., et al. (1996). Oxytocin is hydrolyzed by an enzyme in human placenta that is identical to the oxytocinase of pregnancy serum. *Peptides, 17*(2), 257-261.

Nation, D.A., Szeto, A., Mendez, A.J., Brooks, L.G., Zaias, J., Herderick, E.E., et al. (2010). Oxytocin attenuates atherosclerosis and adipose tissue inflammation in socially isolated ApoE-/- mice. *Psychosom Med, 72*(4), 376-382.

Neumann, I.D. (2001). Alterations in behavioral and neuroendocrine stress coping strategies in pregnant, parturient and lactating rats. *Prog Brain Res, 133*, 143-152.

Neumann, I.D. (2002). Involvement of the brain oxytocin system in stress coping: interactions with the hypothalamo-pituitary-adrenal axis. *Prog Brain Res, 139*, 147-162.

Neumann, I.D. (2008). Brain oxytocin: A key regulator of emotional and social behaviours in both females and males. *J Neuroendocrinol, 20*(6), 858-865.

Neumann, I.D., Wigger, A., Torner, L., Holsboer, F., & Landgraf, R. (2000). Brain oxytocin inhibits basal and stress-induced activity of the hypothalamo-pituitary-adrenal axis in male and female rats: partial action within the paraventricular nucleus. *J Neuroendocrinol, 12*(3), 235-243.

Neve, H.A., Paisley, A.C., & Summerlee, A.J. (1982). Arousal a prerequisite for suckling in the conscious rabbit? *Physiol Behav, 28*(2), 213-7.

Newton, N. (1992). The relation of the milk-ejection reflex to the ability to breast feed. *Ann N Y Acad Sci, 652*, 484-486.

Nishimori, K., Young, L.J., Guo, Q., Wang, Z., Insel, T.R., & Matzuk, M.M. (1996). Oxytocin is required for nursing but is not essential for parturition or reproductive behavior. *Proc Natl Acad Sci U S A, 93*(21), 11699-11704.

Nissen, E., Gustavsson, P., Widstrom, A.M., & Uvnäs-Moberg, K. (1998). Oxytocin, prolactin, milk production and their relationship with personality traits in women after vaginal delivery or Cesarean section. *J Psychosom Obstet Gynaecol, 19*(1), 49-58.

Nissen, E., Lilja, G., Matthiesen, A.S., Ransjo-Arvidsson, A.B., Uvnäs-Moberg, K., & Widstrom, A.M. (1995). Effects of maternal pethidine on infants' developing breast feeding behaviour. *Acta Paediatr, 84*(2), 140-145.

Nissen, E., Lilja, G., Widstrom, A.M., & Uvnäs-Moberg, K. (1995). Elevation of oxytocin levels early post partum in women. *Acta obstetricia et gynecologica Scandinavica, 74*(7), 530-533.

Nissen, E., Uvnäs-Moberg, K., Svensson, K., Stock, S., Widstrom, A.M., & Winberg, J. (1996). Different patterns of oxytocin, prolactin but not cortisol release during breastfeeding in women delivered by caesarean section or by the vaginal route. *Early Hum Dev, 45*(1-2), 103-118.

Nissen, E., Widstrom, A.M., Lilja, G., Matthiesen, A.S., Uvnäs-Moberg, K., Jacobsson, G., et al. (1997). Effects of routinely given pethidine during labour on infants' developing breastfeeding behaviour. Effects of dose-delivery time interval and various concentrations of pethidine/norpethidine in cord plasma. *Acta Paediatr, 86*(2), 201-208.

Nowak, R., Goursaud, A.P., Levy, F., Orgeur, P., Schaal, B., Belzung, C., et al. (1997). Cholecystokinin receptors mediate the development of a preference for the mother by newly born lambs. *Behav Neurosci, 111*(6), 1375-1382.

Nowak, R., Murphy, T.M., Lindsay, D.R., Alster, P., Andersson, R., & Uvnäs-Moberg, K. (1997). Development of a preferential relationship with the mother by the newborn lamb: importance of the sucking activity. *Physiol Behav, 62*(4), 681-688.

Numan, M. (2006). Hypothalamic neural circuits regulating maternal responsiveness toward infants. *Behav Cogn Neurosci Rev, 5*(4), 163-190.

Numan, M., & Sheehan, T.P. (1997). Neuroanatomical circuitry for mammalian maternal behavior. *Ann N Y Acad Sci, 807*, 101-125.

Numan, M., & Woodside, B. (2010). Maternity: neural mechanisms, motivational processes, and physiological adaptations. *Behav Neurosci, 124*(6), 715-741. doi: 10.1037/a0021548.

Nylander, G., Lindemann, R., Helsing, E., & Bendvold, E. (1991). Unsupplemented breastfeeding in the maternity ward. Positive long-term effects. *Acta Obstet Gynecol Scand, 70*(3), 205-209.

Odent, M. (2012). The role of the shy hormone in breastfeeding. *Midwifery Today Int Midwife*(101), 14.

Ohlsson, B., Forsling, M.L, Rehfeld, J.F., & Sjölund, K. (2002). Cholecystokinin stimulation leads to increased oxytocin secretion in women. *Eur J Surg, 168*(2), 114-118.

Ohlsson, B., Truedsson, M., Bengtsson, M., Torstenson, R., Sjölund, K., Björnsson, E.S., Simrèn, M. (2005). Effects of long-term treatment with oxytocin in chronic constipation; a double blind, placebo-controlled pilot trial. *Neurogastroenterol Motil, 17*(5),697-704.

Ohlsson, B., Truedsson, M., Djerf, P., & Sundler, F. (2006). Oxytocin is expressed throughout the human gastrointestinal tract. *Regul Pept, 135*(1-2), 7-11.

Olausson, H., Lamarre, Y., Backlund, H., Morin, C., Wallin, B.G., Starck, G., et al. (2002). Unmyelinated tactile afferents signal touch and project to insular cortex. *Nat Neurosci, 5*(9), 900-904.

Olausson, H., Uvnäs-Moberg, K., & Sohlstrom, A. (2003). Postnatal oxytocin alleviates adverse effects in adult rat offspring caused by maternal malnutrition. *Am J Physiol Endocrinol Metab, 284*(3), E475-480.

Olausson, H., Wessberg, J., Morrison, I., McGlone, F., & Vallbo, A. (2010). The neurophysiology of unmyelinated tactile afferents. *Neurosci Biobehav Rev, 34*(2), 185-191.

Olson, B.R., Drutarosky, M.D., Chow, M. S., Hruby, V.J., Stricker, E.M., & Verbalis, J.G. (1991). Oxytocin and an oxytocin agonist administered centrally decrease food intake in rats. *Peptides, 12*(1), 113-118.

Olson, B.R., Hoffman, G.E., Sved, A.F., Stricker, E.M., & Verbalis, J.G. (1992). Cholecystokinin induces c-fos expression in hypothalamic oxytocinergic neurons projecting to the dorsal vagal complex. *Brain Res, 569*(2), 238-248.

Ostrom, K.M. (1990). A review of the hormone prolactin during lactation. *Prog Food Nutr Sci, 14*(1), 1-43.

Ott, I., & Scott, J.C. (1910). The action of infundibulin upon the mammary secretion. *Proc. Soc. Exp. Biol.Med., 8*, 48-49.

Paterno, M.T., Van Zandt, S.E., Murphy, J., & Jordan, E.T. (2012). Evaluation of a student-nurse doula program: an analysis of doula interventions and their impact on labor analgesia and cesarean birth. *J Midwifery Womens Health, 57*(1), 28-34.

Pauk, J., Kuhn, C.M., Field, T.M., & Schanberg, S.M. (1986). Positive effects of tactile versus kinesthetic or vestibular stimulation on neuroendocrine and ODC activity in maternally-deprived rat pups. *Life Sci, 39*(22), 2081-2087.

Pedersen, C.A., Ascher, J.A., Monroe, Y.L., & Prange, A.J. Jr. (1982). Oxytocin induces maternal behavior in virgin female rats. *Science, 216*(4546), 648-50.

Pedersen, C.A., Caldwell, J.D., Johnson, M.F., Fort, S.A., & Prange, A.J., Jr. (1985). Oxytocin antiserum delays onset of ovarian steroid-induced maternal behavior. *Neuropeptides, 6*(2), 175-182.

Pedersen, C.A., Caldwell, J.D., Peterson, G., Walker, C.H., & Mason, G.A. (1992). Oxytocin activation of maternal behavior in the rat. *Ann N Y Acad Sci, 652*, 58-69.

Pedersen, C.A., & Prange, A.J., Jr. (1979). Induction of maternal behavior in virgin rats after intracerebroventricular administration of oxytocin. *Proc Natl Acad Sci U S A, 76*(12), 6661-6665.

Pernow, B. (1983). Substance P. *Pharmacological reviews, 35*(2), 85-141.

Petersen, W.E., & Ludwick, T.M. (1942). The humoral nature of the factor causing the let-down of milk. *Fed Proc, 1*, 66-67.

Petersson, M., Ahlenius, S., Wiberg, U., Alster, P., & Uvnäs-Moberg, K. (1998). Steroid dependent effects of oxytocin on spontaneous motor activity in female rats. *Brain Res Bull, 45*(3), 301-305.

Petersson, M., Alster, P., Lundeberg, T., & Uvnäs-Moberg, K. (1996a). Oxytocin increases nociceptive thresholds in a long-term perspective in female and male rats. *Neurosci Lett, 212*(2), 87-90.

Petersson, M., Alster, P., Lundeberg, T., Uvnäs-Moberg, K. (1996b). Oxytocin causes a long-term decrease of blood pressure in female and male rats. *Physiology and Behavior, 60*(5), 1311-1315.

Petersson, M., Diaz-Cabiale, Z., Angel Narvaez, J., Fuxe, K., & Uvnäs-Moberg, K. (2005). Oxytocin increases the density of high affinity alpha(2)-adrenoceptors within the hypothalamus, the amygdala and the nucleus of the solitary tract in ovariectomized rats. *Brain Res, 1049*(2), 234-239.

Petersson, M., Eklund, M., & Uvnäs-Moberg, K. (2005). Oxytocin decreases corticosterone and nociception and increases motor activity in OVX rats. *Maturitas, 51*(4), 426-433.

Petersson, M., Hulting, A., Andersson, R., & Uvnäs-Moberg, K. (1999). Long-term changes in gastrin, cholecystokinin and insulin in response to oxytocin treatment. *Neuroendocrinology, 69*(3), 202-208.

Petersson, M., Hulting, A.L., Uvnäs-Moberg, K. (1999). Oxytocin causes a sustained decrease in plasma levels of corticosterone in rats. *Neuroscience Letters, 264*(1-3), 41-44.

Petersson, M., Lundeberg, T., Sohlström, A., Wiberg, U., & Uvnäs-Moberg, K. (1998). Oxytocin increases the survival of musculocutaneous flaps. *Naunyn Schmiedebergs Arch Pharmacol. 357*(6), 701-704.

Petersson, M., Lundeberg, T., & Uvnäs-Moberg, K. (1999a). Oxytocin enhances the effects of clonidine on blood pressure and locomotor activity in rats. *J Auton Nerv Syst, 78*(1), 49-56.

Petersson, M., Lundeberg, T., & Uvnäs-Moberg, K. (1999b). Short-term increase and long-term decrease of blood pressure in response to oxytocin-potentiating effect of female steroid hormones. *J Cardiovasc Pharmacol, 33*(1), 102-108.

Petersson, M., & Uvnäs-Moberg, K. (2003). Systemic oxytocin treatment modulates glucocorticoid and mineralocorticoid receptor mRNA in the rat hippocampus. *Neurosci Lett, 343*(2), 97-100.

Petersson, M., & Uvnäs-Moberg, K. (2004). Prolyl-leucyl-glycinamide shares some effects with oxytocin but decreases oxytocin levels. *Physiol Behav, 83*(3), 475-481.

Petersson, M., & Uvnäs-Moberg, K. (2007). Effects of an acute stressor on blood pressure and heart rate in rats pretreated with intracerebroventricular oxytocin injections. *Psychoneuroendocrinology, 32*(8-10), 959-965.

Petersson, M., & Uvnäs-Moberg, K. (2008). Postnatal oxytocin treatment of spontaneously hypertensive male rats decreases blood pressure and body weight in adulthood. *Neurosci Lett, 440*(2), 166-169.

Petersson, M., Uvnäs-Moberg, K., Erhardt, S., & Engberg, G. (1998). Oxytocin increases Locus Coeruleus alpha 2-adrenoreceptor responsiveness in rats. *Neurosci Lett, 255*(2), 115-118.

Petersson, M., Wiberg, U., Lundeberg, T., & Uvnäs-Moberg, K. (2001). Oxytocin decreases carrageenan induced inflammation in rats. *Peptides, 22*(9), 1479-1484.

Pierrehumbert, B., Torrisi, R., Laufer, D., Halfon, O., Ansermet, F., & Beck Popovic, M. (2009). Oxytocin response to an experimental psychosocial challenge in adults exposed to traumatic experiences during childhood or adolescence. *Neuroscience, 166*(1), 168-177. doi: 10.1016/j.neuroscience.2009.12.016.

Pittman, Q.J., Blume, H.W., & Renaud, L.P. (1981). Connections of the hypothalamic paraventricular nucleus with the neurohypophysis, median eminence, amygdala, lateral septum and midbrain periaqueductal gray: an electrophysiological study in the rat. *Brain Res, 215*(1-2), 15-28.

Porges, S.W. (2009). The polyvagal theory: new insights into adaptive reactions of the autonomic nervous system. *Cleve Clin J Med, 76* Suppl 2, S86-90. doi: 10.3949/ccjm.76.s2.17.

Poulain, D.A., Rodriguez, F., & Ellendorff, F. (1981). Sleep is not a prerequisite for the milk ejection reflex in the pig. *Exp Brain Res, 43*(1), 107-10.

Poulain, D.A., & Wakerley, J.B. (1982). Electrophysiology of hypothalamic magnocellular neurones secreting oxytocin and vasopressin. *Neuroscience, 7*(4), 773-808.

Prime, D.K., Geddes, D.T., Spatz, D.L., Robert, M., Trengove, N.J., & Hartmann, P.E. (2009). Using milk flow rate to investigate milk ejection in the left and right breasts during simultaneous breast expression in women. *Int Breastfeed J, 4*, 10.

Prime, D.K., Geddes, D.T., Hepworth, A.R., Trengove, N.J., & Hartmann, P.E. (2011). Comparison of the patterns of milk ejection during repeated breast expression sessions in women. *Breastfeed Med, 6*(4):183-90. doi: 10.1089/bfm.2011.0014.

Puder, B.A., & Papka, R.E. (2001). Hypothalamic paraventricular axons projecting to the female rat lumbosacral spinal cord contain oxytocin immunoreactivity. *J Neurosci Res. 64*(1), 53-60.

Rahm, V.A., Hallgren, A., Hogberg, H., Hurtig, I., & Odlind, V. (2002). Plasma oxytocin levels in women during labor with or without epidural analgesia: a prospective study. *Acta Obstet Gynecol Scand, 81*(11), 1033-1039.

Ramsay, D.T., Kent, J.C., Owens, R.A., & Hartmann, P.E. (2004). Ultrasound imaging of milk ejection in the breast of lactating women. *Pediatrics, 113*(2), 361-7.

Ramsay, D.T., Mitoulas, L.R., Kent, J.C., Cregan, M.D., Doherty, D.A., Larsson, M., & Hartmann, P.E. (2006). Milk flow rates can be used to identify and investigate milk ejection in women expressing breast milk using an electric breast pump. *Breastfeed Med, 1*(1), 14-23.

Ransjo-Arvidson, A.B., Matthiesen, A.S., Lilja, G., Nissen, E., Widstrom, A.M., & Uvnäs-Moberg, K. (2001). Maternal analgesia during labor disturbs newborn behavior: effects on breastfeeding, temperature, and crying. *Birth, 28*(1), 5-12.

Renaud, L.P., Tang, M., McCann, M.J., Stricker, E.M., & Verbalis, J.G. (1987). Cholecystokinin and gastric distension activate oxytocinergic cells in rat hypothalamus. *Am J Physiol, 253*(4 Pt 2), R661-665.

Renz-Polster, H., David, M.R., Buist, A.S., Vollmer, W.M., O'Connor, E.A., Frazier, E.A., & Wall, M.A. (2005). Caesarean section delivery and the risk of allergic disorders in childhood. *Clin Exp Allergy, 35*(11), 1466-1472.

Richard, P., Moos, F., & Freund-Mercier, M.J. (1991). Central effects of oxytocin. *Physiol Rev, 71*(2), 331-370.

Righard, L., & Alade, M.O. (1990). Effect of delivery room routines on success of first breast-feed. *Lancet, 336*(8723), 1105-1107.

Rinaman, L., Hoffman, G.E., Dohanics, J., Le, W.W., Stricker, E.M., & Verbalis, J.G. (1995). Cholecystokinin activates catecholaminergic neurons in the caudal medulla that innervate the paraventricular nucleus of the hypothalamus in rats. *J Comp Neurol, 360*(2), 246-256.

Risberg, A., Olsson, K., Lyrenas, S., & Sjöquist, M. (2009). Plasma vasopressin, oxytocin, estradiol, and progesterone related to water and sodium excretion in normal pregnancy and gestational hypertension. *Acta Obstet Gynecol Scand, 88*(6), 639-46. doi: 10.1080/00016340902919002.

Robinson, J.E., & Short, R.V. (1977). Changes in breast sensitivity at puberty, during the menstrual cycle, and at parturition. *Br Med J, 1*(6070), 1188-1191.

Roduit, C., Scholtens, S., de Jongste, J.C., Wijga, A.H., Gerritsen, J., Postma, D.S., ...Smit, H.A. (2009). Asthma at 8 years of age in children born by caesarean section. *Thorax, 64*(2), 107-113. doi: 10.1136/thx.2008.100875.

Rogers, R.C., & Hermann, G.E. (1987). Oxytocin, oxytocin antagonist, TRH, and hypothalamic paraventricular nucleus stimulation effects on gastric motility. *Peptides, 8*(3), 505-513.

Rojkittikhun, T., Uvnäs-Moberg, K., & Einarsson, S. (1993). Plasma oxytocin, prolactin, insulin and LH after 24 h of fasting and after refeeding in lactating sows. *Acta Physiol Scand, 148*(4), 413-419.

Rosen, J.M., Wyszomiersky, S.L., & Hadsell, D. (1999). Regulation of milkprotein gene expression. *Annu rev Nutr, 19*, 407-436.

Rosenblatt, D.B., Belsey, E.M., Lieberman, B.A., Redshaw, M., Caldwell, J., Notarianni, L., et al. (1981). The influence of maternal analgesia on neonatal behaviour: II. Epidural bupivacaine. *Br J Obstet Gynaecol, 88*(4), 407-413.

Rosenblatt, J.S. (1994). Psychobiology of maternal behavior: contribution to the clinical understanding of maternal behavior among humans. *Acta Paediatr Suppl, 397*, 3-8.

Rosenblatt, J.S. (2003). Outline of the evolution of behavioral and nonbehavioral patterns of parental care among the vertebrates: critical characteristics of mammalian and avian parental behavior. *Scand J Psychol, 44*(3), 265-271.

Rosenblatt, J.S., Mayer, A.D., & Giordano, A.L. (1988). Hormonal basis during pregnancy for the onset of maternal behavior in the rat. *Psychoneuroendocrinology, 13*(1-2), 29-46.

Rowe-Murray, H.J., & Fisher, J.R. (2001). Operative intervention in delivery is associated with compromised early mother-infant interaction. *BJOG, 108*(10), 1068-1075.

Rowe-Murray, H.J., & Fisher, J.R. (2002). Baby friendly hospital practices: cesarean section is a persistent barrier to early initiation of breastfeeding. *Birth, 29*(2), 124-131.

Ryden, G., & Sjoholm, I. (1969). Half-life of oxytocin in blood of pregnant and non-pregnant women. *Acta Endocrinol (Copenh), 61*(3), 425-431.

Said, S.I, & Mutt, V. (1970). Polypeptide with broad biological activity: Isolation from small intestine. *Science, 169*(3951), 1217-1218.

Salariya, E.M., Easton, P.M., & Cater, J.I. (1978). Duration of breast-feeding after early initiation and frequent feeding. *Lancet, 2*(8100), 1141-1143.

Salt, T.E., & Hill, R.G. (1983). Neurotransmitter candidates of somatosensory primary afferent fibres. *Neuroscience, 10*(4), 1083-1103.

Samson, W.K., Lumpkin, M.D., & McCann, S.M. (1986). Evidence for a physiological role for oxytocin in the control of prolactin secretion. *Endocrinology, 119*(2), 554-560.

Samson, W.K., & Schell, D.A. (1995). Oxytocin and the anterior pituitary gland. *Adv Exp Med Biol, 395*, 355-364.

Samuelsson, B., Uvnäs-Moberg, K., Gorewit, R., & Svennersten-Sjaunja. K. (1996). Profiles of the hormones somatostatin, gastrin, CCK, prolactin, Growth hormone and cortisol. ll. In dairy cows that are milked during food deprivation. *Livest. Prod. Sci, 46*(1), 57-64.

Sarkar, D.K., & Gibbs, D.M. (1984). Cyclic variation of oxytocin in the blood of pituitary portal vessels of rats. *Neuroendocrinology, 39*(5), 481-483.

Sato, A. (1987). Neural mechanisms of somatic sensory regulation of catecholamine secretion from the adrenal gland. *Adv Biophys, 23*, 39-80.

Sato, A., Sato, Y., & Schmidt, R.F. (1997). The impact of somatosensory input on autonomic functions. *Rev Physiol Biochem Pharmacol, 130*, 1-328.

Sato, Y., Hotta, H., Nakayama, H., & Suzuki, H. (1996). Sympathetic and parasympathetic regulation of the uterine blood flow and contraction in the rat. *J Auton Nerv Syst, 59*(3), 151-158.

Sawchenko, P.E., & Swanson, L.W. (1983). The organization and biochemical specificity of afferent projections to the paraventricular and supraoptic nuclei. *Prog Brain Res, 60*, 19-29.

Sawyer, W.H. (1977). Evolution of neurohypophyseal hormones and their receptors. *Fed Proc, 36*(6), 1842-1847.

Schumacher, M., Coirini, H., Flanagan, L.M., Frankfurt, M., Pfaff, D.W., & McEwen, B.S. (1992). Ovarian steroid modulation of oxytocin receptor binding in the ventromedial hypothalamus. *Ann NY Acad Sci, 652*, 374-86.

Schumacher, M., Coirini, H., Johnson, A.E., Flanagan, L.M., Frankfurt, M., Pfaff, D.W., et al. (1993). The oxytocin receptor: a target for steroid hormones. *Regul Pept, 45*(1-2), 115-119.

Scott, K.D., Berkowitz, G., & Klaus, M. (1999). A comparison of intermittent and continuous support during labor: a meta-analysis. *Am J Obstet Gynecol, 180*(5), 1054-1059.

Scott, K.D., Klaus, P.H., & Klaus, M.H. (1999). The obstetrical and postpartum benefits of continuous support during childbirth. *J Womens Health Gend Based Med, 8*(10), 1257-1264.

Seay, B., & Harlow, H.F. (1965). Maternal separation in the rhesus monkey. *J Nerv Ment Dis, 140*(6), 434-441.

Seltzer, L.J., Ziegler, T.E., & Pollak, S.D. (2010). Social vocalizations can release oxytocin in humans. *Proc Biol Sci, 277*(1694), 2661-2666.

Selye, H. (1976). *Stress in health and disease.* Boston: Butterworths.

Sepkoski, C.M., Lester, B.M., Ostheimer, G.W., & Brazelton, T.B. (1992). The effects of maternal epidural anesthesia on neonatal behavior during the first month. *Dev Med Child Neurol, 34*(12), 1072-1080.

Shair, H.N., Masmela, J.R., & Hofer, M.A. (1999). The influence of olfaction on potentiation and inhibition of ultrasonic vocalization of rat pups. *Physiol Behav, 65*(4-5), 769-772.

Shehab, S.A., & Atkinson, M.E. (1986). Vasoactive intestinal polypeptide (VIP) increases in the spinal cord after peripheral axotomy of the sciatic nerve originate from primary afferent neurons. *Brain Res, 372*(1), 37-44.

Sheward, W.J., Coombes, J.E., Bicknell, R.J., Fink, G., & Russell, J.A. (1990). Release of oxytocin but not corticotrophin-releasing factor-41 into rat hypophysial portal vessel blood can be made opiate dependent. *J Endocrinol, 124*(1), 141-150.

Shughrue, P.J., Komm, B., & Merchenthaler, I. (1996). The distribution of estrogen receptor-beta mRNA in the rat hypothalamus. *Steroids, 61*(12), 678-681.

Sikorski, J., Renfrew, M.J., Pindoria, S., & Wade, A. (2003). Support for breastfeeding mothers: a systematic review. Paediatr Perinat Epidemiol, 17(4), 407-17.

Silber, M., Almkvist, O., Larsson, B., & Uvnäs-Moberg, K. (1990). Temporary peripartal impairment in memory and attention and its possible relation to oxytocin concentration. *Life Sci, 47*(1), 57-65.

Silber, M., Larsson, B., & Uvnäs-Moberg, K. (1991). Oxytocin, somatostatin, insulin and gastrin concentrations vis-a-vis late pregnancy, breastfeeding and oral contraceptives. *Acta Obstet Gynecol Scand, 70*(4-5), 283-289.

Sjogren, B., Widstrom, A.M., Edman, G., & Uvnäs-Moberg, K. (2000). Changes in personality pattern during the first pregnancy and lactation. *J Psychosom Obstet Gynaecol, 21*(1), 31-38.

Skuse, D.H., Lori, A., Cubells, J.F., Lee, I., Conneely, K.N., Puura, K., ...Young, L.J. (2014). Common polymorphism in the oxytocin receptor gene (OXTR) is associated with human social recognition skills. *Proc Natl Acad Sci USA, 111*(5), 1987-92. doi: 10.1073/pnas.1302985111.

Smedh, U., & Uvnäs-Moberg, K. (1994). Intracerebroventricularly administered corticotropin-releasing factor releases somatostatin through a cholinergic, vagal pathway in freely fed rats. *Acta Physiol Scand, 151*(2), 241-248.

Soderquist, J., Wijma, B., Thorbert, G., & Wijma, K. (2009). Risk factors in pregnancy for post-traumatic stress and depression after childbirth. *BJOG, 116*(5), 672-680.

Sofroniew, M.W. (1983). Vasopressin and oxytocin in the mammalian brain and spinal cord. *Trends in Neurosciences, 6*, 467-472.

Sohlstrom, A., Carlsson, C., & Uvnäs-Moberg, K. (2000). Effects of oxytocin treatment in early life on body weight and corticosterone in adult offspring from ad libitum-fed and food-restricted rats. *Biol Neonate, 78*(1), 33-40.

Sosa, R., Kennell, J., Klaus, M., Robertson, S., & Urrutia, J. (1980). The effect of a supportive companion on perinatal problems, length of labor, and mother-infant interaction. *N Engl J Med, 303*(11), 597-600.

Spatz, D.L. (2014). Preventing obesity starts with breastfeeding. *J Perinat Neonatal Nurs, 28*(1), 41-50. doi: 10.1097/JPN.0000000000000009.

Stachowiak, A., Macchi, C., Nussdorfer, G.G., & Malendowicz, L.K. (1995). Effects of oxytocin on the function and morphology of the rat adrenal cortex: in vitro and in vivo investigations. *Res Exp Med*

(Berl), 195(5), 265-274.

Stancampiano, R., & Argiolas, A. (1993). Proteolytic conversion of oxytocin in vivo after microinjection in the rat hippocampus. *Peptides, 14*(3), 465-469.

Stancampiano, R., Melis, M.R., & Argiolas, A. (1991). Proteolytic conversion of oxytocin by brain synaptic membranes: role of aminopeptidases and endopeptidases. *Peptides, 12*(5), 1119-1125.

Stark, M., & Finkel, A.R. (1994). Comparison between the Joel-Cohen and Pfannenstiel incisions in cesarean section. *Eur J Obstet Gynecol Reprod Biol, 53*(2), 121-122.

Stern, J.E., & Zhang, W. (2003). Preautonomic neurons in the paraventricular nucleus of the hypothalamus contain estrogen receptor beta. *Brain Res, 975*(1-2), 99-109.

Stocche, R.M., Klamt, J.G., Antunes-Rodrigues, J., Garcia, L.V., & Moreira, A.C. (2001). Effects of intrathecal sufentanil on plasma oxytocin and cortisol concentrations in women during the first stage of labor. *Reg Anesth Pain Med, 26*(6), 545-550.

Stock, S., Fastbom, J., Bjorkstrand, E., Ungerstedt, U., & Uvnäs-Moberg, K. (1990). Effects of oxytocin on in vivo release of insulin and glucagon studied by microdialysis in the rat pancreas and autoradiographic evidence for [3H]oxytocin binding sites within the islets of Langerhans. *Regul Pept, 30*(1), 1-13.

Stock, S., & Uvnäs-Moberg, K. (1985). Oxytocin infusions increase plasma levels of insulin and VIP but not of gastrin in conscious dogs. *Acta Physiol Scand, 125*(2), 205-210.

Stock, S., & Uvnäs-Moberg, K. (1988). Increased plasma levels of oxytocin in response to afferent electrical stimulation of the sciatic and vagal nerves and in response to touch and pinch in anaesthetized rats. *Acta Physiol Scand, 132*(1), 29-34.

Strathearn, L., Fonagy, P., Amico, J., & Montague, P.R. (2009). Adult attachment predicts maternal brain and oxytocin response to infant cues. *Neuropsychopharmacology, 34*(13):2655-66. doi: 10.1038/npp.2009.103.

Strathearn, L., Iyengar, U., Fonagy, P., & Kim, S. (2012). Maternal oxytocin response during mother-infant interaction: Associations with adult temperament. *Horm Behav, 61*(3), 429-435.

Strevens, H., Kristensen, K., Langhoff-Roos, J., & Wide-Swensson, D. (2002). Blood pressure patterns through consecutive pregnancies are influenced by body mass index. *Am J Obstet Gynecol, 187*(5):1343-8.

Strevens, H., Wide-Swensson, D., & Ingemarsson, I. (2001). Blood pressure during pregnancy in a Swedish population; impact of parity. *Acta Obstet Gynecol Scand, 80*(9), 824-9.

Strunecka, A., Hynie, S., & Klenerova, V. (2009). Role of oxytocin/oxytocin receptor system in regulation of cell growth and neoplastic processes. *Folia Biol (Praha), 55*(5), 159-165.

Stuebe, A.M., Kleinman, K., Gillman, M.W., Rifas-Shiman, S.L., Gunderson, E.P., & Rich-Edwards, J. (2010). Duration of lactation and maternal metabolism at 3 years postpartum. J Womens Health (Larchmt), 19(5), 941-50. doi: 10.1089/jwh.2009.1660.

Stuebe, A.M., Rich-Edwards, J.W., Willett, W.C., Manson, J.E., & Michels, K.B. (2005). Duration of lactation and incidence of type 2 diabetes. *JAMA, 294*(20), 2601-10.

Stuebe, A.M., Schwarz, E.B., Grewen, K., Rich-Edwards, J.W., Michels, K.B., Foster, E.M., ...& Forman, J. (2011). Duration of lactation and incidence of maternal hypertension: a longitudinal cohort study. *Am J Epidemiol, 174*(10):1147-58. doi: 10.1093/aje/kwr227.

Su, L.L., Chong, Y.S., & Samuel, M. (2012). Carbetocin for preventing postpartum haemorrhage. *Cochrane Database Syst Rev, 2,* CD005457.

Suva, J., Caisova, D., & Stajner, A. (1980). Modification of fat and carbohydrate metabolism by neurohypophyseal hormones. III. Effect of oxytocin on non-esterified fatty acid, glucose, triglyceride and cholesterol levels in rat serum. *Endokrinologie, 76*(3), 333-339.

Svanstrom, M.C., Biber, B., Hanes, M., Johansson, G., Naslund, U., & Balfors, E.M. (2008). Signs of myocardial ischaemia after injection of oxytocin: a randomized double-blind comparison of oxytocin and methylergometrine during Caesarean section. *Br J Anaesth, 100*(5), 683-689.

Svardby, K., Nordstrom, L., & Sellstrom, E. (2007). Primiparas with or without oxytocin augmentation: a prospective descriptive study. *J Clin Nurs, 16*(1), 179-184.

Svennersten, K., Gorewit, R.C., Sjaunja, L.O., & Uvnäs-Moberg, K. (1995). Feeding during milking enhances milking-related oxytocin secretion and milk production in dairy cows whereas food deprivation decreases it. *Acta Physiol Scand, 153*(3), 309-10.

Svennersten, K., Nelson, L., & Uvnäs-Moberg, K. (1990). Feeding-induced oxytocin release in dairy cows. *Acta Physiol Scand, 140*(2), 295-296.

Swanson, L.W., & Sawchenko, P.E. (1980). Paraventricular nucleus: a site for the integration of neuroendocrine and autonomic mechanisms. *Neuroendocrinology, 31*(6), 410-417.

Swanson, L.W., & Sawchenko, P.E. (1983). Hypothalamic integration: organization of the paraventricular and supraoptic nuclei. *Annu Rev Neurosci, 6,* 269-324.

Szeto, A., McCabe, P. ., Nation, D.A., Tabak, B.A., Rossetti, M.A., McCullough, M.E., et al. (2011). Evaluation of enzyme immunoassay and radioimmunoassay methods for the measurement of plasma oxytocin. *Psychosom Med, 73*(5), 393-400.

Szeto, A., Nation, D.A., Mendez, A.J., Dominguez-Bendala, J., Brooks, L.G., Schneiderman, N., et al. (2008). Oxytocin attenuates NADPH-dependent superoxide activity and IL-6 secretion in macrophages and vascular cells. *Am J Physiol Endocrinol Metab, 295*(6), E1495-1501.

Szyf, M., McGowan, P., & Meaney, M.J. (2008). The social environment and the epigenome. *Environ Mol Mutagen, 49*(1), 46-60.

Szyf, M., Weaver, I.C., Champagne, F.A., Diorio, J., & Meaney, M.J. (2005). Maternal programming of steroid receptor expression and phenotype through DNA methylation in the rat. *Front Neuroendocrinol, 26*(3-4), 139-162.

Takahashi, Y., Tamakoshi, K., Matsushima, M., & Kawabe, T. (2011). Comparison of salivary cortisol, heart rate, and oxygen saturation between early skin-to-skin contact with different initiation and duration times in healthy, full-term infants. *Early Hum Dev, 87*(3), 151-157.

Tancin, V., Kraetzl, W., Schams, D., & Bruckmaier, R.M. (2001). The effects of conditioning to suckling, milking and of calf presence on the release of oxytocin in dairy cows. *Appl Anim Behav Sci, 72*(3), 235-246.

Terenzi, M.G., & Ingram, C.D. (2005). Oxytocin-induced excitation of neurones in the rat central and medial amygdaloid nuclei. *Neuroscience, 134*(1), 345-354.

Thavagnanam, S., Fleming, J., Bromley, A., Shields, M.D., & Cardwell, C.R. (2008). A meta-analysis of the association between Caesarean section and childhood asthma. *Clin Exp Allergy, 38*(4), 629-633. doi: 10.1111/j.1365-2222.2007.02780.x.

Theodosis, D.T. (2002). Oxytocin-secreting neurons: A physiological model of morphological neuronal and glial plasticity in the adult hypothalamus. *Front Neuroendocrinol, 23*(1), 101-35.

Theodosis, D.T., Chapman, D.B., Montagnese, C., Poulain, D.A., & Morris, J.F. (1986). Structural plasticity in the hypothalamic supraoptic nucleus at lactation affects oxytocin-, but not vasopressin-secreting neurones. *Neuroscience, 17*(3), 661-78.

Thomas, J.S., Koh, S.H., & Cooper, G.M. (2007). Haemodynamic effects of oxytocin given as i.v. bolus or infusion on women undergoing Caesarean section. *Br J Anaesth, 98*(1), 116-119.

Todd, K., & Lightman, S.L. (1986). Oxytocin release during coitus in male and female rabbits: effect of opiate receptor blockade with naloxone. *Psychoneuroendocrinology, 11*(3), 367-371.

Tops, M., van Peer, J.M., Korf, J., Wijers, A.A., & Tucker, D.M. (2007). Anxiety, cortisol, and attachment predict plasma oxytocin. Psychophysiology, 44(3), 444-449.

Tornhage, C.J., Serenius, F., Uvnäs-Moberg, K., & Lindberg, T. (1998). Plasma somatostatin and cholecystokinin levels in preterm infants during kangaroo care with and without nasogastric tube-feeding. *J Pediatr Endocrinol Metab, 11*(5), 645-651.

Torvaldsen, S., Roberts, C.L., Simpson, J.M., Thompson, J.F., & Ellwood, D.A. (2006). Intrapartum epidural analgesia and breastfeeding: a prospective cohort study. *Int Breastfeed J, 1,* 24.

Tribollet, E., Barberis, C., Dreifuss, J.J., & Jard, S. (1988). Autoradiographic localization of vasopressin and oxytocin binding sites in rat kidney. *Kidney Int, 33*(5), 959-965.

Triopon, G., Goron, A., Agenor, J., Aya, G.A., Chaillou, A.L., Begler-Fonnier, J., et al. (2010). [Use of carbetocin in prevention of uterine atony during cesarean section. Comparison with oxytocin]. *Gynecol Obstet Fertil, 38*(12), 729-734.

Tsuchiya, T. (1994). Effects of cutaneous mechanical stimulation on plasma corticosterone, luteinizing hormone (LH), and testosterone levels in anesthetized male rats. *Hokkaido Igaku Zasshi, 69*(2), 217-235.

Tsuchiya, T., Nakayama, Y., & Sato, A. (1991). Somatic afferent regulation of plasma corticosterone in anesthetized rats. *Jpn J*

Physiol, 41(1), 169-176.

Tucker, H.A. (2000). Hormones, mammary growth, and lactation: A 41 year perspective. *J. Dairy Sciences, 83*, 874-884.

Tulman, L.J. (1986). Initial handling of newborn infants by vaginally and cesarean-delivered mothers. *Nurs Res, 35*(5), 296-300.

Uvnäs-Moberg, K., Arn, I., & Magnusson, D. (2005). The psychobiology of emotion: the role of the oxytocinergic system. *Int J Behav Med, 12*(2), 59-65.

Uvnäs-Moberg, K. (1985). Mod att föda. *läkartidningen, 82*(1-2), 4524-4528.

Uvnäs-Moberg, K. (1989). The gastrointestinal tract in growth and reproduction. *Sci Am, 261*(1), 78-83.

Uvnäs-Moberg, K. (1994). Role of efferent and afferent vagal nerve activity during reproduction: integrating function of oxytocin on metabolism and behaviour. *Psychoneuroendocrinology, 19*(5-7), 687-695.

Uvnäs-Moberg K. (1996). Neuroendocrinology of the mother-child interaction. *Trends Endocrinol Metab, 7*(4):126-31.

Uvnäs-Moberg, K. (1997). Oxytocin linked anti-stress effects--the relaxation and growth response. *Acta Physiol Scand Suppl, 640*, 38-42.

Uvnäs-Moberg, K. (1998a). Anti-stress Pattern Induced by Oxytocin. *News Physiol Sci, 13*, 22-25.

Uvnäs-Moberg, K. (1998b). Oxytocin may mediate the benefits of positive social interaction and emotions. *Psychoneuroendocrinology, 23*(8), 819-835.

Uvnäs-Moberg, K. (2003). *The Oxytocin Factor, Tapping the Hormone of calm, Love and Healing.* Boston: Da Capo Press. a member of the perseus books group.

Uvnäs Moberg, K. (2009). *Närhetens hormon. Oxytocinets roll i relationer.* Stockholm: Natur och Kultur.

Uvnäs-Moberg, K. (2012). *Oxytocin the hormone of closeness*: Pinter & Martin Ltd.

Uvnäs-Moberg, K., Ahlenius, S., Hillegaart, V., & Alster, P. (1994). High doses of oxytocin cause sedation and low doses cause an anxiolytic-like effect in male rats. *Pharmacol Biochem Behav, 49*(1), 101-106.

Uvnäs-Moberg, K., Alster, P., Hillegaart, V., & Ahlenius, S. (1992). Oxytocin reduces exploratory motor behaviour and shifts the activity towards the centre of the arena in male rats. *Acta Physiol Scand, 145*(4), 429-430.

Uvnäs-Moberg, K., Alster, P., Hillegaart, V., & Ahlenius, S. (1995). Suggestive evidence for a DA D3 receptor-mediated increase in the release of oxytocin in the male rat. *Neuroreport, 6*(9), 1338-1340.

Uvnäs-Moberg, K., Alster, P., Lund, I., Lundeberg, T., Kurosawa, M., & Ahlenius, S. (1996). Stroking of the abdomen causes decreased locomotor activity in conscious male rats. *Physiol Behav, 60*(6), 1409-1411.

Uvnäs-Moberg, K., Alster, P., & Petersson, M. (1996). Dissociation of oxytocin effects on body weight in two variants of female Sprague-Dawley rats. *Integr Physiol Behav Sci, 31*(1), 44-55.

Uvnäs-Moberg, K., Alster, P., Petersson, M., Sohlstrom, A., & Bjorkstrand, E. (1998). Postnatal oxytocin injections cause sustained weight gain and increased nociceptive thresholds in male and female rats. *Pediatr Res, 43*(3), 344-348.

Uvnäs-Moberg, K., Alster, P., & Svensson, T.H. (1992). Amperozide and clozapine but not haloperidol or raclopride increase the secretion of oxytocin in rats. *Psychopharmacology (Berl), 109*(4), 473-476.

Uvnäs-Moberg, K., Bjorkstrand, E., Hillegaart, V., & Ahlenius, S. (1999). Oxytocin as a possible mediator of SSRI-induced antidepressant effects. *Psychopharmacology (Berl), 142*(1), 95-101.

Uvnäs-Moberg, K., Bruzelius, G., Alster, P., & Lundeberg, T. (1993). The antinociceptive effect of non-noxious sensory stimulation is mediated partly through oxytocinergic mechanisms. *Acta Physiol Scand, 149*(2), 199-204.

Uvnäs-Moberg, K., Bystrova, K., Widström, A.M., Ekstrom, A., Handlin, L. Ransjö-Arvidsson, K. (2014). Oxytocin and cortisol levels in mothers and infants having skin to skin contact or nursery care after birth differ 4 days after birth. Unpublished data.

Uvnäs-Moberg, K., Eklund, M., Hillegaart, V., & Ahlenius, S. (2000). Improved conditioned avoidance learning by oxytocin administration in high-emotional male Sprague-Dawley rats. *Regul Pept, 88*(1-3), 27-32.

Uvnäs-Moberg, K., & Eriksson, M. (1996). Breastfeeding: physiological, endocrine and behavioural adaptations caused by oxytocin and local neurogenic activity in the nipple and mammary gland. *Acta Paediatr, 85*(5), 525-530.

Uvnäs-Moberg, K., Hillegaart, V., Alster, P., & Ahlenius, S. (1996). Effects of 5-HT agonists, selective for different receptor subtypes, on oxytocin, CCK, gastrin and somatostatin plasma levels in the rat. *Neuropharmacology, 35*(11), 1635-1640.

Uvnäs-Moberg, K., Johansson, B., Lupoli, B., & Svennersten-Sjaunja, K. (2001). Oxytocin facilitates behavioural, metabolic and physiological adaptations during lactation. *Appl Anim Behav Sci, 72*(3), 225-234.

Uvnäs-Moberg, K., Lundeberg, T., Bruzelius, G., & Alster, P. (1992). Vagally mediated release of gastrin and cholecystokinin following sensory stimulation. *Acta Physiol Scand, 146*(3), 349-356.

Uvnäs-Moberg, K., Marchini, G., & Winberg, J. (1993). Plasma cholecystokinin concentrations after breast feeding in healthy 4 day old infants. *Arch Dis Child, 68*(1 Spec No), 46-48.

Uvnäs-Moberg, K., Nielsen, E., Ahmed, S., & Fianu-Jonasson, A. (2014). A pharmcokinetic analysis of oxytocin levels in postmenopausal women. Unpublished data.

Uvnäs-Moberg K., & Nissen, E. (2005). Hormonell regerling av beteende under amningen. In B. Sjögren (Ed.), *Kropp och själ och barnafödande - Psyciosocial obstetrik på 2000 talet.* Lund: Studentlitteratur.

Uvnäs-Moberg, K., & Petersson, M. (2005). Oxytocin, a mediator of anti-stress, well-being, social interaction, growth and healing. *Z Psychosom Med Psychother, 51*(1), 57-80.

Uvnäs-Moberg, K., & Petersson, M. (2011). Role of oxytocin related effects in manual therapies. In J. H. King, W., Patterson

M.M. (Ed.), *The Science and Application of Manual Therapy.* Amsterdam: Elsevier.

Uvnäs-Moberg, K., Posloncec, B., & Ahlberg, L. (1986). Influence on plasma levels of somatostatin, gastrin, glucagon, insulin and VIP-like immunoreactivity in peripheral venous blood of anaesthetized cats induced by low intensity afferent stimulation of the sciatic nerve. *Acta Physiol Scand, 126*(2), 225-230.

Uvnäs-Moberg, K., & Prime, D. (2013). Oxytocin effects in mothers and infants during breastfeeding. *Infant, 9*(6), 201-206.

Uvnäs-Moberg, K., Sjögren, C., Westlin, L., Andersson, P.O., & Stock, S. (1989). Plasma levels of gastrin, somatostatin, VIP, insulin and oxytocin during the menstrual cycle in women (with and without oral contraceptives). *Acta Obstet Gynecol Scand, 68*(2), 165-169.

Uvnäs-Moberg, K., Stock, S., Eriksson, M., Linden, A., Einarsson, S., & Kunavongkrit, A. (1985). Plasma levels of oxytocin increase in response to suckling and feeding in dogs and sows. *Acta Physiol Scand, 124*(3), 391-398.

Uvnäs-Moberg, K., Widstrom, A.M., Marchini, G., & Winberg, J. (1987). Release of GI hormones in mother and infant by sensory stimulation. *Acta Paediatr Scand, 76*(6), 851-860.

Uvnäs-Moberg K, Widstrom, A.M., Nissen E, & Björvell H. (1990). Personality traits in women 4 days postpartum and their correlation with plasma levels of oxytocin an prolactin. *J. Psychosom. Obstet. Gynaecol, 11*, 261-273.

Uvnäs-Moberg, K., Widstrom, A.M., Werner, S., Matthiesen, A. S., & Winberg, J. (1990). Oxytocin and prolactin levels in breast-feeding women. Correlation with milk yield and duration of breast-feeding. *Acta Obstet Gynecol Scand, 69*(4), 301-306.

Uvnäs-Wallensten, K., Efendic, S., Johansson, C., Sjodin, L., & Cranwell, P.D. (1980). Effect of intraluminal pH on the release of somatostatin and gastrin into antral, bulbar and ileal pouches of conscious dogs. *Acta Physiol Scand, 110*(4), 391-400.

Uvnäs-Wallensten, K., Efendic, S., & Luft, R. (1977). Inhibition of vagally induced gastrin release by somatostatin in cats. *Horm Metab Res, 9*(2), 120-123.

Uvnäs-Wallensten, K., Efendic, S., Roovete, A., & Johansson, C. (1980). Decreased release of somatostatin into the portal vein following electrical vagal stimulation in the cat. *Acta Physiol Scand, 109*(4), 393-398.

Vallbo, A., Olausson, H., Wessberg, J., & Norrsell, U. (1993). A system of unmyelinated afferents for innocuous mechanoreception in the human skin. *Brain Res, 628*(1-2), 301-304.

Vallbo, A.B., Olausson, H., & Wessberg, J. (1999). Unmyelinated afferents constitute a second system coding tactile stimuli of the human hairy skin. *J Neurophysiol, 81*(6), 2753-2763.

Valros, A., Rundgren, M., Spinka, M., Saloniemi, H., Hultén, F., Uvnäs-Moberg, K., ...Algers, B. (2004). Oxytocin, prolactin and somatostatin in lactating sows; associations with body resources, mobilisation and maternal behaviour *Livest Prod Sci, 2004*(85), 1-13.

Van Bockstaele, E.J., Colago, E.E., & Valentino, R.J. (1998). Amygdaloid corticotropin-releasing factor targets Locus Coeruleus dendrites: substrate for the co-ordination of emotional and cognitive limbs of the stress response. *J Neuroendocrinol, 10*(10), 743-757.

van Oers, H.J., de Kloet, E.R., Whelan, T., & Levine, S. (1998). Maternal deprivation effect on the infant's neural stress markers is reversed by tactile stimulation and feeding but not by suppressing corticosterone. *J Neurosci, 18*(23), 10171-10179.

Varendi, H., Porter, R. H., & Winberg, J. (1994). Does the newborn baby find the nipple by smell? *Lancet, 344*(8928), 989-990.

Velandia, M., Matthisen, A.S., Uvnäs-Moberg, K., & Nissen, E. (2010). Onset of vocal interaction between parents and newborns in skin-to-skin contact immediately after elective cesarean section. *Birth, 37*(3), 192-201.

Velandia, M., Uvnäs-Moberg, K., & Nissen, E. (2011). Sex differences in newborn interaction with mother or father during skin-to-skin contact after Caesarean section. *Acta Paediatr.*

Velandia, M., Uvnäs-Moberg, K., & Nissen, E. (2014a). Oxytocin levels after skin to skin contact and suckling in mothers after elective cesarean section; influence of exogenous oxytocin. Unpublished data.

Velandia, M., Uvnäs-Moberg, K., & Nissen, E. (2014b). Maternal KSP profile 2 days after elective cesarean section; influence of skin to skin contact and exogenous oxytocin. Unpublished data.

Velmurugan, S., Brunton, P.J., Leng, G., & Russell, J.A. (2010). Circulating secretin activates supraoptic nucleus oxytocin and vasopressin neurons via noradrenergic pathways in the rat. *Endocrinology, 151*(6), 2681-2688.

Verbalis, J.G., Blackburn, R.E., Hoffman, G.E., & Stricker, E.M. (1995). Establishing behavioral and physiological functions of central oxytocin: insights from studies of oxytocin and ingestive behaviors. *Adv Exp Med Biol, 395*, 209-225.

Verbalis, J.G., McCann, M.J., McHale, C.M., & Stricker, E.M. (1986). Oxytocin secretion in response to cholecystokinin and food: differentiation of nausea from satiety. *Science, 232*(4756), 1417-1419.

Verbalis, J.G., Stricker, E.M., Robinson, A.G., & Hoffman, G.E. (1991). Cholecystokinin activates C-fos expression in hypothalamic oxytocin and corticotropin-releasing hormone neurons. *J Neuroendocrinol, 3*(2), 205-13. doi: 10.1111/j.1365-2826.1991.tb00264.x.

Veronesi, M.C., Kubek, D.J., & Kubek, M.J. (2011). Intranasal delivery of neuropeptides. *Methods Mol Biol, 789*, 303-312.

Voloschin, L M., & Tramezzani, J.H. (1979). Milk ejection reflex linked to slow wave sleep in nursing rats. *Endocrinology, 105*(5), 1202-1207.

Vrachnis, N., Malamas, F. M., Sifakis, S., Deligeoroglou, E., & Iliodromiti, Z. (2011). The oxytocin-oxytocin receptor system and its antagonists as tocolytic agents. *Int J Endocrinol, 2011*, 350546.

Wakerley, J.B., Poulain, D.A., & Brown, D. (1978). Comparison of firing patterns in oxytocin- and vasopressin-releasing neurones during progressive dehydration. *Brain Res, 148*(2), 425-40.

Wakshlak, A., & Weinstock, M. (1990). Neonatal handling reverses behavioral abnormalities induced in rats by prenatal stress. *Physiol Behav, 48*(2), 289-292.

Waldenstrom, U., & Schytt, E. (2009). A longitudinal study of women's memory of labour pain--from 2 months to 5 years after the birth. *BJOG, 116*(4), 577-583. doi: 10.1111/j.1471-0528.2008.02020.x.

Wathes, C., & Swann, R.W. (1982). Is oxytocin an ovarian hormone. *Nature, 297,* 225-227.

Weber, B.C., Manfredo, H.N., & Rinaman, L. (2009). A potential gastrointestinal link between enhanced postnatal maternal care and reduced anxiety-like behavior in adolescent rats. *Behav Neurosci, 123*(6), 1178-84. doi: 10.1037/a0017659.

Weller, A., & Blass E.M. (1988). Behavioral evidence for cholecystokinin-opiate interactions in neonatal rats. *Am J Physiol, 255*(6 Pt 2):R901-907.

Weller, A., & Weller, L. (1993). Menstrual synchrony between mothers and daughters and between roommates. *Physiol Behav, 53*(5), 943-949.

Weller, A., & Weller, L. (1997). Menstrual synchrony under optimal conditions: Bedouin families. *J Comp Psychol, 111*(2), 143-151.

Weng, M., & Walker, W.A. (2013). The role of gut microbiota in programming the immune phenotype. *J Dev Orig Health Dis, 4*(3). doi: 10.1017/S2040174412000712.

Wex, J., Abou-Setta, A. M., Clerici, G., & Di Renzo, G.C. (2011). Atosiban versus betamimetics in the treatment of preterm labour in Italy: clinical and economic importance of side-effects. *Eur J Obstet Gynecol Reprod Biol, 157*(2), 128-135.

White-Traut, R., Watanabe, K., Pournajafi-Nazarloo, H., Schwertz, D., Bell, A., & Carter, C.S. (2009). Detection of salivary oxytocin levels in lactating women. *Dev Psychobiol, 51*(4), 367-73. doi: 10.1002/dev.20376.

Wiberg, B., Humble, K., & de Chateau, P. (1989). Long-term effect on mother-infant behaviour of extra contact during the first hour post partum. V. Follow-up at three years. *Scand J Soc Med, 17*(2), 181-191.

Widstrom, A.M., Christensson, K., Ransjo-Arvidson, A.B., Matthiesen, A.S., Winberg, J., & Uvnäs-Moberg, K. (1988). Gastric aspirates of newborn infants: pH, volume and levels of gastrin- and somatostatin-like immunoreactivity. *Acta Paediatr Scand, 77*(4), 502-508.

Widstrom, A.M., Marchini, G., Matthiesen, A.S., Werner, S., Winberg, J., & Uvnäs-Moberg, K. (1988). Nonnutritive sucking in tube-fed preterm infants: effects on gastric motility and gastric contents of somatostatin. *J Pediatr Gastroenterol Nutr, 7*(4), 517-523.

Widstrom, A.M., Matthiesen, A.S., Winberg, J., & Uvnäs-Moberg, K. (1989). Maternal somatostatin levels and their correlation with infant birth weight. *Early Hum Dev, 20*(3-4), 165-174.

Widstrom, A.M., Ransjo-Arvidson, A.B., Christensson, K., Matthiesen, A.S., Winberg, J., & Uvnäs-Moberg, K. (1987). Gastric suction in healthy newborn infants. Effects on circulation and developing feeding behaviour. *Acta Paediatr Scand, 76*(4), 566-572.

Widstrom, A.M., Wahlberg, V., Matthiesen, A.S., Eneroth, P., Uvnäs-Moberg, K., Werner, S., et al. (1990). Short-term effects of early suckling and touch of the nipple on maternal behaviour. *Early Hum Dev, 21*(3), 153-163.

Widstrom, A.M., Werner, S., Matthiesen, A.S., Svensson, K., & Uvnäs-Moberg, K. (1991). Somatostatin levels in plasma in nonsmoking and smoking breast-feeding women. *Acta Paediatr Scand, 80*(1), 13-21.

Widstrom, A.M., Winberg, J., Werner, S., Hamberger, B., Eneroth, P., & Uvnäs-Moberg, K. (1984). Suckling in lactating women stimulates the secretion of insulin and prolactin without concomitant effects on gastrin, growth hormone, calcitonin, vasopressin or catecholamines. *Early Hum Dev, 10*(1-2), 115-122.

Widstrom, A.M., Winberg, J., Werner, S., Svensson, K., Posloncec, B., & Uvnäs-Moberg, K. (1988). Breast feeding-induced effects on plasma gastrin and somatostatin levels and their correlation with milk yield in lactating females. *Early Hum Dev, 16*(2-3), 293-301.

Wiesenfeld, A.R., Malatesta, C.Z., Whitman, P.B., Granrose, C., & Uili, R. (1985). Psychophysiological response of breast- and bottle-feeding mothers to their infants' signals. *Psychophysiology, 22*(1), 79-86.

Wijma, K., Soderquist, J., & Wijma, B. (1997). Posttraumatic stress disorder after childbirth: a cross sectional study. *J Anxiety Disord, 11*(6), 587-597.

Wiklund, I., Norman, M., Uvnäs-Moberg, K., Ransjo-Arvidson, A.B., & Andolf, E. (2009). Epidural analgesia: breast-feeding success and related factors. *Midwifery, 25*(2), e31-38.

Wilde, C.J., Addey, C.V., Boddy, L.M., & Peaker, M. (1995). Autocrine regulation of milk secretion by a protein in milk. *Biochem J, 305 (Pt 1),* 51-58.

Wilde, C.J., Addey, C.V., Bryson, J.M., Finch, L.M., Knight, C.H., & Peaker, M. (1998). Autocrine regulation of milk secretion. *Biochem Soc Symp, 63,* 81-90.

Winberg, J. (2005). Mother and newborn baby: mutual regulation of physiology and behavior--a selective review. *Dev Psychobiol, 47*(3), 217-229.

Witt, D.M., Winslow, J.T., & Insel, T.R. (1992). Enhanced social interactions in rats following chronic, centrally infused oxytocin. *Pharmacol Biochem Behav, 43*(3), 855-861.

Wu, H., Hu, K., & Jiang, X. (2008). From nose to brain: understanding transport capacity and transport rate of drugs. *Expert Opin Drug Deliv, 5*(10), 1159-1168.

Yamashita, H., Kannan, H., Kasai, M., & Osaka, T. (1987). Decrease in blood pressure by stimulation of the rat hypothalamic paraventricular nucleus with L-glutamate or weak current. *J Auton Nerv Syst, 19*(3), 229-234.

Yokoyama, Y., Ueda, T., Irahara, M., & Aono, T. (1994). Releases of oxytocin and prolactin during breast massage and suckling in puerperal women. *Eur J Obstet Gynecol Reprod Biol, 53*(1), 17-20.

Young, W.S., 3rd, Shepard, E., Amico, J., Hennighausen, L., Wagner,

K.U., LaMarca, M.E., et al. (1996). Deficiency in mouse oxytocin prevents milk ejection, but not fertility or parturition. *J Neuroendocrinol, 8*(11), 847-853.

Yurth, D.A. (1982). Placental transfer of local anesthetics. *Clin Perinatol, 9*(1), 13-28.

Zerihun, L., & Harris, M. (1983). An electrophysiological analysis of caudally-projecting neurones from the hypothalamic paraventricular nucleus in the rat. *Brain Res, 261*(1), 13-20.

Zhou, A. W., Li, W.X., Guo, J., & Du, Y.C. (1997). Facilitation of AVP(4-8) on gene expression of BDNF and NGF in rat brain. *Peptides, 18*(8), 1179-1187.

Zimmerman, E.A., Nilaver, G., Hou-Yu, A., & Silverman, A.J. (1984). Vasopressinergic and oxytocinergic pathways in the central nervous system. *Fed Proc, 43*(1), 91-96.

List of Abbreviations

ACTH - adrenococorticotrophic hormone

BDNF - brain-derived growth factor

BNST - Bed Nucleus Stria Terminalis

CCK - cholecystokinin

CGRP - calcitonin gene-related peptide

CNS - central nervous system

CRF - corticotrophin-releasing factor

CRH - corticotrophin-releasing hormone

CSF - cerebrospinal fluid

CT fibers - C-Tactile fibers

DAG - diacylglycerol

DMX - vagal motor nucleus, dorsal motor nucleus of the vagus nerve

DVC - dorsal vagal complex

EEG - electroencephalogram test)

EIA - enzyme-linked immunoassay (also abbreviated as ELISA)

E.Q. - emotional intelligence

FIL - inhibitory factor

FMRI—functional magnetic resonance imaging

FSH - follicle stimulating hormone

GABA—Gamma amino butyric acid

GNRH - gonadotrophin-releasing hormone

GR receptor - glucocorticoid receptor

HCL - hydrochloric acid

HPA axis - hypothalamic-pituitary-adrenal axis

HPLC - high performance liquid chromatography

HRT - hormone replacement therapy

HRV - heart rate variability

ICV - intracerebroventricular

IU - international units

IV - intravenous

KSP - Karolinska Scales of Personality

LC - Locus Coeruleus

LH - luteinizing hormone

mcg - microgram

MPOA—medial preoptic area

MR - mineralocorticoid receptor

NA - nucleus accumbens

NEFA - non-esterified fatty acids

NGF - nerve growth factor

NPY - Neuropeptide Y

NTS - nucleus tractus solitarius

PAG - periaqueductal grey

PCERA - Parent-Child Early Relational Assessment

pH—"potential of hydrogen"—a measure of acidity or alkalinity

PTSD - post traumatic stress disorder

PVN - paraventricular nucleus

RIA - radioimmunoassay

RN - raphe nuclei

RVLM - rostroventral lateral medulla

SC - subcutaneous

SON - supraoptic nucleus

SP - substance P

SSRI - serotonin uptake inhibitors

TRH - thyrotropin releasing hormone

TSH - thyroid stimulating hormone

VIP - vasoactive intestinal peptide

INDEX

S

Satiety Hormone 130

Secretion of Gastric Acid In Utero 126

Secretion of Hormones In Utero 126

Self-Confidence 144

Sensitivity to Touch 76

Sensory Cues 51, 76

Sensory Interaction 42

Sensory Nerves 19

Sensory Stimulation 39, 40, 133

Separation 96, 169

Separation Anxiety 97

Serotonin 112

Sex Differences 76

Sexual Activity 38

Short-Term Satiety 131

Signaling Substance 18, 37

Skin 70, 107

Skin as a Sensory Organ 19

Skin Hunger 68

Skin Temperature 50, 76, 78, 83, 154, 161

Skin-to-Skin Contact 40, 56, 60, 73, 75, 79, 82, 83, 84, 85, 97, 106, 137, 138, 140, 148, 169, 171

Smoking Women 119

Social Interaction 31, 34, 82, 88, 89, 134, 138, 161

Somatic Nervous System 18

Somatosensory Nerves 103

Somatosensory Stimulation 41

Somatosensory-Vagal Reflexes 133

Somatostatin 114, 126

Somatostatin Levels 112, 119

State vs Trait 91

Steroid Hormones 21

Storing of Energy 118

Stress 55, 82, 88, 90, 96, 101, 102, 134

Stress Buffering 103

Stress Levels 83, 161

Stress of Being Born 79, 84

Stress of Giving Birth 84

Stress Patterns 42

Stress System 41

Sucking 70

Suckling 38, 46, 55, 58, 102, 103, 105, 106, 113, 124, 125, 127, 137, 138, 140, 148, 161

Suckling-Induced Effects 124

Suckling-Related Anti-stress Effects 106

Support 144

Sympathetic Nerve Activity 55, 114

Sympathetic Nerve Fibers 137

Sympathetic Nervous System 18, 55, 101, 102

Sympathetic Nervous Tone 83, 107, 108, 120

Sympathetic Tone 41, 91

Synchronization of Birth 95

Synthesis of Oxytocin 27

Synthetic Oxytocin 15

T

Tactile and Vocal Interaction 78

Tactile Interaction 71

Tactile Stimulation 39, 67

Time to Suck 65

Touch 131

Trait 119

Transfer of Energy 113

Transfer of Nutrients 114

Treatment of Premature Infants 85

Trust 144

U

Unfamiliar Environments 96

Unfamiliar Surrounding(s) 96, 98

Uterine Contractions 153

V

Vagal Nerve Activity 83, 114

Vagal Nerves 112, 126, 131, 132

Vagal Nerve Tone 120

Vaginal Delivery 168

Vasopressin 23

About the Author

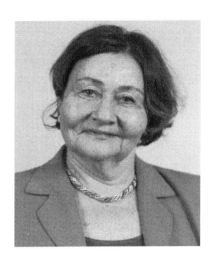

Dr. Kerstin Uvnäs-Moberg is a physician, with a PhD in pharmacology. She is presently working as a professor in physiology. She has researched oxytocin for the past 30 years. Her interest in oxytocin derives from a deep interest in issues around women's health.

She has written two books about oxytocin and published 450 papers in peer-reviewed journals. Dr. Uvnäs-Moberg has supervised more than 30 PhD students within a broad range of professions: physicians, psychologists, veterinarians, midwives, agronomists, and students of biomedicine. She is still very active supervising experimental studies and writing scientific papers and books.

Dr Uvnäs-Moberg lives in Sweden. She has four children and six grandchildren. When she is not working, she enjoys spending time with her friends, and above all, with her children and grandchildren.

Dear Reader,

Thank you for purchasing and reading this book. I hope you enjoyed it.

If so, you can help me reach other readers by writing a review of the book on Amazon.com, ibreastfeeding.com, and/or on any appropriate website.

Sincerely,

Kerstin Uvnäs Moberg

Made in the USA
Charleston, SC
19 January 2017